Operative Thoracic Surgery

SERIES EDITORS

R C G Russell MS FRCS FRCPS
Consulting Surgeon, University College Hospitals, London

Henry A Pitt MD
Professor and Vice Chairman, Department of Surgery, Indiana University, Indianapolis, Indiana

ART EDITOR

Gillian Lee FMAA HonFIMI AMI RMIP
Gillian Lee Illustrations, 15 Little Plucketts Way, Buckhurst Hill, Essex

Operative Thoracic Surgery

FIFTH EDITION

Edited by

Larry R Kaiser MD
The John Rhea Barton Professor and Chairman
Department of Surgery
University of Pennsylvania
Surgeon-in-Chief
University of Pennsylvania Health System
Philadelphia, Pennsylvania, USA

Glyn G Jamieson MS MD FRACS FRCS FACS
Dorothy Mortlock Professor and Chairman
Department of Surgery
University of Adelaide
Royal Adelaide Hospital
Adelaide, South Australia, Australia

Hodder Arnold
www.hoddereducation.com

First published in Great Britain in 1956 by
Butterworth Heinemann
Second edition 1968
Third edition 1976
Fourth edition 1982

This fifth edition published in 2006 by
Hodder Arnold, an imprint of Hodder Education and a member of the Hodder
Headline Group, 338 Euston Road, London NW1 3BH

http://www.hoddereducation.com

Distributed in the United States of America by
Oxford University Press Inc.,
198 Madison Avenue, New York, NY10016
Oxford is a registered trademark of Oxford University Press

Whilst the advice and information in this book are believed to be true and
accurate at the date of going to press, neither the author[s] nor the publisher
can accept any legal responsibility or liability for any errors or omissions that
may be made. In particular (but without limiting the generality of the
preceding disclaimer) every effort has been made to check drug dosages;
however it is still possible that errors have been missed. Furthermore, dosage
schedules are constantly being revised and new side-effects recognized. For
these reasons the reader is strongly urged to consult the drug companies'
printed instructions before administering any of the drugs recommended in
this book.

British Library Cataloguing in Publication Data
A catalogue record for this book is available from the British Library

Library of Congress Cataloging-in-Publication Data
A catalog record for this book is available from the Library of Congress

ISBN-10   0 340 75973 9
ISBN-13   978 0 340 759 738

1 2 3 4 5 6 7 8 9 10

Commissioning Editor: Sarah Burrows
Project Manager: Nora Naughton
Production Controller: Joanna Walker
Cover Designer: Nichola Smith
Art Editor: Gillian Lee

Typeset in 10 on 12pt Minion by Phoenix Photosetting, Chatham, Kent
Printed and bound in Italy by Printer Trento

What do you think about this book? Or any other Hodder Arnold title?
Please send your comments to www.hoddereducation.com

Contents

Contributors

Rudolf Bumm MD
Assistant Professor, Department of Surgery, Technical University of Munich, Munich, Germany

Raul Burgos MD PhD
Associate Professor, Autonomous University of Madrid, Department of Cardiovascular and Thoracic Surgery, Hospital Puerta de Hierro, Madrid, Spain

Evaristo Castedo MD
Professor of Surgery, Autonomous University of Madrid, Department of Cardiovascular and Thoracic Surgery, Hospital Puerta de Hierro, Madrid, Spain

Robert J Cerfolio MD FACS FACCP
Associate Professor of Surgery, Chief of Section of Thoracic Surgery, University of Alabama at Birmingham; Department of Surgery, Division of Cardiothoracic Surgery, Birmingham, Alabama, USA

Annamaria Ciccone MD
Division of Thoracic Surgery, Universita La Sapienza, Rome, Italy

Ara A Chalian MD FACS
Specialist Associate Professor, Director Head and Neck Reconstructive Surgery Service, Department of Otorhinolaryngology – Head and Neck Surgery, University of Pennsylvania Health System, Philadelphia, Pennsylvania, USA

C Peter Clarke MB BS FRACS FACS
Professorial Fellow, Department of Surgery, University of Melbourne; Senior Thoracic Surgeon, Austin Health, Heidelberg, Victoria, Australia

John Dark
Professor, Regional Cardiothoracic Centre, Freeman Hospital, Newcastle upon Tyne, UK

Tiziano De Giacomo MD
Division of Thoracic Surgery, Universita La Sapienza, Rome, Italy

Maher Deeb MD
Fellow, Hospital of the University of Pennsylvania, Philadelphia, Pennsylvania, USA; Shaare Zedek Medical Center, Jerusalem, Israel

Claude Deschamps MD
Professor of Surgery, Mayo College of Medicine, Rochester, Minnesota, USA

Jean Deslauriers MD FRCS(C)
Professor of Surgery at Laval University, Sainte-Foy, Quebec, Canada

André Duranceau MD
Professor of Surgery, Chair, Division of Thoracic Surgery, Centre hospitalier de l'Université de Montréal, Montréal, Quebec, Canada

Joseph S Friedberg MD FACS
Associate Professor of Surgery, Division of Thoracic Surgery, Penn-Presbyterian Medical Center, Philadelphia, Pennsylvania, USA

J Alex Haller Jr MD
Emeritus Professor of Pediatric Surgery, Department of Surgery, The Johns Hopkins University School of Medicine; Emeritus Chief of Pediatric Surgery, Department of Surgery, Johns Hopkins Hospital, Baltimore, Maryland, USA

Peter H Hollaus MD
Consultant, General and Thoracic Surgeon, Department of Thoracic Surgery, Pulmologisches Zentrum Wien, Vienna, Austria

Arnulf H Hölscher MD FACS FRCS
Professor of Surgery and Chairman, Department of Visceral and Vascular Surgery, University of Cologne Medical School; Director, Department of Visceral and Vascular Surgery, Medical Center University of Cologne, Cologne, Germany

Olivier Huber MD
Associate Professor, Department of Surgery, University of Geneva; Head, Foregut Surgery, University Hospital of Geneva, Geneva, Switzerland

John Hunter MD
Professor and Chairman, Department of Surgery, Oregon Health Sciences University, Portland, Oregon, USA

Peter Goldstraw FRCS
Consultant Thoracic Surgeon, Royal Brompton Hospital, London; Professor of Thoracic Surgery, Imperial College, London, UK

Glyn G Jamieson MS MD FRACS FRCS FACS
Dorothy Mortlock Professor and Chairman, Department of Surgery, University of Adelaide, Royal Adelaide Hospital, Adelaide, South Australia, Australia

David P Jenkins BSC MS FRCS
Formerly Specialist Registrar, Department of Thoracic Surgery, Harefield Hospital, Middlesex, UK; Consultant Cardiothoracic Surgeon, Papworth Hosptial, Cambridge, UK

Sarah H Kagan PhD RN
Associate Professor of Gerontological Nursing; School of Nursing, Gerontology Clinical Nurse Specialist, Hospital of the University of Pennsylvania; Secondary Faculty, Department of Otorhinolaryngology – Head and Neck Surgery, University of Pennsylvania, Philadelphia, Pennsylvania, USA

Larry R Kaiser MD
The John Rhea Barton Professor and Chairman, Department of Surgery, University of Pennsylvania; Surgeon-in-Chief, University of Pennsylvania Health System, Philadelphia, Pennsylvania, USA

Jamie Kelly BM BSC MRCS FRCS(GEN SURG)
Upper Gastro Intestinal Fellow, University of Adelaide, Department of Surgery, Royal Adelaide Hospital, Adelaide, South Australia, Australia

Baiya Krishnadasan MD
Assistant Professor, Department of Surgery, Division of Cardiothoracic Surgery, University of Washington School of Medicine, Seattle, Washington, USA

John C Kucharczuk MD
Assistant Professor of Surgery, Division of Cardiothoracic Surgery, Hospital of the University of Pennsylvania, Philadelphia, Pennsylvania, USA

Bernard Launois MD FACS
Professor of Digestive and Transplantation Surgery, Hospital Pontchaillou, Rennes, France

Luiz Eduardo V Leão MD PhD
Professor and Chairman, Department of Surgery, Division of Thoracic Surgery, Escola Paulista de Medicina – Universidade Federal de São Paulo, São Paulo, Brazil

Alex G Little MD
Elizabeth Berry Gray Chair and Professor, Department of Surgery, Wright State University School of Medicine, Dayton, Ohio, USA

Jun-Feng Liu PhD
Professor and Doctor in Chief, Department of Thoracic Surgery, Fourth Hospital, Hebei Medical University, The People's Republic of China

Robert Ludemann MD PhD
Research Fellow, University of Adelaide, Department of Surgery, Royal Adelaide Hospital, Adelaide, South Australia, Australia

Paolo Macchiarini MD PhD
Professor of Surgery, University of Barcelona Medical School; Chairman, Department of General Thoracic Surgery, Hospital Clinic of Barcelona, Spain

Tomás Angelillo Mackinlay MD
British Hospital of Buenos Aires, Capital Federal, Buenos Aires, Argentina

Guy J Maddern PhD MS FRACS
R. P. Jepson Professor of Surgery, Department of Surgery, University of Adelaide, Adelaide, South Australia, Australia; Director, Division of Surgery, The Queen Elizabeth Hospital, Woodville, South Australia, Australia

Michael T Marrinan FRCS(ED)
Consultant Cardiothoracic Surgeon, King's College Hospital, London, UK

M Blair Marshall MD
Chief, Division of Thoracic Surgery, Georgetown University Medical Center, Washington, District of Columbia, USA

Christopher John Martin MB BS MSC FRACS
Professor of Surgery, University of Sydney; Head of Surgery, Nepean Hospital, Sydney, Australia

Kenneth L Mattox MD
Professor and Vice Chair, Michael E. DeBakey Department of Surgery, Baylor College of Medicine, Houston, Texas, USA

Reza Mehran MD FRCS(C)
Assistant Professor of Surgery, University of Ottawa, Ottawa, Ontario, Canada

Shinichiro Miyoshi MD PhD
Professor and Chairman, Department of Cardiothoracic Surgery, Dokkyo University School of Medicine, Mibu, Tochigi, Japan

Francis C Nichols MD
Assistant Professor of Surgery and Consultant Division of General Thoracic Surgery, Mayo Clinic College of Medicine, Rochester, Minnesota, USA

Mark B Orringer MD FRCS
Professor and Head, Section of Thoracic Surgery, University of Michigan Medical Center, Ann Arbor, Michigan, USA

Charles N Paidas MD
Associate Professor Surgery, Pediatrics, Oncology and Anesthesiology and Critical Care Medicine, Department of Surgery, Division of Pediatric Surgery, The Johns Hopkins University School of Medicine, Baltimore, Maryland, USA

Carlos Pellegrini MD
The Henry N. Harkins Professor and Chairman, Department of Surgery, University of Washington School of Medicine, Seattle, Washington, USA

Erino Angelo Rendina
Division of Thoracic Surgery, Universita La Sapienza, Rome, Italy

Joseph B Shrager MD
Associate Professor, Department of Surgery, University of Pennsylvania School of Medicine; Chief of Thoracic Surgery, Hospital of the University of Pennsylvania and Pennsylvania Hospital, Philadelphia, Pennsylvania, USA

J Rüdiger Siewert MD
Professor, Director, and Chairman, Department of Surgery, Technical University of Munich, Munich, Germany

Edward R Townsend FRCS
Consultant Thoracic Surgeon, Thoracic Surgery Unit, Royal Brompton and Harefield Hospital NHS Trust, Harefield, Middlesex, UK

Victor F Trastek MD
Professor of Surgery, Consultant Division of General Thoracic Surgery and Chair, Board of Governors Mayo Clinic Arizona, Scottsdale, Arizona, USA

Noriaki Tsubota MD PhD
Clinical Professor, Department of Thoracic and Cardiovascular Surgery, Kobe University School of Medicine, Kobe, Hyogo, Japan; Vice President, Department of General Thoracic Surgery, Hyogo Medical Center, Akashi, Hyogo, Japan

Ryosuke Tsuchiya MD
Chief, Division of Thoracic Surgery, National Cancer Center Hospital, Tokyo, Japan

Harold Clifton Urschel Jr MD
Chair; Cardiovascular and Thoracic Surgical Research, Education and Clinical Excellence, Baylor University Medical Center; Professor of Cardiothoracic Surgery (Clinical), University of Texas Southwestern Medical Center at Dallas Southwestern Medical School, Dallas, Texas, USA

Andres Varela PhD
Professor, Department of Surgery, Autonomous University of Madrid;
Section Chief of Thoracic Surgery and Lung Transplantation,
Department of Cardiovascular and Thoracic Surgery, Hospital Puerta
de Hierro, Madrid, Spain

Federico Venuta MD
Division of Thoracic Surgery, Universita La Sapienza, Rome, Italy

Jon-Cecil M Walkes MD
Cardiothoracic Resident, Michael E. DeBakey Department of Surgery,
Baylor College of Medicine, Houston, Texas, USA

David Ian Watson MB BS MD FRACS
Professor and Head, Flinders University Department of Surgery;
Senior Consultant Surgeon and Head of Gastrointestinal Services,
Flinders Medical Centre, Bedford Park, South Australia, Australia

Randal S Weber MD FACS
Hubert L. and Oliver Stringer Distinguished Professor of Cancer
Research, Chairman Department of Head and Neck Surgery,
University of Texas; MD Anderson Cancer Center, Houston, Texas,
USA

Contributing medical artists

Angela Christie FMAA
14 West End Avenue, Pinner, Middlesex

Peter Cox RDD, MMAA, RMIP
25 Hampton Close, Worcester

Gillian Lee FMAA, HonFIMI, AMI, RMIP
Gillian Lee Illustrations, 15 Little Plucketts Way, Buckhurst Hill, Essex

Gillian Oliver FMAA
7 Princes Street, Stotfold, Hitchin, Hertfordshire

Preface

It is with considerable pride that the editors are able to present this volume of Operative Surgery which covers the whole of Thoracic Surgery in one volume joining the skills of the lung surgeon and the oesophageal surgeon together for the benefit of many who practice this as a single specialty. Nearly twenty years have passed since the previous volume was published, and during this time, quite dramatic changes have occurred in the management of thoracic and esophageal diseases. The editors' believe that each of these advances has been adequately described in this volume to reflect the major changes in management. Of particular note has been the development of thoracoscopic surgery, which has brought considerable benefits in both the management of certain lung and oesophageal diseases. Perhaps, the greatest change in surgical practice has been the development of even more specialised units with the objective of achieving a sufficient volume of surgical caseload which current evidence based data predict will improve the results of surgical morbidity, mortality and the long term survival. The results of our colleagues from China have certainly led the field in the reduction of mortality of oesophageal resection, and is an example of the benefits of surgical volume with great technical skill.

The series of Operative Surgery was founded in the middle of the 1950s when surgical technique was beginning to crystallise into what we know today as the correct technique and in the contribution of the skill of the surgeon to outcome. Performance of the correct operation at the correct time and in the correct way have been the hallmark of the series. It is to Charles Robb and Rodney Smith that many surgeons owe a debt for pioneering this classic series of surgical operative texts with their ability to display an operation by the use of excellent illustration with short descriptive notes. No doubt more technically advanced media will take over from the written page but, to date, the general editors have yet to find a medium which will enable the surgeons to flip through a few pages and be enlightened about the technical aspect of an operative technique. For this reason we persist with this series hoping that many will find this volume as useful as the others.

No illustrative text on Operative Surgery would be possible without the skill, the quite incredible artistry, of Gillian Lee and her team who have produced a most beautiful series of operative illustrations which will not date with time. We editors owe our great thanks to her, and hope that all our readers will find this form of presentation to their liking. Finally, our contributors, our technical editors and our publishers should be thanked for what has been a mammoth task of cooperation, which we hope our readers will appreciate.

The Editors

SECTION I

Thoracic surgery

Repair of pectus excavatum

CHARLES N. PAIDAS MD
Associate Professor of Surgery, Pediatrics, Oncology and Anesthesiology and Critical Care Medicine, Department of Surgery, Division of Pediatric Surgery, The Johns Hopkins University School of Medicine, Baltimore, Maryland, USA

J. ALEX HALLER, JR. MD
Emeritus Professor of Pediatric Surgery, Department of Surgery, The Johns Hopkins University School of Medicine; Emeritus Chief of Pediatric Surgery, Department of Surgery, Johns Hopkins Hospital, Baltimore, Maryland, USA

HISTORY

Pectus excavatum, or funnel chest, is the most common congenital anomaly of the thorax in children. Although descriptions of repair of pectus excavatum were given in the early 1900s, it was not until the late 1930s that Ochsner and De Bakey described and repaired the anomaly, taking into account an overgrowth of cartilage that resulted in a posterior displacement of the sternum. In 1949, Mark Ravitch provided a detailed description of the defect and suggested the operation that is in common use to this day. Ravitch observed a central depressed sternum, rounded shoulders, potbelly, sloped ribs, and paradoxical movement of the chest wall inward on deep inspiration. His operation focused on removal of the deformed, overgrown costal cartilages with preservation of the perichondrium and stabilization of the sternum. For nearly 50 years, the Ravitch procedure, with minor modifications such as the use of stainless steel bar supports for the sternum, has been the benchmark procedure for pectus excavatum. In 1998, Donald Nuss introduced a minimally invasive technique for repair of pectus excavatum. This technique (Nuss procedure) has received growing acceptance as an alternative method of repair, but evidence-based long-term follow-up is needed.

PRINCIPLES AND JUSTIFICATION

The majority of children with pectus excavatum are asymptomatic and are referred for the anatomical deformity and cosmetic concerns. A small subset complains of nonspecific chest pain. The constellation of physical findings include rounded shoulders, sloped ribs, potbelly, and sunken chest. The excavatum defect does not cause scoliosis of the spine. The heart can be displaced into the left hemithorax, and in severe cases the point of maximum intensity may be in the midaxillary line.

PREOPERATIVE ASSESSMENT AND PREPARATION

Chest computed tomographic scan provides the most accurate assessment of heart displacement and lung volumes. The ratio of the distance between the sternum and vertebral bodies and the transverse diameter of the chest through the deepest portion of the defect may be used to calculate an index of severity. In normal children, this index is less than 2.5, whereas the index may range from 3 to 7 in those with severe deformities.

Simultaneous pulmonary and cardiac evaluation has shown that a severe deformity can cause compression of the right side of the heart. Right ventricular outflow distortion causes decreased cardiac output during strenuous exercise. Thus, a sunken sternum causes cardiovascular symptoms that are best characterized as decreased cardiac output during exercise. Nevertheless, the problem of appropriate selection of children who will benefit from correction of the defect still remains. Indications for operative correction include chest pain on exertion, dyspnea on exertion, cosmetic concerns, psychological stress, and future need for sternotomy for replacement of cardiac valves in children with Marfan syndrome who have both pectus excavatum and aortic valve insufficiency. Reconstruction should not be performed during a growth spurt. Rather, repair is best performed in the school-age child after a pubertal growth spurt (typically 9–12 years of age).

Exercise stress pulmonary function tests provide baseline data for symptomatic and asymptomatic patients. The vast majority of children show normal pulmonary function at rest. Some with severe deformities may have mild restrictive pulmonary function. Exercise pulmonary function studies in older children (10–12 years old) who are very athletic have demonstrated measurable decreases in cardiopulmonary function. A computed tomographic scan is helpful in the older patient to evaluate the degree of sternal rotation and position of the heart. We no longer use preoperative echocardiography in asymptomatic patients. We reserve cardiac evaluation for those patients with elastic cartilage deformities such as Marfan or Ehlers-Danlos syndrome.

ANESTHESIA

Chest wall reconstruction should be performed under general anesthesia with or without a thoracic epidural. If an epidural is used, a urinary bladder catheter is also recommended.

OPERATION

Modified Ravitch repair of pectus excavatum

The general concept of the modified Ravitch operation is resection of all abnormal costal cartilages. The sternum is displaced by the overgrowth in length of the cartilages and, therefore, needs only to be fractured on its anterior table to restore a normal position once it has been freed from the costal cartilages.

INCISION

1 A transverse, rather than vertical, incision through the deepest portion of the defect is the most appealing from a cosmetic perspective.

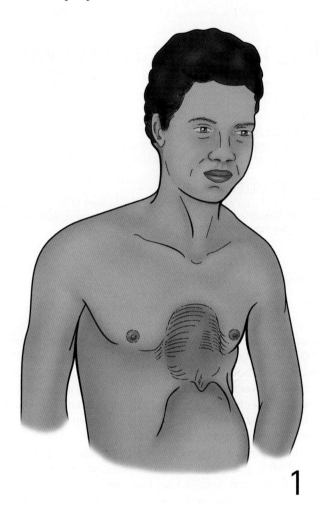

1

SKIN AND MUSCLE FLAPS

2 Superiorly and inferiorly based skin flaps at the level of, but not including, the pectoralis major fascia are raised. Pectoralis muscle flaps are created by dissecting from the midline to a position lateral enough to expose the costochondral junction. The entire defect may involve ribs 3–8, but most commonly the anomaly alters cartilages 5–8 bilaterally. A minimum of four cartilages bilaterally should be excised.

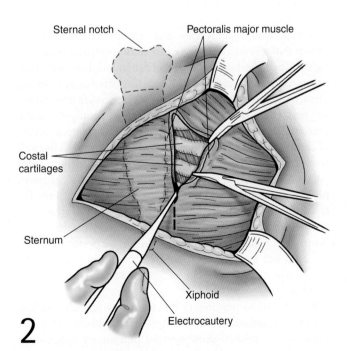

Sternal notch — Pectoralis major muscle

Costal cartilages

Sternum

Xiphoid

Electrocautery

2

SUBPERICHONDRIAL RESECTION OF THE DEFORMED CARTILAGES

3a–c

The perichondrium is incised anteriorly along each cartilage, and cephalad and caudad flaps are created to expose the defective cartilage (Figure 3a). Meticulous care is needed for the posterior portion of the dissection to avoid entering the pleural space. Each deformed cartilage is resected sharply from its junction with rib laterally to the attachment with the sternum (Figure 3b). The perichondrium must be preserved in its entirety because it is from this tissue that new cartilage and subsequent bone are generated (Figure 3c). Moreover, devascularization of the perichondrium may be a major cause for an acquired thoracodystrophy years later after pectus reconstruction.

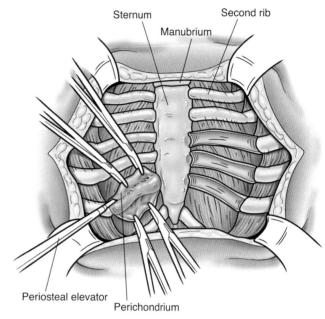

Sternum
Second rib
Manubrium
Periosteal elevator
Perichondrium

3a

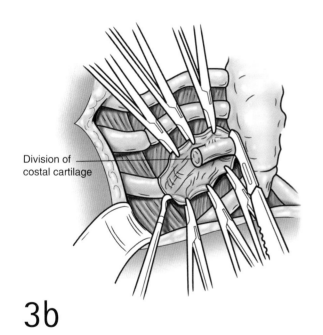

Division of costal cartilage

3b

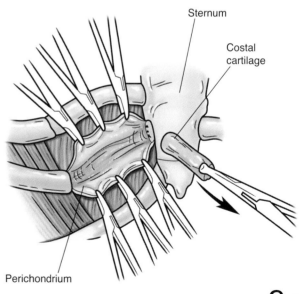

Sternum
Costal cartilage
Perichondrium

3c

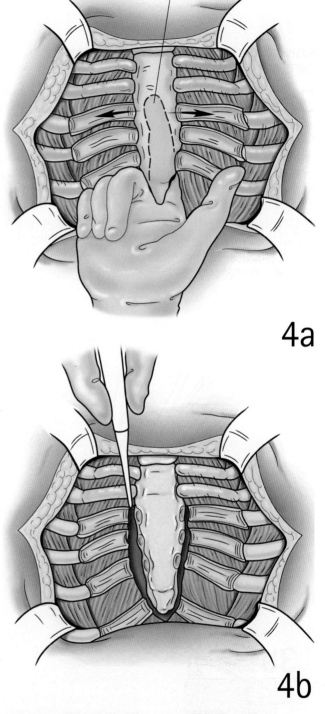

Pleura and pericardium
freed from sternum

4a

4b

MOBILIZATION OF THE STERNUM

4a, b The xiphoid is exposed and elevated, and a retrosternal plane is bluntly developed with the finger (Figure 4a). The pleura and pericardium are freed from the sternum using further finger dissection. The sternum is mobilized by dividing the intercostals and perichondrial bundles from their junction with the sternum (Figure 4b). Detachment begins at the xiphoid and proceeds just above the highest involved perichondrial bundle.

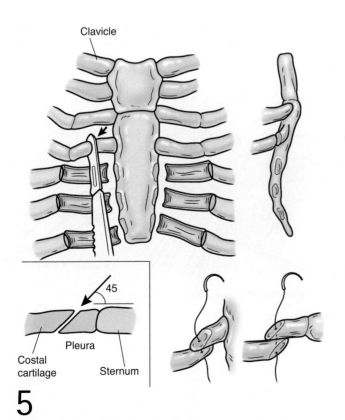

Clavicle

45

Costal
cartilage

Pleura

Sternum

5

STERNAL 'TRIPOD' SUPPORT

5 The sternum is then lifted into a more neutral position and supported by the lowest of the normal costal cartilages. Subperichondral exposure of this normal cartilage is performed bilaterally. This normal cartilage is divided obliquely (45 degrees) from medial to lateral so the medial portion (anterior) sits atop the lateral (posterior). To complete the tripod support of the sternum, the medial segment of cartilage is then sutured atop the lateral half.

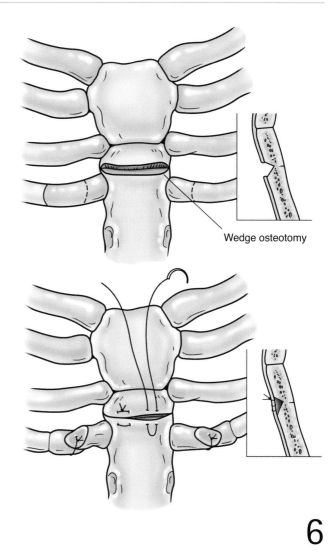

Wedge osteotomy

6

6 A single oblique or transverse wedge osteotomy of the anterior table of the sternum facilitates resolving the rotation of the sternum and adds to its support. Occasionally, a second anterior table osteotomy is required. A wedge of bone is removed, and the periosteum of the sternum is then sutured to further secure the sternum in its neutral position.

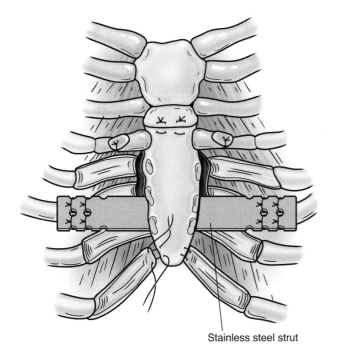

Stainless steel strut

7

7 For children older than 10–12 years, or those with elastic cartilage abnormalities (Marfan syndrome, Ehlers-Danlos syndrome), additional sternal support is recommended with a substernal stainless steel bar placed beneath the distal third of the sternum and secured to the ribs. Detached intercostal bundles need not be sutured to the sternum. If the distance between the sternum and resected bundle is no more than 2–3 cm, however, the defect may be closed with approximation of these tissues.

WOUND CLOSURE

8 A substernal drain is positioned to include decompression of any violated pleural space. Pectoralis flaps are closed over the sternum. A subcutaneous drain is inserted. Finally, skin flaps are reapproximated with subcuticular sutures.

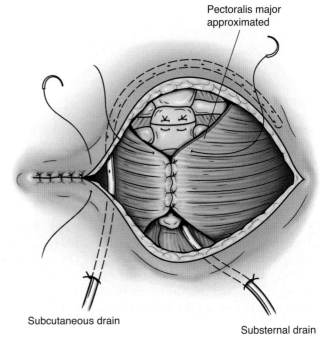

Pectoralis major approximated

Subcutaneous drain

Substernal drain

8

POSTOPERATIVE CARE

Perioperative antibiotics are discontinued at 24 hours. Incentive spirometry is vital to avoid atelectasis and possible pneumonia. Urinary retention is common in the teenager and older patient. Therefore, a bladder catheter is recommended for postoperative days 1 and 2. Costal cartilages regenerate within 6–8 weeks. Contact sports should be avoided during this regenerative interval. In children older than 10–12 years who undergo strut placement via the modified Ravitch repair, the strut is usually removed in 6–8 months.

OUTCOME

All reconstructions should yield a satisfactory cosmetic result. Modest physiological benefit can be documented in athletic teenagers at the peak of their fitness. In other cases, additional studies have demonstrated no physiological effect. Recurrence rates are reported as less than 5%. Recurrence seems to be more prevalent if the operation was done at a very early age (younger than 5–7 years) or during the older teen years (15–17 years). An acquired form of Jeune syndrome (thoracic chondrodystrophy) has been described in children repaired younger than 3 years old. These children underwent

extensive resection of the chest wall such that cartilage and perichondrium were devascularized. This problem is not a recurrence of the defect but rather represents a failure of the chest wall to grow. Over time, no growth occurred in the resected areas, which led to the chondrodystrophy. A floating sternum has also been described. In this condition, cartilage is resorbed, which leaves a fibrous or unstable connection between the sternum and ribs. The unstable sternum must be supported by struts to facilitate stable chest wall dynamics.

OPERATION

Modified minimally invasive repair of pectus excavatum (Nuss procedure)

A number of modifications have been made to the Nuss procedure since it was introduced in 1998. However, the basic concept is unchanged. A substernal bar is used to elevate the sternum and reposition the deformed costal cartilages. We use a modified Nuss procedure at the Johns Hopkins Children's Center. Currently, with the exception of a large bone hook and *in situ* bar benders, all equipment necessary for this reconstruction is supplied by Walter Lorenz Surgical in Jacksonville, Florida.

INCISION AND SKIN FLAPS

9 The patient should be positioned with arms abducted to allow access to the lateral chest wall. Placement of the skin incisions depends on the geography of the defect. If the defect is very low, care must be taken not to position the bar under the xiphoid. Similarly, in the older teenager the defect may extend to cartilages 3 and 4, which thus necessitates more superior chest wall incisions. In general, two 2.5- to 4.0-cm lateral thoracic incisions are made, each beginning below the nipple and extending laterally. The distance below the nipple is determined by which interspace the bar will traverse. Skin flaps are mobilized to include one intercostal space above and below the incision. Sufficient mobilization is necessary to allow for placement of bar stabilizers (see Figure 15).

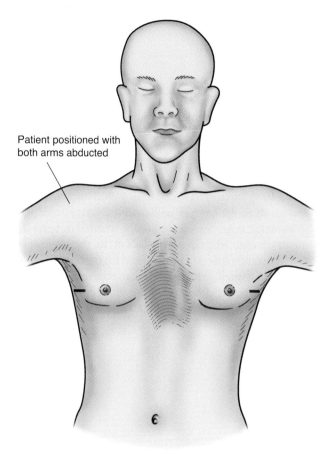

Patient positioned with both arms abducted

9

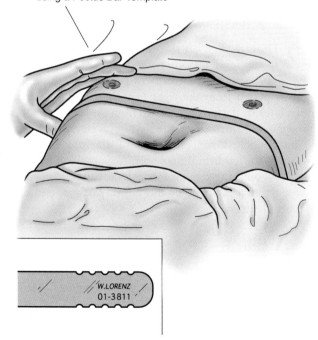

Confirming preoperative measurements using a Pectus Bar Template

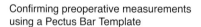

W.LORENZ
01-3811

10

TEMPLATE MEASUREMENTS

10 A bar template is used to determine the appropriate Lorenz bar. The template should be positioned in each of the lateral chest wall wounds and bent to the arc of the desired repair. The templates are numbered to facilitate use of the corresponding bar. We recommend overcorrection with a more angular arc, because the sternum invariably rests atop the bar in a position somewhat lower than that which the surgeon perceives. The segment of the bar directly underneath the sternum should be kept as flat as possible, however, to maintain as much sternal surface area in contact with the bar as possible. This maneuver facilitates a sturdy substernal support. In addition, the left side of the bar is not bent to the extent that the right side is conformed to the shape of the template. This maneuver facilitates easier passage of the bar through the substernal tunnel.

HEMITHORAX DISSECTION

11 The chest is entered, using electrocautery, in the intercostal space corresponding to the optimal position for sternal support. Typically, this position is at one intercostal space above the deepest portion of the defect. Each hemithorax must be entered in the area where the ribs begin to move from anterior to lateral chest wall. This point usually corresponds to the anterior axillary line. Next, a subxiphoid skin puncture is made. A bone hook is inserted into the sternum or ribcage immediately adjacent to the xiphisternal junction through this skin puncture. With the bone hook, the sternum is elevated anteriorly. This maneuver increases the distance between the sternum and pericardium, and facilitates safe substernal passage of the Crafoord clamp.

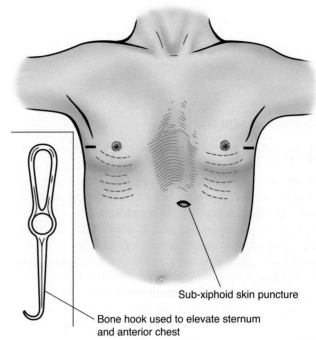

Sub-xiphoid skin puncture

Bone hook used to elevate sternum and anterior chest

11

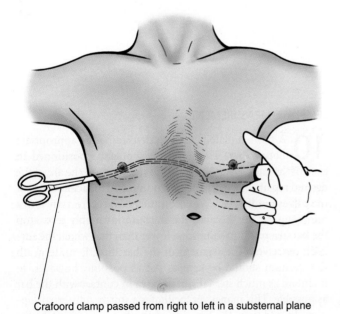

Crafoord clamp passed from right to left in a substernal plane

12

PASSAGE OF SUBSTERNAL CLAMP

12 Through the left-side incision in the intercostal space, finger dissection can be used in a substernal plane to a point as far medially as possible. The Crafoord clamp is passed from the right hemithorax and advanced until it is felt by the fingertip passed from the left hemithorax. Throughout this maneuver, the sternum is elevated by using the bone hook. Once the Crafoord clamp is advanced through to the left hemithorax hole, two umbilical tapes are caught and pulled retrograde through the tunnel. Some centers use a thoracoscope to doubly ensure safe passage of the Crafoord clamp.

INSERTION OF PECTUS BAR

13 The appropriate, previously bent Lorenz bar is tied to one of the umbilical tapes and passed from the right to left of the hemithorax in a concave-up position. Again, the anterior chest is elevated using the bone hook to ensure safe passage through the tunnel. Once the left side of the bar is through the chest, it can be bent to conform to the left side of the template.

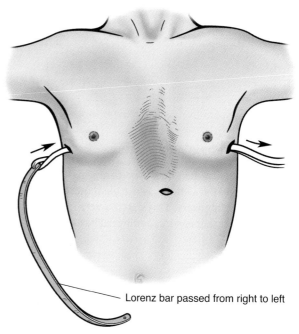

Lorenz bar passed from right to left

13

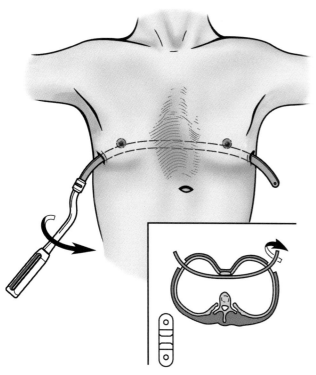

14

BAR FLIPPING AND APPLICATION OF STABILIZERS

14 The bar (concave up) is now flipped from a cranial to caudal direction. The bar should never be flipped in the reverse direction because the xiphoid can be injured and a less than optimal substernal support created. The bar is held in this position (concave down), and the surgeon immediately observes the desired position of the sternum and anterior chest. Bilateral bar stabilizers should be fastened to the bar.

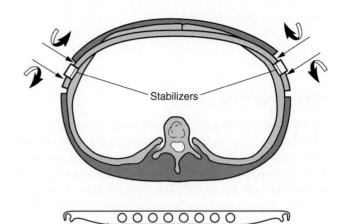

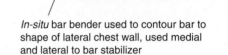

In-situ bar bender used to contour bar to shape of lateral chest wall, used medial and lateral to bar stabilizer

IN SITU BAR BENDING AND FIXATION

15 *In situ* bar bending now conforms the bar to the ribcage. Bar bending is usually required on each side of the vertical stabilizers. This step is a very important in the procedure because it ensures additional bar support.

15

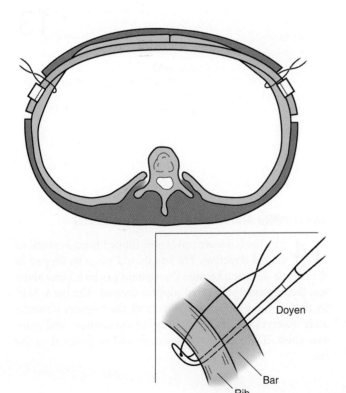

16 The bar is wired (No. 5 gauge) to the rib that it crossed over on each side of the chest just medial to the stabilizers using a tapered Doyen with a hole in the tip.

16

WOUND CLOSURE

Subcutaneous tissue is closed in the presence of 35–40 cm of peak inspiratory pressure. This maneuver facilitates removal of air contained in each hemithorax. A small red rubber catheter can also be inserted into each hemithorax and removed at the completion of wound closure. Last, the skin is closed.

POSTOPERATIVE CARE

A chest radiograph is obtained in the recovery room. Generally, 20–30% pneumothorax is well tolerated and does not require tube decompression. As with the Ravitch repair, older patients may require insertion of a Foley catheter. Despite a more minimal chest wall dissection, duration of narcotic requirement is longer than with the modified Ravitch repair. No contact sports are allowed for 8 weeks. Afterward, return to full activities is permitted. Children younger than 12 years may undergo bar removal at 2 years, whereas older teenagers, adolescents, and adults may require bar stabilization for 3–4 years.

OUTCOME

Complications include flipped bar, pneumothorax, pleural effusions, and chest wall asymmetry; one episode of cardiac puncture has been reported. Long-term results have yet to be determined. A significant learning curve is associated with the introduction of this new technique. Thoracoscopy or finger dissection and displacement of the sternum using a bone hook such as described herein have facilitated bar insertion. *In situ* bar bending and wiring have prevented flipping and displacement. Although published series show that this procedure is best performed between the ages of 8 and 12, we have used this modified technique ($n = 65$) at the Johns Hopkins Children's Hospital for adolescents and adults with excellent early results (age range, 8–42 years). We have also used the modified Nuss procedure for reoperation after a Ravitch-type repair ($n = 6$) with similar excellent early results.

FURTHER READING

Haller J. History of the operative management of pectus deformities. Surgical treatment of anterior chest wall deformities. *Chest Surgery Clinics of North America* 2000; 10: 227–35.

Haller J. Complications of surgery for pectus excavatum. Surgical treatment of anterior chest wall deformities. *Chest Surgery Clinics of North America* 2000; 10(2): 415–26.

Haller JA, Loughlin GM. Cardiorespiratory function is significantly improved following corrective surgery for severe pectus excavatum. *Journal of Cardiovascular Surgery* 2000; 41: 125–30.

Hebra A, Swoveland B, Egbert M, *et al.* Outcome analysis of minimally invasive repair of pectus excavatum: review of 251 cases. *Journal of Pediatric Surgery* 2000; 35: 252–8.

Morshuis W, Folgering H, Barentsz J, Van Lier H, Lacquet L. Pulmonary function before surgery for pectus excavatum and at long-term follow-up. *Chest* 1994; 105: 1646–52.

Nuss D, Kelly RE, Croitoru DP, Katz ME. A 10-year review of a minimally invasive technique for the correction of pectus excavatum. *Journal of Pediatric Surgery* 1998; 33: 545–52.

Thoracic trauma

KENNETH L. MATTOX, MD
Professor & Vice Chair, Michael E. DeBakey Department of Surgery, Baylor College of Medicine, Houston, Texas, USA

JON-CECIL M. WALKES, MD
Cardiothoracic Resident, Michael E. DeBakey Department of Surgery, Baylor College of Medicine, Houston, Texas, USA

HISTORY

For all countries of the world, throughout history, trauma is the leading cause of premature years of life lost, accounting for more years of life lost than the next three causes of death (cancer, cardiovascular disease, infectious diseases) combined. Thoracic trauma is responsible for up to 25% of the immediate deaths from trauma and is either responsible or contributes to an additional 25% of delayed trauma deaths. Among the trauma patients who die after reaching a health care facility, up to 33% of these deaths are preventable with appropriate systems applications, rapid transport, early diagnosis, appropriate therapy, expeditious indicated operation, and applications of surgical critical care principles postoperatively. A variety of thoracic operations are performed for specific conditions or injuries, and this chapter will focus on representative thoracic trauma operations. Although sporadic references to isolated injuries are made throughout history, the operations for thoracic trauma are a function of the twentieth century and principally the last half of the twentieth century.

PRINCIPLES AND JUSTIFICATION

Up to 80% of patients with thoracic trauma do not require a formal operation and are managed by observation, tube thoracostomy, and/or pain control. The most common operations following thoracic trauma are tube thoracostomy and exploratory thoracotomy. Indications for an operation for thoracic trauma are relatively well defined (Tables 2.1–2.3). Several historical thoracic trauma operations require careful justification prior to application. These procedures include subxyphoid pericardiotomy, thoracic exploration for simple mediastinal traverse, and "book" or "trapdoor" thoracotomy.

During the last decade of the twentieth century, advances in imaging, thoracoscopy, and endovascular therapies rapidly began to alter both the evaluation and treatment of thoracic trauma. In addition, advances in surgical critical care, anesthesia, and drugs altered the preoperative and postoperative care of patients with thoracic injury. As an example, bullet embolism and transthoracic injection of industrial solvents are no longer absolute indications for thoracotomy

Table 2.1 *Indications for acute thoracotomy*

Hemopericardium
Traumatic thoracotomy
Continuing hemothorax
Radiological evidence of thoracic great vessel injury
Esophageal injury
Massive air leak
Major bronchus injury
Witnessed traumatic arrest

Table 2.2 *Considerations for further evaluation following thoracic trauma*

Chest wall penetration of industrial solvents
Bullet embolism
Systemic air embolism
Mediastinal traverse

Table 2.3 *Indications for chronic thoracotomy*

Retained clotted hemothorax
Traumatic lung abscess
Delayed discovery of pseudoaneurysm
Traumatic cardiac valve or septal injury
Nonclosure of a chylous fistula
Biliary–bronchial fistula

PREOPERATIVE ASSESSMENT AND PREPARATION

Evaluation of any trauma patient involves prehospital assessment and transport, primary and secondary surveys in the emergency center, including trauma and thoracic surgeon evaluation and decision-making with regard to operation and continuing reassessment. To avoid missing an injury, a tertiary survey (repeat and re-repeat of the secondary survey) is recommended by many surgeons. The importance of injury background history, past medical history, and physical examination cannot be overemphasized.

Laboratory evaluation

For any trauma patient, minimum laboratory studies are required, such as dipstick urinalysis, hematocrit and, possibly, arterial blood gas evaluation. Should an operation be anticipated, type and cross match is considered. If angiography is anticipated, blood urea nitrogen (BUN) and creatinine are useful to the angiographer. Many of the routinely ordered biochemical tests do not alter the surgical decision-making, and include tests such drug screening, electrolytes, clotting studies, and liver function tests.

Routine and special imaging

The single most helpful evaluation of a patient with thoracic trauma is routine supine chest X-ray. A "funny looking mediastinum" suggests numerous signs that have been described and indicates a need for additional tests. Up to 5% of patients later found to have an injured aorta do not have any of these signs, nor a mediastinal hematoma on chest CT scanning. Hemothorax, pneumothorax, pneumomediastinum, bullet tract trajectories, mediastinal hematomas, missile fragments, broken bones, subcutaneous emphysema, thoracic outlet hematomas, and many other conditions can be readily diagnosed on this initial X-ray, and follow-up routine chest X-rays. Technological advances in imaging are randomly used by evaluating physicians, often without eliciting any additional or new information other than that already demonstrated on initial chest X-ray. These newer tests include computed tomography (CT), ultrasonography, magnetic resonance imaging (MRI), magnetic resonance angiography (MRA), and echocardiography, especially transesophageal echocardiography. Some digitizing machines provide 3-D reconstructed structures.

Spiral computed tomography

For a number of reasons, CT has been used with increased frequency for patients with thoracic trauma. Specifically, many emergency center physicians are using CT to look for mediastinal hematomas in patients with blunt thoracic injuries. Application of CT in this instance consumes both financial and personnel resources for a test that rarely alters the necessity for thoracic arteriography. CT often fails to demonstrate many of the more than 12 common congenital anatomical variants, which may be present in this subset of patients. CT scanning is critical to the evaluation of thoracic trauma patients with delayed or infectious pulmonary complications. The technology of enhanced CT is ever changing. New technology allowing for 3-D reconstruction of vascular structures is impressive, but often confusing. Many radiologists are reporting new spiral CT findings for which no clear understanding of the anatomical, histopathological, or physiological significance exists. It is important that any surgeon making a surgical decision fully understands the variances of emerging technology and is assured of specific injury patterns prior to an operation.

Focused abdominal sonogram for trauma (FAST)

The use of ultrasound imaging of the heart allows the surgeon to diagnose hemopericardium, oftentimes before it becomes clinically evident. As such, ultrasound is an invaluable screening tool in patients with suspected hemopericardium. Typically, the surgeon will obtain a subxyphoid or subcostal view of the heart and pericardial space coupled with a three-view ultrasonogram of the abdomen. The main limitation of the FAST exam is the learning curve of the examiner. Once mastered, one may expect a specificity of 95%. The most utilitarian application of FAST is in the patient with a hemopericardium.

Magnetic resonance imaging (MRI)/magnetic resonance angiography (MRA)

MRI and MRA are rarely used in the evaluation of thoracic trauma. Some spinal cord injuries require MRI, and MRA might be indicated for evaluation of thoracic outlet vascular injury in patients with dye allergies.

Arteriography

Arteriography is the gold standard for diagnosis of vascular injury. Even with a transesophageal echocardiography (TEE) or enhanced spiral CT scan demonstrating hemomediastinum, most surgeons will not operate on a thoracic vascular injury until the arteriogram has demonstrated the specific anatomy and injury location. For blunt injury to the thoracic aorta, aortography should follow a suspicious initial plain chest X-ray. For suspected penetrating injury to the aorta, aortography may not demonstrate the injury due to the dense dye column. For suspected thoracic outlet vascular injury, arteriography in the stable patient is essential in selecting the incision and planning treatment.

Transesophageal echocardiography (TEE)

TEE has been used electively by cardiac surgeons to assess the adequacy of cardiac septal and valvular repairs. TEE may be used to diagnose such septal and valvular injury following trauma. TEE has been used in some trauma centers to demonstrate an aortic injury. Like spiral CT, TEE is inconsistent in diagnosing with accuracy aortic injuries outside the usual location of the proximal descending thoracic aorta. At times, the TEE is also extremely sensitive, demonstrating shadows also shown with echo findings at thoractomy.

Esophagoscopy/tracheoscopy/bronchoscopy

Endoscopy is often used in penetrating thoracic trauma. In penetrating injuries, the blast effects often caused by missiles are frequently associated with extensive tissue destruction surrounding the area of penetration. Endoscopy allows the trauma surgeon to identify injuries to the aerodigestive tract and then operatively address such injuries in an appropriate manner.

ANESTHESIA

Most trauma centers require a board certified anesthesiologist to be on duty for trauma cases needing an operation. This requirement is especially important for a patient needing a thoracic operation. Often, special airway tubes, such as double lumen ventilatory tubes (Robertshaw and Carlin) are requested. If airway reconstruction is necessary, use of anode tubes might be necessary. By far the most important elements for successful management of the trauma patient is the need for constant communication between the anesthesiologist and the surgeon. The equipment is especially important with regard to blood pressure levels, crystalloid fluid management, use of paralytics, and pain control.

OPERATION

"Minor procedures"

TUBE THORACOSTOMY

Tube thoracostomy in thoracic trauma patients is a fundamental procedure and essential skill in the surgeon's armamentarium. Tube thoracostomies are used to evacuate air or fluid from the chest. They may be lifesaving in the case of the tension pneumothorax. They effectively evacuate blood and provide a means of monitoring blood loss, thereby aiding in the decision for formal thoracotomy (see Chapter 12).

PERICARDIOCENTESIS

Pericardiocentesis has traditionally been used in patients suffering from cardiac tamponade. With the advent of subxyphoid cardiac ultrasonography, hemopericardium is now diagnosed before it becomes clinically evident. As a result, patients are frequently taken to the operating room for formal evacuation. However, pericardiocentesis carries the risk for iatrogenic cardiac injury when performed by an inexperienced individual.

SUBXYPHOID PERICARDIOTOMY

With the advent of the FAST examination, subxyphoid pericardiotomy has virtually no indications. On rare occasions, when abdominal exploration reveals no explanation for continuing hypotension, a transabdominal pericardiotomy might be considered.

ENDOVASCULAR RECONSTRUCTION

Increasingly, transvascular stenting, including stented grafts, is being used to treat thoracic vascular injury, including subclavian, innominate, and even descending thoracic injury, both blunt and penetrating. For thoracic outlet vascular injury, some such treatment is being accomplished at the time of initial diagnostic arteriography. However, most endovascular treatment is still being performed under research protocols.

"Major" exploratory procedures

POSITIONING

Supine and lateral decubitus positions are essentially the only ones used in thoracic trauma. Oblique positions often compromise exposure and repair.

INCISIONS

The utility incision for thoracic trauma is an anterolateral thoracotomy, usually through the fourth or fifth interspace. Occasionally, a bilateral transternal anterolateral thoracotomy is required, taking care to ligate the transected internal mammary arteries. With a transternal thoracotomy, the incision is curved upward exposing a sufficient amount of sternum for good closure. A median sternotomy should be reserved for stab wounds between the nipples and for suspected ascending aorta and thoracic outlet injury. Posterolateral thoracotomy is used for injury to the lung, esophagus, descending aorta, azygous vein, and thoracic duct injury.

EMERGENCY CENTER (RESUSCITATIVE) THORACOTOMY

Indications for emergency center thoracotomy have been narrowed over recent years. Numerous studies have demonstrated that the majority of unintubated patients requiring prehospital external cardiac massage for 4 minutes die, while the majority of intubated patients die if administered prehospital cardiopulmonary resuscitation for greater than 10 minutes. Ideally, a patient requiring resuscitative thoracotomy has been intubated by prehospital personnel.

1 For emergency thoracotomy the patient should be placed supine and the incision drawn in an inframammary location at the level of the left fifth interspace. In women, the breast must be retracted cephalad to open up the interspace.

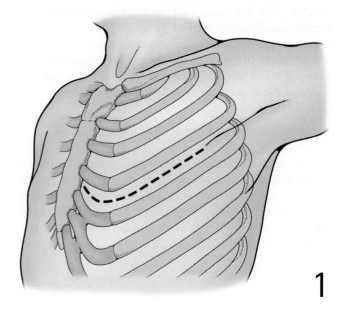

1

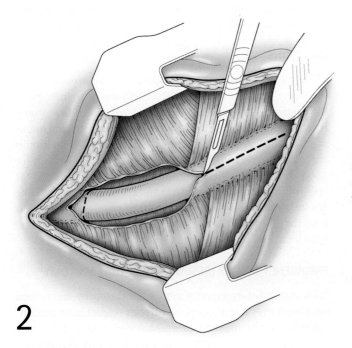

2

2 The intercostal muscles are divided with Mayo scissors, and the interspace opened using a standard rib retractor with ratchets away from the sternum.

3 Scissors are used to open the pericardium anterior to the phrenic nerve.

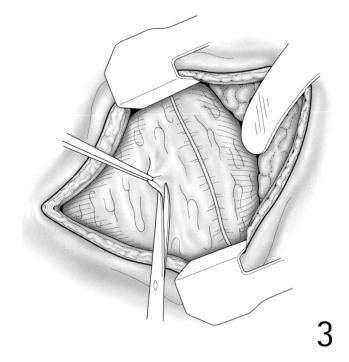

3

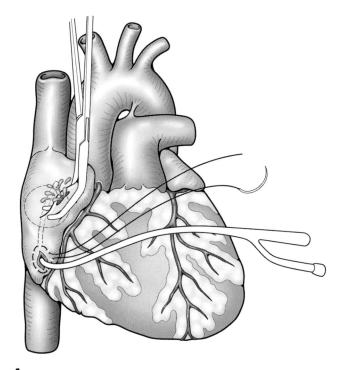

4

4 Blood clots are removed, and bleeding is controlled with direct digital pressure. The lung is retracted anteriorly, and the descending thoracic aorta is occluded with a large vascular clamp. In a nonbeating heart with penetrating injury, cardiorrhaphy is accomplished prior to defibrillation. When the heart is distended, inflow occlusion is accomplished, and the heart is compressed to facilitate cardiorrhaphy.

For injuries of the right atrial appendage, a curved vascular clamp may be applied to control hemorrhage, and the defect is closed using a running 4-0 polypropylene suture.

CARDIORRHAPHY

Whether part of an emergency center (resuscitative) or operating room thoracotomy, cardiorrhaphy is performed in the same manner. Cardiorrhaphy is required more often for penetrating wounds. In the beating heart, cardiorrhaphy is delayed until other aspects of a resuscitation have been accomplished, such as cross clamping the aorta, securing an airway, and assuring vascular access. Intermittent cardiac compressions assure forward aortic blood flow during this process.

Temporary control of cardiac hemorrhage may be accomplished using standard or extra wide skin stapling devices. Glove perforation may be as high as 80% in urgent post-traumatic cardiorrhaphy.

5 Definitive control and repair of cardiac wounds is accomplished with 3-0 or 4-0 polypropylene suture.

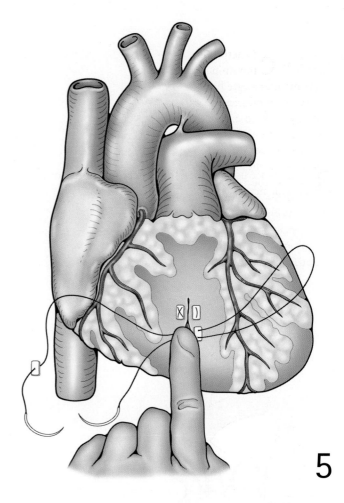

5

Injuries to the right and left ventricle are repaired using horizontal mattress sutures. Vascular clamps are usually not applied to the ventricles. Some surgeons use Teflon pledgets to reinforce the repair, although we find that pledgets are not required. Pledgeted sutures are not routinely used on the left ventricle. Care is taken while placing horizontal mattress stitches near the left anterior descending coronary artery (or other major arteries) so as not to occlude an injured vessel. Cardiopulmonary bypass for the repair of an injured left anterior descending coronary artery by aorto-coronary bypass has been successfully reported in less than six cases. After cardiorrhaphy is completed, internal cardiac massage may be re-instituted if necessary. Intracardiac injections may be accomplished. Cardiac resuscitation is aided by gentle saline lavage of the heart using fluid warmed to 110°F (43.5°C).

REPAIR OF INJURY TO THE ASCENDING AORTA

For suspicious injury to the thoracic outlet (blunt or penetrating), a median sternotomy is extended to the neck to assure that control can be achieved. Injuries to the ascending aorta are more common in penetrating trauma, although the authors have repaired six blunt ascending aortic injuries in the past 4 years. Single, anteriorly located wounds might be repaired by simple aortorrhaphy with 4-0 polypropylene. Very proximal and posterior ascending aortic injury often requires the patient to be placed on cardiopulmonary bypass.

In cases of injury that involve both anterior and posterior walls of the aorta, a Dacron tube graft is inserted using a running 4-0 polypropylene suture, while on cardiopulmonary bypass.

REPAIR OF AORTIC ARCH/INNOMINATE ARTERY INJURY

Blunt injury to the aortic arch is often confused with a proximal innominate artery injury, as the intima from the orifice of the innominate artery rolls up and presents on the arteriogram at 1–3 cm beyond this orifice. Cardiopulmonary bypass is almost never required for innominate artery reconstruction.

6a–c Penetrating injuries to the entirety of the innominate artery are reconstructed in the same manner as are blunt aortic arch and innominate artery injury. Such injuries are approached through a median sternotomy with an anterior neck extension. For ease in exposure, the innominate vein might require purposeful division. Injuries are reconstructed by simple bypass exclusion technique with the appropriately sized knitted Dacron graft sutured to the ascending aorta in an end-to-side fashion, prior to the interruption of flow through the innominate artery. With vascular clamps on either side of the injury, the distal anastomosis is accomplished without heparinization, shunts, or hypothermia. When the distal anastomosis is completed, the base of the innominate at the aorta is oversewn.

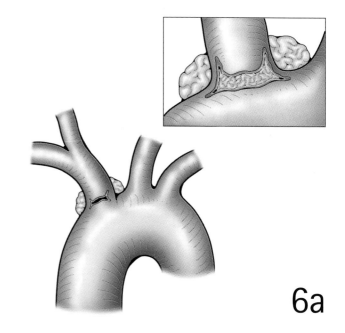

6a

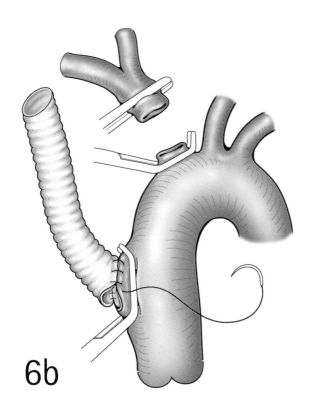

6b

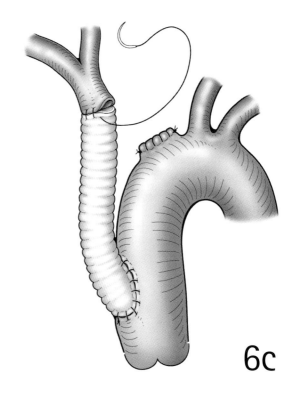

6c

REPAIR OF DESCENDING THORACIC AORTIC INJURY

Within the next 5 years, changing therapy for "stable" proximal descending aortic injuries will shift to endovascular stented grafts, up to and including acute injury. Increasingly, "stable" aortic injury will have purposeful delay of reconstruction. Reconstruction is accomplished via a fourth interspace posterolateral thoractomy. After entering the chest, the initial objective with injury of this location is to gain control of the thoracic aorta, both distal to the site of hematoma and at the aortic arch. The transverse aortic arch is exposed and encircled, using umbilical tapes between the left carotid and left subclavian arteries. The surgeon may consider any one of several standard and accepted techniques to address circulation distal to the vascular clamps. Should either active or passive shunting (with or without heparinization) be considered, the cannulae are inserted and bypass instituted. Whether shunting or simple clamp and repair techniques are chosen, the proximal and distal clamps are applied to the proximal aorta, left subclavian artery, and distal thoracic aorta. The aorta is entered at the point of maximum hematoma, and the degree of injury is assessed. A Dacron interposition graft is required in more than 85% of the cases. The preferred suture material for primary or graft interposition is 4-0 polypropylene.

PULMONARY TRACTOTOMY

When a through and through injury to the lung is encountered, uncontrolled bleeding often occurs from both holes. One option is to perform an anatomical resection, either lobectomy or pneumonectomy. As these injuries are often nonanatomical and post-traumatic pneumonectomy is not well tolerated, pulmonary tractotomy is a recommended option.

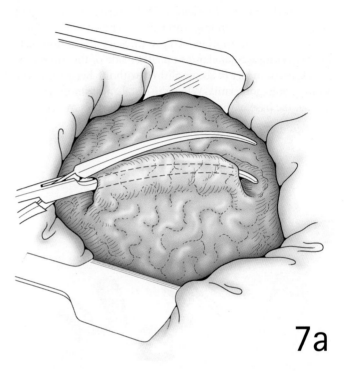

7a

7a,b A pulmonary tractotomy is an alternative approach. Two large vascular clamps are passed through the parenchymal defect. The tissue is divided and then oversewn. However, oversewing entry and exit holes at the surface of the lung may result in uncontrollable hemoptysis or the development of a large pulmonary hematoma, which might require a later pneumonectomy.

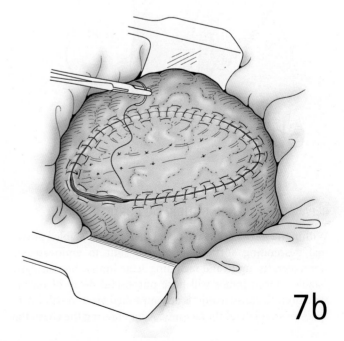

7b

8 The surgeon may place two large vascular clamps or pulmonary stapling devices through the lung injury, entering into one of the puncture holes. The entrance and exit sites are then joined using a knife or scissors.

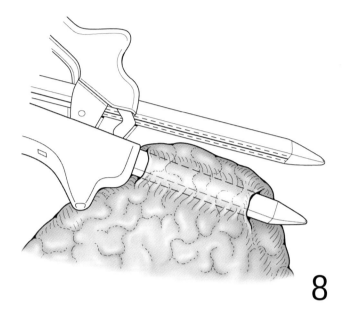

8

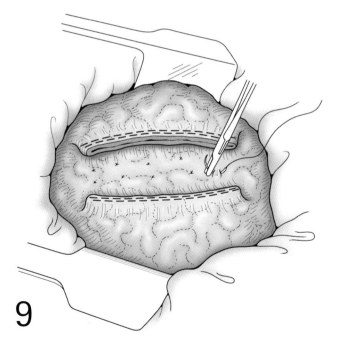

9

9 The base of the opened tract is oversewn with 0-polypropylene on a large needle, and the two clamped sides of the tract are stapled with a GIA stapler or oversewn with 0-polypropylene suture. 4-0 polypropylene suture is used to selectively ligate bleeding vessels and control air leaks.

TRACHEOPLASTY/BRONCHORRHAPHY

Tracheal and bronchus injury are extremely rare and are most often encountered within 2 cm of the carina. Management and approach to trachea and bronchus injury depends on the size and location of injury. Most cervical tracheal injuries can be repaired through a transverse cervical incision. Thoracic tracheal and right bronchial injuries are approached through a right fourth posterolateral incision. Left mainstem bronchial injury is approached through a left fourth postero-lateral incision.

10a–c The extent of mucosal injury is identified and the muscularis opened to expose the entire mucosal layer. The injury is closed in two layers. Repair of the injury is performed with 3-0 interrupted absorbable sutures, with knots tied outside the bronchus or trachea. After completion, the repair may be buttressed with a vascularized intercostals pedicle flap.

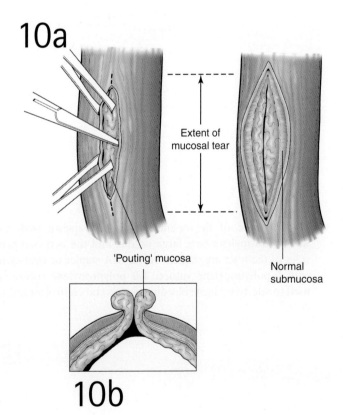

10a

Extent of mucosal tear

'Pouting' mucosa

Normal submucosa

10b

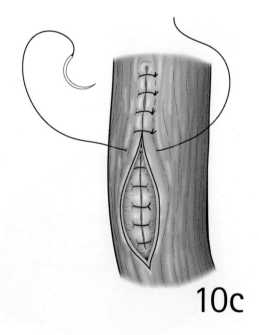

10c

ESOPHAGORRHAPHY

Patients with an esophageal injury may present insidiously or in profound septic shock. Pain is the most common symptom of esophagus perforation. Esophagography with barium contrast should be performed judiciously. These authors do not recommend water-soluble contrast material because it is less sensitive in confirming a diagnosis and, if aspirated, can contribute to a significant pulmonary reaction. Exposure of the upper esophagus is facilitated by division of the azygous vein. After the injury is identified, any necrotic mediastinal pleura is excised, and the repair is performed in two layers. After repair is completed, a musculopleural flap is mobilized based on the intercostals neurovascular bundle and used to buttress the repair. The area should be widely drained. In instances of a longstanding mediastinal abscess and/or in a septic unstable patient, the esophageal injury may be simply drained with the aid of a very large T-tube placed into the esophagus and brought out the side.

LUNG TWIST FOR HEMORRHAGE CONTROL

When uncontrolled bleeding from the lung is encountered during an emergency center or operating room thoracotomy and the patient is hemodynamically unstable, a damage control maneuver known as, "lung twisting" can control the bleeding.

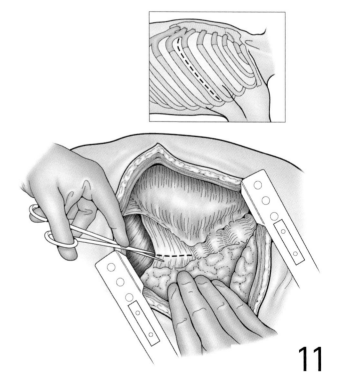

11 To begin, the inferior pulmonary ligament must be released up to the level of the inferior pulmonary vein. Any adhesions between the parietal and visceral pleura are lysed.

11

12 One hand is placed on the anterior aspect of the upper lobe and the other on the posterior aspect of the lower lobe. The apex of the lung is twisted 180 degrees to the base of the pleural cavity, and the base of the lung is rotated 180 degrees to lie at the apex of the cavity.

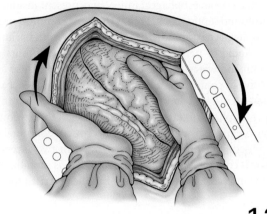

12

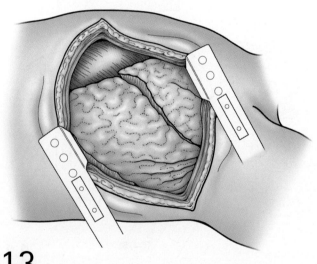

13

13 Once twisted, the apex of the lung will lie along the diaphragm. Bleeding from the lung will completely cease. Laparotomy pads to hold the twisted lung in position might be required.

14 As circulation to the lung also is impaired because the vascular structures will be twisted around the bronchus, lung twisting is analogous to a "medical pneumonectomy." A formal pulmonary resection is performed when the patient is stable.

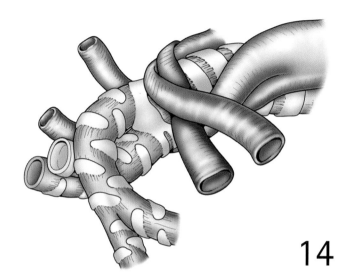

14

POSTOPERATIVE CARE

Patients with thoracic trauma requiring an operation need monitoring in a surgical intensive care unit. Antibiotic and deep vein thrombosis (DVT) prophylaxis for high-risk patients must be considered. Ventilatory management is carefully monitored and controlled. Extubation is accomplished using appropriate weaning protocols. Postoperative complications are similar to those for other operations on the organs which had been injured.

OUTCOME

The mortality and complications of the various operations cited is variable, depending on specific organ(s) injured. For patients surviving the initial traumatic insult and the first 3 days in the surgical intensive care unit, long-term survival is good and usual. Some injuries, such as injury to the esophagus, have a higher morbidity and mortality rate.

FURTHER READING

Ahn SH, Cutry A, Murphy TP, Slaiby JM. Traumatic thoracic aortic rupture: treatment with endovascular graft in the acute setting. *Journal of Trauma* 2001; **50**: 949–51.

Cohn SM, Heid MP, Augenstein JS, Bowen JC, McKenney MG, Duncan Horton TG. Identification of trauma patients at risk of thoracic aortic tear by mechanism of injury. *Journal of Trauma* 2000; **48**: 1008–14.

Grocott HP, Scales G, Schinderle D, King K. A new technique for lung isolation in acute thoracic trauma. *Journal of Trauma* 2000; **49**: 940–2.

Hix WR, Mills M. The management of esophageal wounds. *Annals of Surgery* 1970; **172**: 1002–6.

Kiser C, O'Brien SM, Detterbeck FC. Blunt tracheobronchial injuries: treatment and outcomes. *Annals of Thoracic Surgery* 2001; **71**: 2059–65.

Shin DD, Jr, Wall MJ, Mattox KL. Combined penetrating injury of the innominate artery, left common carotid artery, trachea, and esophagus. *Journal of Trauma* 2000; **49**: 780–3.

Chest wall tumors

ANNA MARIA CICCONE
Division of Thoracic Surgery, Universita La Sapienza, Rome, Italy

TIZIANO DE GIACOMO
Division of Thoracic Surgery, Universita La Sapienza, Rome, Italy

ERINO ANGELO RENDINA
Division of Thoracic Surgery, Universita La Sapienza, Rome, Italy

FEDERICO VENUTA
Division of Thoracic Surgery, Universita La Sapienza, Rome, Italy

HISTORY

The first known chest wall resection was reported by Aimar in 1778. Rehn at the beginning of this century reported a very high incidence of complications and quoted a 20% mortality rate, similar to that reported by Quenue and Longuet in 1989. The first report of chest wall resection in the United States was by Parham in 1889. From the early to the middle years of the twentieth century, limited numbers of resections of chest wall tumors were reported. In 1921, Hedgeblom described his experience of 313 cases, of which 73% were malignant. Twenty years later, O'Neal and Ackerman reported 96 cases of tumors of the ribs and of the sternum. Another large experience was reported by Hockemberg in 1953, who observed and treated 205 cases of chest wall tumors. Respiratory complications and sepsis were the most common and serious problems at that time. The modern era of chest wall resection began late in the 1960s, thanks to the improvement in surgical techniques and anesthesia, the introduction of antibiotics and intensive care units, and the development of new methods of reconstruction. Extensive resection of the chest wall became possible with more acceptable morbidity and mortality. Furthermore, better understanding of the natural history, biological variability of the cell types, and the use of radiation and chemotherapy, allowed for better treatments and improved results.

PRINCIPLES AND JUSTIFICATION

Primary chest wall tumors have been estimated to represent less than 1% of all tumors. The majority of them originate from the cartilage or bone, but they can develop in any of the histological elements of the thorax including muscle, nerve, and soft tissue. Moreover, neoplasms of the external thorax could be a metastatic lesion from a previously treated or occult primary tumor. Approximately 60% of the time, primary chest wall tumors are malignant. The principal requirement for adequate local control of chest wall tumors remains wide local excision. With the available skeletal and soft tissue reconstructive techniques, even large lesions can be successfully resected with safe margins. Although the primary purpose of these operations is a curative resection, a significant number of symptomatic patients can benefit from palliative resection. A key element is a multidisciplinary approach by the thoracic surgeon, the reconstructive surgeon, the medical oncologist, and the radiotherapist.

Epidemiology and classification

Although chest wall tumors are uncommon, they consist of a variety of both benign and malignant lesions. They may be primary or metastatic or may involve the chest wall by contiguous spread from adjacent disease, most often lung or breast cancer. Approximately 60% of all primary chest wall tumors are malignant.

MALIGNANT PRIMARY TUMORS

In adults, the most common primary malignant lesions are chondrosarcoma, plasmacytoma, and fibrosarcoma. **Chondrosarcoma** frequently appears as a large lobulated excrescent mass arising from a rib, with scattered calcification.

As with other cartilaginous tumors, chondrosarcomas commonly develop from the costo-chondral junction, and radiographically they may be indistinguishable from an osteochondroma or chondroma. **Plasmacytoma** is less frequent than chondrosarcoma, but the systemic disease, multiple myeloma, is frequently seen to involve several ribs as well as the sternum. The lesions of plasmacytoma or multiple myeloma typically appear as well-defined lytic lesions associated with extrapleural soft masses, similar to most metastatic lesions. In advanced plasmacytoma, marked erosion, expansion, and destruction of the bony cortex is often present, sometimes with a thick ridging around the periphery, causing the "soap bubble" appearance. **Fibrosarcoma** is the most common malignant tumor of the chest wall arising from the soft tissue in adults. However, as reported in most earlier series, the term fibrosarcoma probably includes many cases that now would be classified as malignant fibrous histiocytoma, as well as spindle cell tumors such as malignant schwannoma or synovial sarcoma. Fibrosarcoma often presents as a mass of soft tissue density associated with necrotic low density areas; foci of calcification may be present. Approximately 15% of malignant schwannomas develop in the trunk, and about one-third are on the anterior chest wall. Like their benign counterpart, they appear as rounded or elliptical masses adjacent to the rib. Any radiographic evidence of bony destruction is indicative of a malignant process. Other less common primary chest wall tumors seen in the adult population are **osteosarcoma, liposarcoma, and angiosarcoma.**

In children and adolescents, the most common primary tumor of the chest wall is **Ewing's sarcoma** that generally presents as a lytic and sometimes expansive lesion of a rib or clavicle with associated new bone formation and a soft tissue mass. Frequently, pleural effusion, fever and general symptoms are present. Ewing's sarcoma is also seen as the common metastatic tumor of the bony thorax.

Other less common primary malignant tumors in the pediatric age group are osteosarcoma, rhabdomyosarcoma, and mesenchymoma.

BENIGN TUMORS

Approximately half of all chest wall tumors are benign, and the majority of them are of cartilaginous origin, namely **chondromas, enchondromas, and osteochondromas.** These lesions are often incidentally found on chest X-ray done for unrelated purposes. Malignant degeneration is rare in solitary lesions, but it may occur in as many as 5–20% of cases in inherited syndromes such as multiple osteochondromatosis or enchondromatosis. **Fibrous dysplasia** is the most common bone tumor or tumor-like condition of the ribs, accounting for 20–30% of all benign bone tumors of the chest wall. Fibrous dysplasia probably originates from the bone-forming mesenchyme. The disease usually presents as a painless, lytic lesion, often with a localized area of bone expansion, located in the posterior aspect of the rib. Less common benign bone tumors of the chest wall include

eosinophilic granuloma, osteoblastoma, haemangioma usually located in a vertebral body, and **chondroblastoma.**

The most common benign soft tissue tumor of the chest wall is the **lipoma,** that generally occurs deep in the soft tissue, just outside the parietal pleura and often with an intrathoracic and extrathoracic component connected by an isthmus of tissue between the ribs.

Neurofibromas and **schwannomas** most commonly occur in the posterior mediastinum, but they can originate from the intercostal or other nerves of the chest wall. These tumors usually appear as well-circumscribed spherical or elongated masses, causing sometimes widening of the neural foramina, as well as pressure, erosion, and rib spreading of adjacent ribs. Evident bone destruction indicates a malignant differentiation.

METASTATIC DISEASE

Metastatic lesions are the most common tumors of the chest wall and are seen more frequently than either primary malignant or benign tumors. In the adult population, the most common metastatic diseases are lung, breast, kidney, and prostate carcinomas. With the exceptions of prostate and breast cancer, the large majority of metastatic tumors to the chest wall are lytic. In children, neuroblastoma, leukemia, and Ewing's sarcoma are the most common metastatic lesions.

PREOPERATIVE ASSESSMENT AND PREPARATION
Symptoms and physical findings

Approximately 20% of patients with chest wall tumor are asymptomatic. The most common referred symptom is pain, present in 50–60% of patients with enlarging masses. General symptoms (weight loss, asthenia, fever) are inconstant. Physical examination should be aimed to evaluate the tumor location and size and the possible involvement of contiguous organs. Malignant tumors are usually fixed to the bony thorax. Location of the lesion may suggest the histological type of the tumor. Usually, cartilaginous tumors arise along the costo-chondral junctions in the anterior wall of the chest. Masses away from the osteo-cartilaginous structures are usually of soft tissue origin.

Diagnosis

Radiographic evaluation of the chest wall tumor is crucial to determine the origin of the mass (cartilage, bone, soft tissue), as well as planning for surgical or nonsurgical therapy. A standard **chest X-ray** can be used to localize the lesion and to obtain some information about the status of the lung fields and the pleural cavity (pleural effusion). **Computed tomography** (CT) is the most valuable tool in the evaluation of chest wall neoplasms, because of its excellent contrast resolution and the images in the axial plane. CT defines, albeit incompletely, the relations between the tumor and the contiguous structures. Examination of the lung windows will help to discover eventual synchronous metastatic disease. Mediastinal or bone windows provide the best information on the dimensions and density of the tumor and bone destruction. CT is also valuable to assess the relation of the tumor to the chest wall musculature, helping in chest wall reconstruction planning. **Magnetic resonance imaging** (MRI) can add significant information because of greater contrast resolution and ability to image in multiple planes. Useful data can also be recorded on the nature of the tumor. Bone scan should be performed in all cases of chest wall tumor.

Current opinion suggests that all chest wall tumors should be considered malignant until proven to be otherwise; and when possible, wide excision should be carried out. Usually, small lesions can be resected totally without preliminary biopsy. For larger lesions, preoperative histological diagnosis should be obtained. Fine needle aspiration biopsy or core cutting biopsy is used. The latter has higher accuracy (96%) than fine needle aspiration. If these techniques do not yield a definitive diagnosis, an incisional biopsy is justified and performed through a transverse incision which can easily be excised at the time of the definitive resection.

Preoperative evaluation

Chest wall resection and reconstruction is a major procedure with a risk of life-threatening complication. Accurate preoperative assessment is therefore crucial, because it allows detection and treatment of correctable problems and permits the surgeon to individualize the postoperative management. Risk factors may be cardiovascular, pulmonary, or nutritional.

CARDIAC EVALUATION

In general, the cardiac risk for a chest wall operation is similar to that of any major surgical procedure. A history of recent myocardial infarction or poorly congestive heart failure is a contraindication to elective chest wall resection.

PULMONARY EVALUATION

A good history is essential and should include questioning for smoking, chronic conditions, infections, dyspnea on exertion, and any other symptoms suggesting respiratory impairment. All patients undergoing chest wall resection have some degree of postoperative ventilatory dysfunction. Routine preoperative evaluation should include chest X-ray, arterial blood gas analysis, and spirometry before and after bronchodilation.

NUTRITIONAL ASSESSMENT

Malnourished patients have a higher incidence of postoperative complications. In general, it is advisable to delay the operation as long as is required to correct malnutrition. Body weight, serum protein levels, serum transferrin, and total lymphocyte count can be useful.

CHEST WALL RESECTION AND RECONSTRUCTION

Planning the operation is dependent on the assessment of several factors:

1 Exact histological diagnosis
2 The extent of chest wall involvement
3 History of previous radiation or surgical operation at the site of the disease
4 Medical conditions of the patient
5 Aim of the treatment: cure or palliation.

A combined preoperative evaluation by both the thoracic surgeon and the plastic surgeon is advisable to discuss the need, the availability, and the feasibility of soft tissue coverage in cases of wide chest wall resection.

In patients for whom palliative resection is planned and who have incurable tumor, two main points should be considered: first, although long term survival is not expected, local excision and tumor control can improve the quality of life; second, patients whose symptoms are correlated to compression of the lung or other organs clearly show improvement in symptoms and quality of life after palliative resection. These findings justify surgical treatment, especially when nonsurgical options are of little or no benefit.

Patient's position

Positioning of the patient for a chest wall resection depends on the location of the chest wall tumor. The patient is positioned and draped on the operating table so that both resection and reconstruction are facilitated. For anterior lesions, the patient may be kept in the supine position, with slight lateral elevation to assist in thoracotomy. The majority of the chest wall lesions are most easily resected with the patient positioned as for posterolateral thoracotomy.

ANESTHESIA

Standard inhalation and narcotic techniques can be used for chest wall operations. Selective ventilation using a double lumen tracheal tube is extremely useful, especially to define any adhesions between the chest wall tumor and the underlying lung and to aid the exploration of the chest cavity as well as the resection. Epidural analgesia is usually very useful in the management of postoperative pain.

OPERATION

Tumor resection

Traditionally, the **skin incision** was placed to avoid the tumor, but it is well known nowadays that the incision can safely be done over the tumor to improve the exposure and reduce the vascular damage to the cutaneous area if the skin is spared. In fact, resection of skin and subcutaneous tissues is necessary only if the tumor is adherent to or has penetrated these structures or to excise previous scars, including biopsy sites. The skin overlying previous irradiated tumors should be resected. During the dissection, it is preferable to include one normal musculofascial plane between the skin and the lesion. However, muscle not adherent to the chest wall (latissimus dorsi, pectoralis major, scapular muscles) should be spared if not involved.

1 The pleural cavity is usually entered one intercostal space below or above the first uninvolved rib, and the intrathoracic extension of the tumor is evaluated by finger palpation. The presence or absence of adhesions to the lung and pleural effusion can also be assessed by this initial thoracotomy, as well as the relation of the tumor to the ribs that will serve as the superior, medial and lateral margins. Adhesions between the lung and the chest wall should not be violated; they can be easily divided after complete or almost complete mobilization of the chest wall mass.

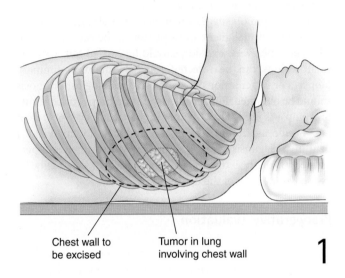

Chest wall to be excised

Tumor in lung involving chest wall

1

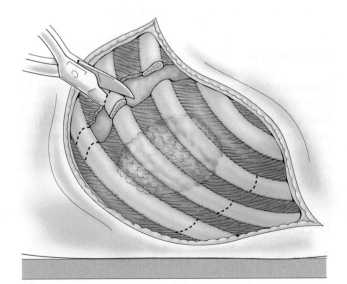

2

2 After the chest has been assessed, and the rib above which the intercostal incision was made is judged to be clear of tumor, the incision is extended anteriorly and posteriorly. The cephalad and caudad margins of the resection are one normal rib superiorly and inferiorly. The extent of lateral margins is controversial. Usually, 3–4 cm of grossly normal tissue with microscopic evaluation of the margins by frozen section is considered sufficient. The ribs are most easily divided using a costotome or a guillotine bone cutter; the intercostal bundle is encircled and divided between ties of nonabsorbable suture. The intercostal muscle may be divided between ribs using diathermy. When a rib is clearly involved by the tumor, it should be completely excised with its cartilaginous articulation, because it is not possible to predict the marrow extension of the tumor.

3 After all of the rib segments are resected and all intercostal bundles are secured, the portion of the chest wall should be completely free except for any attachments to the lung or diaphragm. Segments of pleura and pericardium are included in the resection if involved. With TA or GIA stapling devices, the lung can be divided so the resection will include any adhesions. The diaphragm can be widely excised and re-approximated using mattress sutures. Involvement of the subscapular muscle or the scapula itself can be approached by removing the scapula partially or totally, with re-suturing of the uninvolved muscles to the residual chest wall. En bloc removal of the tumor is an important criterion for a complete resection.

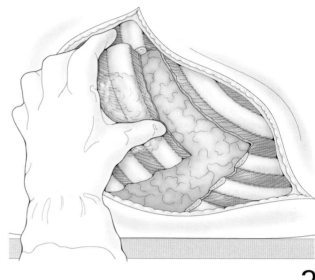

3

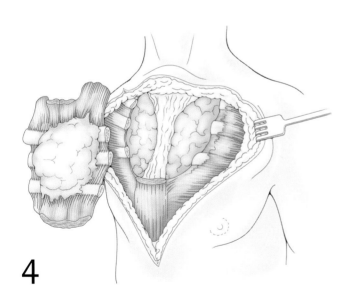

4

4 Tumors of the sternum are evaluated preoperatively for involvement of underlying structures. The skeletal resection of sternal tumors encompasses 2–4 cm of rib in addition to the affected portion of the sternum. It is preferable to keep part of the sternum intact if the margin of resection is safe. It is advisable to save one or both superior epigastric vessels to retain the option of using the rectus abdominis muscle flap for the reconstruction.

Reconstruction

After completion of the resection, skeletal stabilization is carried out, followed by the soft tissue coverage if needed. Basic surgical principles include adequate hemostasis and drainage of the pleural cavity, protection of the pedicle flap from extrinsic compression, approximation of tissues without tension, and measures that prevent air-leak.

In planning the reconstruction of chest wall defects several factors should be considered:

1 The structure of the underlying defect
2 The location and size of the defect
3 The aim of the operation (palliation or cure)
4 The general condition of the patient
5 Previous surgical operation that may interfere with the choice of the flap for reconstruction
6 Prior radiation therapy that may change the quality of the skin and may require full thickness resection of the irradiated field.

SKELETAL RECONSTRUCTION

For limited resections of 5 cm or less, no rigid replacement is necessary because usually no physiological effects will occur after the resection. Larger defects can require some rigid support to obtain sufficient chest wall stabilization in a vulnerable area for respiratory function, to provide additional support for the heart and lungs, to reduce the paradoxical respiration, and to maintain optimal chest function in patients with a long life expectancy. Anterior or inferior defects of more than three ribs usually need skeletal reconstruction.

Posterior defects under the scapula and the large muscles of the back usually do not require bony stabilization. Sternal and sternoclavicular resection causes significant paradox, and reconstruction should be carried out also to protect the underlying mediastinal structures.

Many different types of autogenous or synthetic materials have been used over the years for skeletal reconstruction. The ideal characteristics of the material for skeletal reconstruction should be durability, availability, adaptability to any size and shape, nonreactivity, resistance to infections, translucency to X-rays, incorporation by body tissue, and ease of use. **Bone grafts** have proved to be very durable. The ribs offer the best bone grafts for chest wall reconstruction, they are rigid and not rejected by the body. The disadvantages of using autogenous bone grafts are pain and the possible instability in the area of the harvesting. A variety of **alloplastic materials** have been used such as metal, stainless steel, tantalum, lucite, and fiberglass. Although all these prostheses are able to prevent flail chest, they are extremely rigid, in contrast to the chest wall, and this issue creates special problems (erosion, destruction of the contiguous structure) and even extrusion through the overlying skin or interiorly. Recently, **synthetic materials** have been preferred, in the form of flexible meshes (Prolene, Marlex). These prostheses differ in caliber and construction. Marlex is a single knit fabric, rigid in only one direction and stretchable in the opposite direction. Prolene is a double stitch knit and is rigid in all directions. These meshes can be sutured to the defect margins, tightly enough to be semirigid. The mesh is incorporated into the chest wall by infiltration of its interstices with fibrous tissue. Goretex is a soft tissue patch impervious to air and water, ideal for a large defect associated with pneumonectomy.

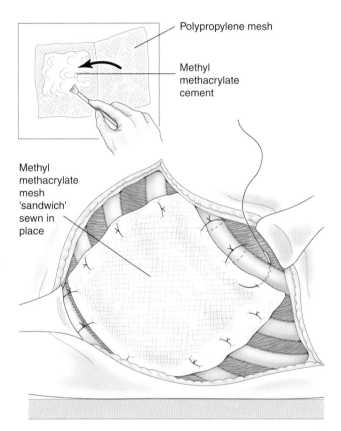

5 When a rigid chest wall replacement is necessary, the **Marlex sandwich** can be used. Two pieces of Marlex mesh are prepared slightly larger than the defect. Methyl methacrylate is then activated and mixed until it begins to gel and then is spread over the one layer to a size smaller than the defect. The second layer of mesh is placed over the methyl methacrylate. The composite is now complete, and it will take 5–10 minutes to harden. During this time, the mesh can be molded to the shape of the defect and sutured to the edges. Muscle and skin closure are then performed. Seroma formation requiring long-term drainage has been associated with the Marlex sandwich technique. Infection, if it occurs in alloplastic materials, dictates immediate removal of the prosthesis. In the meshes or the composite, infections first can be treated conservatively using drainage and irrigation which is usually effective most of the time. If removal is required after 6–8 weeks, a thick fibrous capsule formed by the body can be rigid enough to prevent flail chest in most of the cases.

Polypropylene mesh

Methyl methacrylate cement

Methyl methacrylate mesh 'sandwich' sewn in place

5

SOFT TISSUE RECONSTRUCTION

After completion of the skeletal stabilization, if primary closure cannot be performed, muscle transposition is best to accomplish soft tissue reconstruction. The most commonly used muscle flaps are pectoralis major, latissimus dorsi, and transverse rectus abdominis muscle (TRAM). Size and location of the chest wall defect and preservation of the blood supply to the flap dictate the appropriate reconstruction. Schematically, the thorax can be divided into three areas:

6a–c In the **sternal region** the defects are usually full thickness and require skeletal and soft tissue reconstruction because of the proximity of the skin to the underlying bone. **Pectoralis major** is the most frequent flap used in such defects. The pectoralis can be taken as a muscle flap or as a myocutaneous flap because of the multiple perforators entering the skin through the muscle. The pectoral branch of the thoracoacromial artery is the major blood supply. Release of the humeral tendon of the muscle provides a wider mobilization and rotation. For larger defects located over the mid sternum, pectoral muscle can be used bilaterally. When the pectoralis major is not available and one of the superior epigastric vessels is preserved, a transverse or vertical rectus abdominis flap is a good alternative.

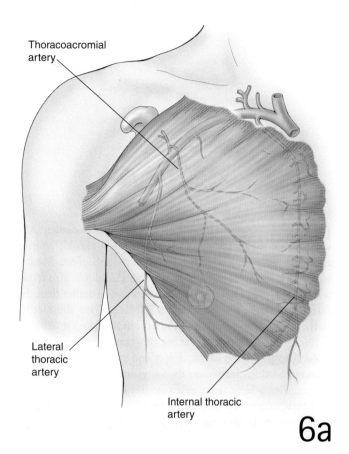

Thoracoacromial artery

Lateral thoracic artery

Internal thoracic artery

6a

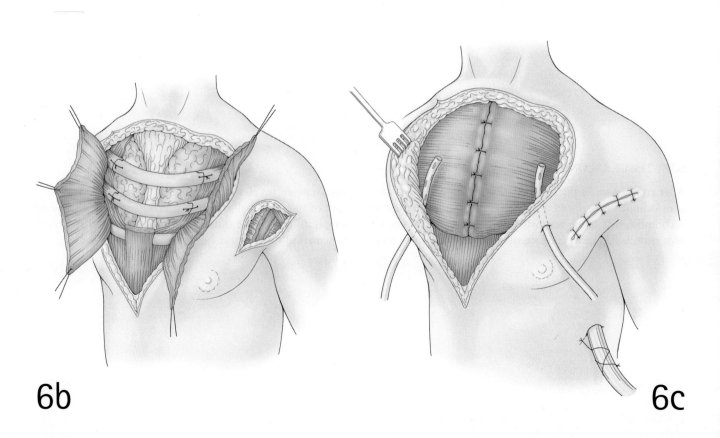

6b

6c

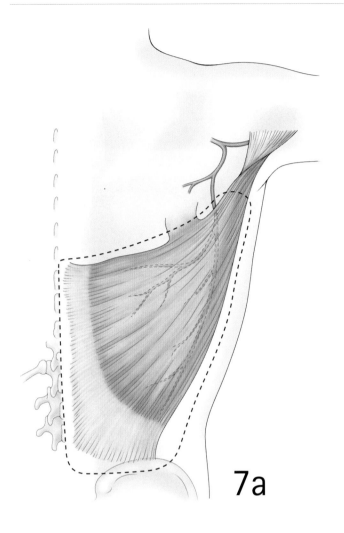

7a,b **Anterior and lateral defects** are the most common after chest wall tumor resection. The flap of choice is the **latissimus dorsi** that can be used as a myocutaneous flap or as a muscular flap. The thoracodorsal artery, a terminal branch of the subscapular artery, is the major blood supply, but it can be carried on the serratus collateral vascular plexus. Because of its long pedicle, a latissimus dorsi flap can be used to cover any area of the chest.

7a

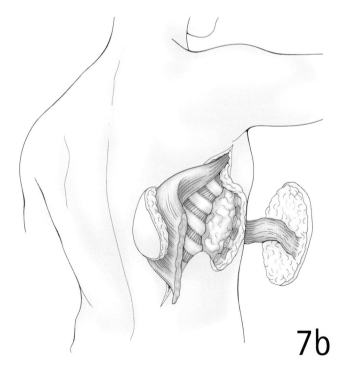

7b

8 **Posterior defects** are infrequent because of the small number of primary chest wall lesions in this area. Moreover, more than one musculofascial layer separates the skin from the chest wall, decreasing the need for additional soft tissue coverage. The flap of choice is the latissimus dorsi. The **trapezius** remains an alternative to cover small defects located over the upper half of the back.

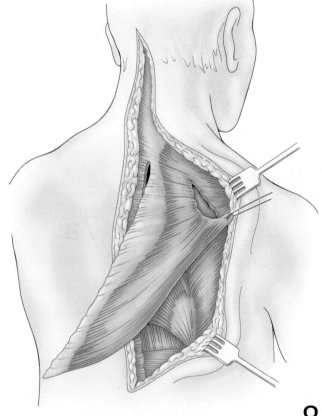

8

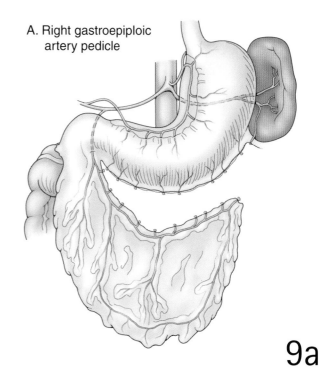

A. Right gastroepiploic
artery pedicle

9a

9a–d When muscle flaps are not available or large enough, the **omentum** based on the right or left epiploic vessels can be placed over bone grafts or mesh. This tissue is very vascular; and when adequately mobilized, it can reach any area of the thorax. The main disadvantage is the need to open the abdomen to prepare it. Omentum will not provide chest wall stability.

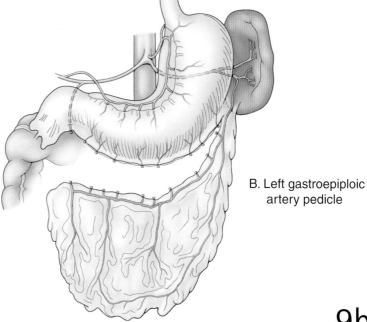

B. Left gastroepiploic
artery pedicle

9b

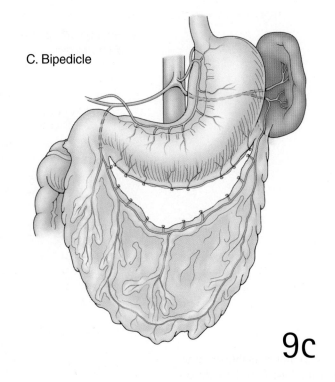

C. Bipedicle

9c

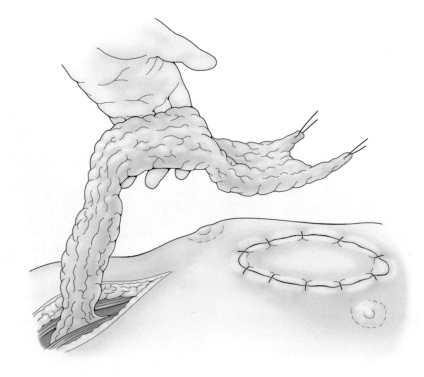

9d

POSTOPERATIVE CARE

Although these patients generally require major chest wall resection and reconstruction, the postoperative morbidity and mortality rate are low. Complications are usually due to infection and partial graft failure. Total graft failure is uncommon. In the postoperative management three areas require special attention: cardiovascular, respiratory, and nutritional.

Common cardiovascular problems are blood pressure irregularities, arrhythmias, congestive heart failure, and myocardial infarction. Hypotension should be avoided and can result in irreversible ischemia of the flaps used in reconstruction. Arrhythmias are common, especially in older patients and are usually correlated to electrolyte imbalances, hypoxia, and fluid overload. Congestive heart failure is usually the result of fluid overload. Pulmonary management is directed to maintaining adequate respiratory function and to recognizing and treating eventual complications. Early extubation, aggressive pulmonary toilet and physiotherapy, pain control and prophylaxis for deep venous thrombosis represent the goals of postoperative care. The patient must be provided with excellent nutritional support; and if necessary, supplemental parenteral or enteral nutrition can be employed.

OUTCOME

Once the histological type of the tumor has been determined, the appropriate therapeutic plans must be prepared. Most of the primary chest wall tumors can be treated by surgical resection as first line of treatment. In selected cases, preoperative or adjuvant chemotherapy, radiation, or a combination of both can play an important role.

Chondrosarcoma is the most common malignant tumor, representing 20% of all chest wall tumors. Chondrosarcomas are usually solitary and localized at the level of the costochondral or sterno-chondral junction. The natural history of this tumor usually consists of slow growth and local recurrence after resection. The 10-year overall survival rate of a series from Memorial Sloan Kettering was 64%; 96% for patients undergoing wide excision, 65% after local excision, and only 14% after palliative resection. This tumor is extremely radio- and chemo-resistant.

Osteogenic sarcoma occurs mainly during childhood and adolescence, and it is associated with typical cortical destruction, periosteal elevation, and extra-osseous extension. This tumor is highly vascularized; and when vascular invasion occurs, it leads to early pulmonary metastases. For these rea-

sons, protocols of neoadjuvant chemotherapy and adjuvant chemotherapy plus radiation protocols have been proposed. Although survival advantages have not been documented, a decrease in local recurrence rate has been observed with a multi-modality therapy regimen.

Plasmacytoma represents 15–30% of all chest wall tumors, presenting often in middle-age to older patients. This tumor is very responsive to chemotherapy and radiation, and the only role for surgery is the diagnosis. The majority of patients unfortunately develop multiple myeloma. Overall 5-year survival rate ranges from 37% to 45%.

Soft-tissue sarcomas represent 20% of malignant lesions of the chest wall. Surgery alone is associated with a high rate of local recurrence (20%). Recent investigations have evaluated the impact of adjuvant therapies (radiation with or without chemotherapy). In the National Cancer study, the overall survival after a multimodality approach was 59% at 5 years with a local recurrence rate of 16%.

Desmoid tumors (low grade fibrosarcoma) are well-differentiated fibrosarcomas. After radical resection, the 10-year survival rate is 95% with a recurrence rate of 30% at 5 years.

Ewing's sarcoma is relatively radiation-sensitive. This tumor is markedly vascular with large areas of necrosis. Despite radiosensitivity, the prognosis before the advent of chemotherapy was poor (5–15% 5-year survival). Currently, surgery is considered the first line therapy followed by local radiation and chemotherapy. Local control of the disease is usually excellent, and disease-free survival rate is about 50% after 3 years.

FURTHER READING

Abbas AE, Deschamps C, Cassivi SD, Nichols FC 3rd, Allen MS, Schleck CD, Pairolero PC Chest-wall desmoid tumors: results of surgical intervention. *Annals of Thoracic Surgery* 2004; **78:** 1219–23; discussion 1219–23.

Allen MS. Chest wall resection and reconstruction for lung cancer. *Thoracic Surgery Clinics* 2004; **14:** 211–16.

Gross JL, Younes RN, Haddad FJ, Deheinzelin D, Pinto CA, Costa ML. Soft-tissue sarcomas of the chest wall: prognostic factors. *Chest* 2005; **127:** 902–8.

Mansour KA, Thourani VH, Losken A, Reeves JG, Miller JI Jr, Carlson GW, Jones GE. Chest wall resections and reconstruction: a 25-year experience. *Annals of Thoracic Surgery* 2002; **73:** 1720–5; discussion 1725–6.

Shrager JB, Wain JC, Wright CD, et al. Omentum is highly effective in the management of complex cardiothoracic surgical problems. *Journal of Thoracic and Cardiovascular Surgery* 2003; **125:** 526–32.

Warzelhan J, Stoelben E, Imdahl A, Hasse J. Results in surgery for primary and metastatic chest wall tumors. *European Journal of Cardiothoracic Surgery* 2001; **19:** 584–8.

Anterior mediastinal lesions

SHINICHIRO MIYOSHI MD, PhD

Professor and Chairman, Department of Cardiothoracic Surgery, Dokkyo University School of Medicine, Mibu, Tochigi, Japan

Anterior mediastinal lesions requiring surgical treatment are usually myasthenia gravis (MG) or thymic tumors. A thymectomy is most frequently used, and occasionally a resection of the surrounding organs is performed in advanced malignancy. This chapter describes extended thymectomy for MG patients and surgical treatment for an invasive thymoma, with special reference to resection and reconstruction of the great vessels.

HISTORY

The effectiveness of a thymectomy for MG was first reported by Blalock in 1939. Because he used a median sternotomy, this approach was adopted and used for a long period of time. A transcervical thymectomy was later advocated in 1966 by the Mount Sinai Hospital group as a less invasive procedure. In 1973, at Osaka University Hospital, Masaoka et al. established the 'extended thymectomy' – en bloc resection of anterior mediastinal adipose tissue, including the thymus, by means of a median sternotomy. Since then, extended thymectomies have been performed as a standard procedure at our institution.

PRINCIPLES AND JUSTIFICATION FOR MYASTHENIA GRAVIS

Although the exact role of the thymus gland in the pathogenesis of MG has not been elucidated, several lines of evidence suggest that it plays a central role in MG, and a thymectomy has been reported to be effective in treating the disease.

A transcervical thymectomy yields a favorable outcome in terms of the cosmetic results of the incision, low morbidity, and minimal hospital stay required. This approach, however, achieves a less complete thymectomy than a transsternal thymectomy. Masaoka et al. reported that repeated operations after ineffective cervical thymectomies revealed a residual thymus in all cases, and complete removal produced clinical improvement in MG. In 1975, they also noted the frequent existence of thymic tissue in anterior mediastinal adipose tissue around the thymus and advocated an extended thymectomy through a median sternotomy. In 1981, the results of this procedure were compared with those for a transsternal thymectomy without adipose tissue resection and a transcervical thymectomy. That study demonstrated the superiority of an extended thymectomy over other procedures.

Since 1987, Jaretzki and colleagues have advocated a 'maximal thymectomy', which adds a resection of fatty tissue in the cervical and hilar regions through a T-shaped cervical/sternal incision. We do not favor enlarging the amount of adipose resection beyond that of an extended thymectomy, because maximal thymectomy has not been shown to produce better results than extended thymectomy.

Controversy remains regarding the indication of thymectomy for elderly patients, pediatric patients, patients with an ocular type of lesion, or patients with a long duration of disease. An extended thymectomy has been reported to be effective in these patients; however, and those factors do not seem to be a contraindication. An extended thymectomy through a median sternotomy can also be used for thymoma resection, which is frequently performed in MG patients.

PREOPERATIVE ASSESSMENT AND PREPARATION FOR MYASTHENIA GRAVIS

Weakness and fatigue with activity are the hallmarks of MG. The ocular muscles are most frequently affected, which leads to blepharoptosis and diplopia. Skeletal and bulbar muscles gradually become affected, which is manifested by weakness in the extremities, impaired chewing, dysarthria, and nasal speech. The diagnosis is confirmed by a Tensilon test, single-fiber electromyography, and determination of acetylcholine receptor antibody levels. All patients should have a chest radiogram with posteroanterior and lateral views, as well as a computerized tomographic (CT) examination to determine whether thymus enlargement or an associated thymoma is present.

Preoperative treatment including steroid administration or plasmapheresis has been recommended by several groups to permit safer surgery, especially for patients with bulbar symptoms. Our current preference, however, is to perform the extended thymectomy first and then to provide steroid pulse therapy only when mechanical ventilation becomes mandatory. Oral medication with an anticholinesterase agent should be continued up to 1 day before the operation.

ANESTHESIA FOR MYASTHENIA GRAVIS

Emotional stress can be a cause of myasthenic crisis; thus, preoperative sedation may be given with due consideration of the depressant effect on respiration. Anticholinergics such as atropine sulfate or scopolamine may be given. Anesthesia is induced by short-acting barbiturates and maintained with N_2O and volatile anesthetics, such as isoflurane and sevoflurane. In most cases, endotracheal intubation and muscle relaxation during the operation can be achieved by deepening of the level of general anesthesia and topical use of local anesthetics without muscle relaxants. Because of the wide variety of muscle strength conditions among MG patients, however, the use of muscle relaxants is sometimes indicated. Both succinylcholine chloride and nondepolarizing agents can be used under strict monitoring with a nerve stimulator.

OPERATION FOR MYASTHENIA GRAVIS

Extended thymectomy

INCISION AND EXPLORATION

1 An extended thymectomy may be performed through a partial median sternotomy. A vertical skin incision is made from 2 cm beneath the sternal notch to 2 cm above the lowest portion of the sternum. The sternum is then divided carefully along the midline, using an electric saw, from the sternal notch to the level of the fifth intercostal space. A small sternal retractor is first positioned, and the sternum is opened slowly to avoid fracture. Bleeding from the sternal periosteum is stopped, and the connective tissue covering the thymus gland is divided along the midline from the pericardium to the neck. Further, the thymus is separated from the posterior surface of the connective tissue by a bilateral blunt dissection. Then, a standard-sized sternal retractor is substituted for the small one. In young women, supramammary or inframammary skin incisions are favored because these incisions leave a cosmetically acceptable scar.

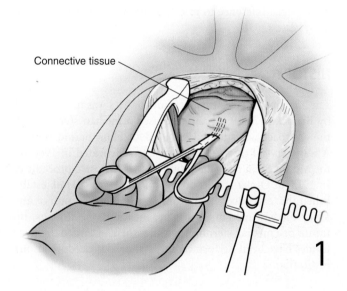

Connective tissue

1

DISSECTION OF THE THYMUS IN ASSOCIATION WITH ADIPOSE TISSUES

2 The lower pole of the gland is dissected from the anterior aspect of the pericardium; the dissection starts at the midline and moves toward the pleural space. The pleural reflections on the thymus gland are gently pushed to the sides by blunt dissection. Thus, the lower pole can be easily mobilized together with the surrounding adipose tissue.

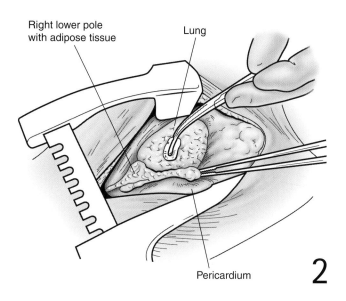

2

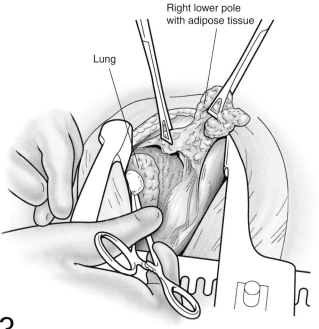

3

3 The lower pole is held in place by a tissue forceps, and mobilization is continued upward, until the small arterial branch from the internal mammary artery is identified and divided between the ligatures. This process is repeated on the contralateral side.

By retraction of the upper end of the wound and dissection from the surrounding connective tissue, the two upper poles of the gland can be identified. A small arterial branch usually enters the uppermost end; it can be caught in a clamp and ligated before the upper poles are finally freed.

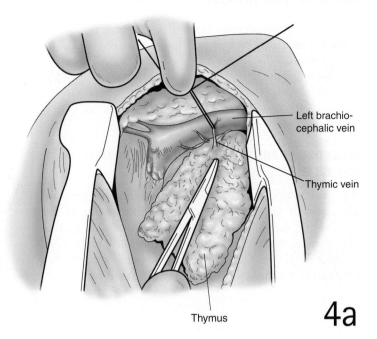

Left brachio-
cephalic vein

Thymic vein

Thymus

4a

4a, b The gland is then separated from the left brachiocephalic vein, and two or three thymic veins can be identified. These veins are divided between the ligatures, and the thymus is removed.

The adipose tissues around the upper poles of the thymus and both brachiocephalic veins, as well as those on the pericardium, should be resected meticulously. The borders of the resection are the diaphragm caudally, the thyroid orally, and the phrenic nerves laterally. After hemostasis is accomplished, a chest tube is positioned in the anterior mediastinum. If the pleural space has been entered, the tip of the chest tube may be advanced into that pleural space. The sternum is repositioned with wire sutures, and the wound is closed in layers.

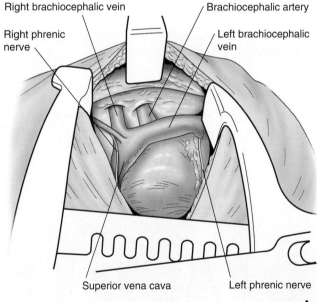

Right brachiocephalic vein

Brachiocephalic artery

Right phrenic nerve

Left brachiocephalic vein

Superior vena cava

Left phrenic nerve

4b

POSTOPERATIVE CARE FOR MYASTHENIA GRAVIS

The decision as to when to extubate the patient is based largely on the preoperative condition. A chest radiograph is usually taken in the operating room before extubation. Most patients, with or without mild symptoms, are extubated in the operating room using routine criteria. A patient with more severe MG presenting bulbar symptoms may spend one night on a ventilator in the intensive care unit. The patient is extubated the next morning after normal arterial blood gas data are confirmed under T-piece breathing. An anticholinesterase agent at half dose is usually restarted on postoperative day 2 or 3, and the dosage is adjusted by observing the condition of the patient. The patient must be watched carefully, as a deterioration of ventilatory status may occur several days postoperatively. When the patient is determined to need ventilatory support for a long period, steroid pulse therapy is given. Sufficient nutrition should be provided by total parenteral nutrition or intragastric tube feeding, depending on the attending physician's preference.

OUTCOME FOR MYASTHENIA GRAVIS

In general, patients with nonthymomatous MG have a better remission rate (RR) than those with thymomatous MG. At our institution, the RR in patients with nonthymomatous MG was found to continue to rise, even after 5 years (45.9% at 5 years, 55.8% at 10 years, 68.4% at 15 years). The palliation rate (PR) was stable after 3 years (91.6% at 3 years, 92.3% at 5 years, 95.2% at 10 years, and 98.2% at 15 years). In a series reported by Mulder, the RR was 51% and the PR was 87%. The RR was 37.9% and the PR was 87.3% in a series described by Maggi. Jaretzki et al. have advocated 'maximal thymectomy', which adds an additional resection of fatty tissues in the cervical and hilar regions through a T-shaped cervical/sternal incision. Their results showed an RR of 46% and a PR of 94% in 72 cases of MG without thymoma.

Among our patients with thymomatous MG, RR was approximately 30% and PR was approximately 80%. The RR of a thymoma series reported by Papatestas was 10%. In Maggi's series, RR was 15.7% and PR was 76.0%, whereas Evoli's series showed a PR of 64%. The results of our series are superior to those of the others cited here. This difference is probably because the others included transcervical and transsternal thymectomies, without adipose tissue resection. These findings suggest the importance of a more extensive elimination of thymic tissue in thymomatous MG patients as well.

Many factors such as age at the time of operation, duration of disease, or MG type have been reported to influence the effects of a thymectomy. With regard to age at the time of operation, among our patients with nonthymomatous MG, younger subjects showed better results than older subjects, which is consistent with other reports. Duration of disease is an important prognostic factor. Our investigation showed superior results among patients with disease of short duration for both nonthymomatous and thymomatous MG. Whether a thymectomy is indicated for patients with the ocular type of MG has been controversial. A long-term follow-up study we conducted, however, showed the effectiveness of an extended thymectomy for patients with the ocular type of MG, both with and without a thymoma.

PRINCIPLES AND JUSTIFICATION FOR THYMOMA

A thymoma is a neoplasm arising from the epithelial cells of the thymus. Most thymomas are slow-growing tumors and are frequently associated with MG; however, the tumor cells do not show a malignant appearance, despite their invasive nature. Although thymomas invade surrounding structures such as the pericardium, lungs, or great vessels, distant metastasis is quite rare. Therefore, local resectability is considered to be an important prognostic factor. Although one of the main reasons for an incomplete resection of invasive thymomas is infiltration to the superior vena cava (SVC), recently, resection and reconstruction of the SVC have been aggressively used. On the other hand, patients with other malignant thymic tumors, such as thymic cancer or malignant germ cell tumor, may not be good candidates for this procedure, as distant metastasis is frequently present at the advanced stage.

PREOPERATIVE ASSESSMENT FOR THYMOMA

5 Patients with an invasive thymoma often complain of symptoms such as coughing, chest pain, or SVC syndrome. The disease is first detected by a chest radiograph. The extent of the tumor can be well evaluated by conventional chest CT and magnetic resonance imaging. Further, venography is useful to demonstrate infiltration of the brachiocephalic veins and SVC. An exact histological diagnosis is very important to differentiate thymomas from other malignant thymic tumors, especially at the advanced stage. A CT-guided biopsy, anterior mediastinotomy, or thoracotomy is used for this purpose.

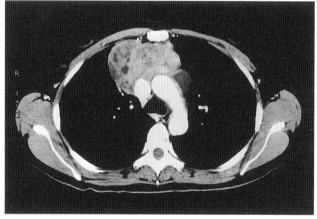

5

ANESTHESIA FOR THYMOMA

If an airway stenosis exists, endotracheal intubation while the patient is awake should be considered. Otherwise, general anesthesia can be induced in the usual manner. A double-lumen endotracheal tube is indicated for procedures such as a partial lung resection. Central venous pressure should be carefully monitored if the venous return is impaired. A thoracic epidural catheter is placed for intraoperative and postoperative pain management. In cases of MG, the anesthesia should be managed accordingly.

OPERATION FOR THYMOMA

Preparation for tumor resection

6 An extended thymectomy, including the tumor in conjunction with resection of the invaded organ, is the final goal. The anterior mediastinum is entered through a full median sternotomy. The intact part of the thymus is first dissected as much as possible, then the invaded pericardium is easily resected. When the mediastinal pleura is invaded by the tumor, the pleura is incised, and the pleural cavity is observed. If an invasion into the lung is present, partial resection is performed with a linear stapler. Thus, the thymus and the tumor can be freed from the surrounding structures, except for the SVC and brachiocephalic veins.

The right and left brachiocephalic veins should be dissected sufficiently distal to the tumor invading site and encircled with cotton umbilical tape. The SVC is also mobilized and encircled with tape, either inside or outside the pericardium, depending on the extent of tumor invasion to the SVC. The azygos vein above the pulmonary hilum and the internal mammary vein are separated and divided between the ligatures. The phrenic nerve is often sacrificed.

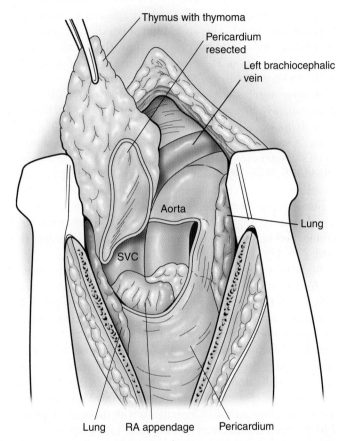

Thymus with thymoma

Pericardium resected

Left brachiocephalic vein

Aorta

Lung

SVC

Lung   RA appendage   Pericardium

6

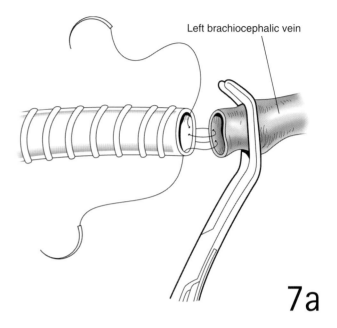

Left brachiocephalic vein

7a

Reconstruction of the left brachiocephalic vein and the superior vena cava

7a, b In general, reconstruction is first performed between the left brachiocephalic vein and the right atrium, followed by reconstruction between the right brachiocephalic vein and the SVC. After heparin sodium is intravenously administered, the left brachiocephalic vein is occluded distally with an atraumatic vascular clamp and ligated proximally, and then divided between them. An anastomosis between the distal stump of the left brachiocephalic vein and the appendage of the right atrium is performed using a ringed Gore-Tex 8.0-mm graft secured with a 5/0 monofilament polypropylene suture by a simple continuous technique.

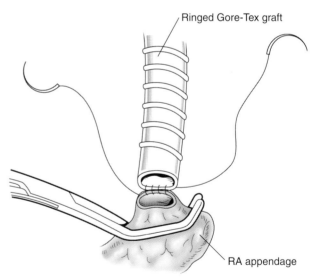

Ringed Gore-Tex graft

RA appendage

7b

8 The right brachiocephalic vein is occluded distally and the SVC proximally, and both veins are divided on the tumor side. Thus, the thymus, including the tumor, is completely removed. The SVC is reconstructed in the same manner as the left brachiocephalic vein using a ringed Gore-Tex 10.0-mm graft. When the clamps are released, bleeding may occur from the suture lines, but these usually seal promptly.

Some surgeons believe that one brachiocephalic vein is adequate to return blood from the upper half of the body to the heart. Reconstruction of the right brachiocephalic vein can be abandoned without major complications, except for transient swelling in the right upper extremity. In this instance, effort should be made to leave the azygos vein intact. The stumps are closed with over-and-over continuous sutures.

After hemostasis is accomplished, a chest tube is positioned in the anterior mediastinum. A second chest tube is sometimes inserted in the right pleural space through the fifth or sixth intercostal space. The sternum is then repositioned with wire sutures, and the wound closed in layers.

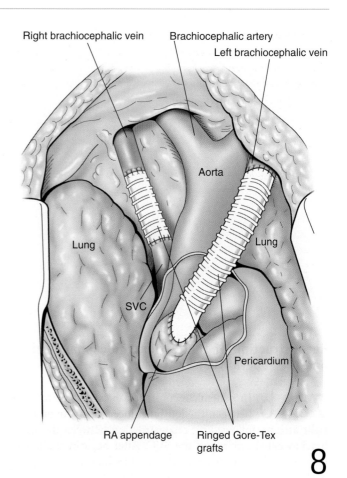

Right brachiocephalic vein • Brachiocephalic artery • Left brachiocephalic vein • Aorta • Lung • Lung • SVC • Pericardium • RA appendage • Ringed Gore-Tex grafts

8

Complications

Major complications are rarely encountered. Occlusion of the graft, particularly that used for the left brachiocephalic vein, sometimes occurs, because it is long and could be compressed by the sternum and ascending aorta. When both veins are reconstructed, however, occlusion of only one graft may not cause a problem. Postoperative respiratory failure may be related to the severity of the associated MG and complicated by phrenic nerve injury. Because patients with MG have a relatively early stage thymoma, this ominous combination is quite rare.

OUTCOME FOR THYMOMA

The clinical staging system for thymomas devised by Masaoka, which is based on the local extension of the tumor, has been shown to reflect the prognosis, and the significance of staging by this system as a prognostic factor has been confirmed by several other institutions. A brief description of Masaoka's criteria follows:

Stage I: macroscopically completely encapsulated with no capsular invasion
Stage II: 1. macroscopic invasion into surrounding fatty tissue or mediastinal pleura, or
2. microscopic invasion into capsule
Stage III: macroscopic invasion into a neighboring organ, that is, pericardium, great vessels, or lung
Stage IVa: pleural or pericardial dissemination
Stage IVb: lymphogenous or hematogenous metastasis

Among 194 consecutively treated patients with thymoma who underwent a complete resection or subtotal resection at our institution, the 10-year and 20-year survival rates were 99% and 90% for stage I disease, 94% and 90% for stage II tumors, 88% and 56% for stage III disease, 30% and 15% for stage IVa lesions, and 0% and 0% for stage IVb tumors. In addition, the 10-year and 20-year survival rates for patients with stage III disease were 97% and 75% when no involvement of the great vessels was present, and 70% and 29% when these vessels were involved. Thus, involvement of the great vessels was the single independent prognostic factor in patients with stage III disease, by multi-variate analysis.

An invasive thymoma with involvement of the great vessels, especially involvement of the SVC, is a challenging case. Because thymomas are usually sensitive to radiation or chemotherapy, preoperative induction therapy may improve the prognosis of these advanced thymomas.

FURTHER READING

Evoli A, Batocchi AP, Provenzano C, Ricci E, Tonali P. Thymectomy in the treatment of myasthenia gravis: report of 247 patients. *Journal of Neurology* 1988; **235:** 272–6.

Jaretzki A III, Penn AS, Younger DS, *et al*. 'Maximal' thymectomy for myasthenia gravis. Results. *Journal of Thoracic Cardiovascular Surgery* 1988; **95:** 747–57.

Kirschner PA, Osserman KE, Kark AE. Studies in myasthenia gravis. Transcervical total thymectomy. *Journal of the American Medical Association* 1969; **209:** 906–10.

Maggi G, Casadio C, Cavallo A, Cianci R, Molinatti M, Ruffini E. Thymectomy in myasthenia gravis. Results of 662 cases operated upon in 15 years. *European Journal of Cardiothoracic Surgery* 1989; **3:** 504–11.

Masaoka A, Monden Y. Comparison of the results of transsternal simple, transcervical simple, and extended thymectomy. *Annals of the New York Academy of Sciences* 1981; **377:** 755–65.

Masaoka A, Monden Y, Nakahara K, Tanioka T. Follow-up study of thymomas with special reference to their clinical stages. *Cancer* 1981; **48:** 2485–92.

Masaoka A, Monden Y, Seike Y, Tanioka T, Kagotani K. Reoperation after transcervical thymectomy for myasthenia gravis. *Neurology* (NY) 1982; **32:** 83–5.

Masaoka A, Yamakawa Y, Niwa H, *et al*. Extended thymectomy for myasthenia gravis patients: a 20-year review. *Annals of Thoracic Surgery* 1996; **62:** 853–9.

Mulder DG, Graves M, Herrmann C. Thymectomy for myasthenia gravis: recent observations and comparisons with past experience. *Annals of Thoracic Surgery* 1989; **48:** 551–5.

Okumura M, Miyoshi S, Takeuchi Y, *et al*. Results of surgical treatment of thymoma with special reference to the involved organs. *Journal of Thoracic and Cardiovascular Surgery* 1999; **117:** 605–13.

Papatesta AE, Genkins G, Kornfeld P, *et al*. Effects of thymectomy in myasthenia gravis. *Annals of Surgery* 1987; **206:** 79–88.

Shimizu N, Moriyama S, Aoe M, *et al*. The surgical treatment of invasive thymoma: resection with vascular reconstruction. *Journal of Thoracic and Cardiovascular Surgery* 1992; **103:** 414–20.

Younger DS, Jaretzki A, Penn AS. Maximum thymectomy for myasthenia gravis. *Annals of the New York Academy of Sciences* 1987; **505:** 832–5.

Thymectomy

LARRY R. KAISER, MD
The John Rhea Barton Professor and Chairman, Department of Surgery, University of Pennsylvania; Surgeon-in-Chief, University of Pennsylvania Health System, Philadelphia, PA, USA

HISTORY

Over the past few decades, complete removal of the thymus gland has been shown to improve the clinical course of patients with myasthenia gravis (MG). However, the precise relationship between the thymus and the generation of MG has not been completely elucidated. Blalock performed a thymectomy via median sternotomy in 1936 for a woman with thymoma and MG and noted an improvement in her myasthenic symptoms. He subsequently reported on a series of patients without thymoma who underwent thymectomy, noting similar improvement in the clinical course of the disease. In this report of 20 thymectomies, he observed improvement in 13 of 17 survivors. To date, a prospective randomized trial to assess the role of surgery on the clinical course of MG has not been performed, but a number of carefully controlled cohort studies comparing thymectomy with standard medical management have been completed. Essentially all of these studies have shown a significantly greater incidence of remission in the operated group versus those treated with medication alone.

PRINCIPLES AND JUSTIFICATION

The presence of myasthenia gravis constitutes the most common indication for the performance of elective thymectomy. The other main indication is the presence of a mass within the thymus gland. Approximately 15% of patients with MG have thymoma, while approximately 35% of patients with thymoma have MG. Patients presenting with a thymoma should be thoroughly evaluated for symptoms of MG, and likewise those presenting with MG should have a computed tomographic (CT) scan of the chest to evaluate the anterior mediastinum. The relationship between MG and the thymus gland

has been well established, though the precise mechanism for the improvement of symptoms following thymectomy has not been established. Following thymectomy, up to 40% of patients with MG can be expected to have a complete response as measured by no requirement for medication. The time course of the improvement may vary, and continued resolution of symptoms may occur for up to 18 months following thymectomy. Further improvement would not be expected to occur after this time period. An additional 30–40% of patients will achieve a partial response usually manifest by a significant reduction in the amount and type of medication required for symptom control. A small percentage of patients fail to achieve any symptomatic relief from their disease. Patients should understand the likelihood of achieving a response so that an informed decision regarding thymectomy may be made. With the development and refinement of minimally invasive approaches to thymectomy, the risk–benefit ratio seems to be tilted toward the performance of thymectomy even in the older patient or those with minimal symptoms. In the past when a median sternotomy was required for thymectomy many neurologists were hesitant about referring patients for such an extensive operation. However, especially with the transcervical approach, such hesitation is no longer warranted.

PREOPERATIVE ASSESSMENT AND PREPARATION

Put simply, any patient with MG is a candidate for thymectomy, but this principle certainly does not imply that all patients with the disease are referred for resection. No laboratory test or other diagnostic maneuver exists that will predict the response to thymectomy – this only can be assessed following the procedure. Likely, this unpredictability is one of the reasons that many neurologists refer only the occasional patient for thymectomy despite the recognition that many patients have a beneficial response. Much of this reluctance is predicated on the "size" and perceived magnitude of the operation, namely a median sternotomy, which is the procedure most commonly employed for thymectomy. Less invasive approaches to thymectomy, specifically the transcervical approach as presented in this chapter, should go a long way toward addressing many of these concerns.

Specific preoperative testing prior to thymectomy is limited to CT scanning of the chest and measurement of pulmonary function. The CT scan of the chest is used to assess for the presence of a thymoma, a finding that could dictate the operative approach. The key finding, in addition to whether or not a thymoma is present, is an assessment of size and whether the mass appears to be encapsulated or invasive. The definitive assessment of invasion can only be made at the time of operation, but often a fairly reliable assumption regarding encapsulation can be made. A CT scan of the chest should be obtained in all patients following a diagnosis of MG to specifically exclude a thymoma, a finding present in up to 30–40 per cent of these patients. A measurement of forced vital capacity (as a minimum) should be made to ascertain whether any involvement of respiratory muscles exists, a finding that could have implications following general anesthesia and the operation. Respiratory muscle involvement, if severe, could be predictive of a postoperative mechanical ventilation requirement and would clearly mandate the need for more intensive preoperative preparation.

Prior to thymectomy, patients should be managed with optimal medical therapy following establishment of the specific diagnosis of MG. First-line therapy in MG usually consists of pyridostigmine, an anticholinesterase inhibitor, given as a single agent. The majority of patients experience significant relief of symptoms following initiation of this drug, and in most patients it is the only drug needed. Corticosteroids, specifically prednisone, is the most commonly used immunosuppressive agent for treating the symptoms of MG and may be necessary in the occasional patient who responds less than optimally to pyridostigmine. Other immunosuppressants, specifically azathioprine, may also be used. Prior to operation, depending on the judgment of the referring neurologist, plasmapheresis may be performed that usually consists of three plasma exchanges carried out during the week preceding the operation. This procedure significantly reduces the level of circulating antiacetylcholine receptor antibodies. Depending on venous access, this procedure may be done on an outpatient basis. Following plasmapheresis, patients usually report feeling better than they have done in many months. Plasmapheresis should be performed for patients with reduced vital capacity, though this procedure becomes less important when the thymectomy is performed via the transcervical approach.

ANESTHESIA

General anesthesia can be performed safely in patients with MG following optimal preparation and adequate monitoring of neuromuscular transmission during and following the surgical procedure. Patients are requested to take their medication on the morning of the operative procedure just as they would normally. Because of the decreased number of acetylcholine receptors or their functional blockade by antibodies directed against them, the use of succinylcholine or other nondepolarizing muscle relaxants is avoided. Other types of muscle relaxants can be used in smaller amounts as part of a balanced technique of anesthesia. It is important that an anesthesiologist experienced in the care of patients with MG be part of the team in order to avoid postoperative problems. Neuromuscular transmission should be monitored during the operation by peripheral nerve stimulation to aid in titrating the dose of muscle relaxants and to ensure complete reversal of neuromuscular block at the conclusion of the procedure. A detailed discussion of anesthetic technique is beyond the scope of this chapter but may be found in the paper by Bazaka.

OPERATION

The standard operation for thymectomy in patients with MG consists of a median sternotomy with total removal of all thymic tissue. This operation is essentially the same operation as described for excision of an anterior mediastinal mass in Chapter 3, so that a detailed description will not be provided in this chapter. The critical factor for thymectomy in the patient with MG is complete removal of the thymus gland. Some have argued that aberrant rests of thymic tissue are so common that more radical operations are justified.

1 Masaoka first described the extended trans-sternal thymectomy where not only the gross thymus but also the surrounding adipose tissue in the anterior mediastinum is removed.

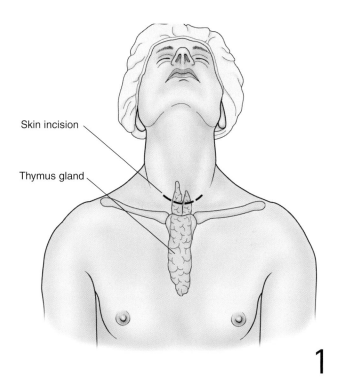

Skin incision

Thymus gland

1

This procedure removes all thymic tissue as well as adipose tissue from the lower poles of the thyroid (superior extent) to the diaphragm (inferior) and from phrenic nerve to phrenic nerve (posterior). A modification of this procedure, the maximal thymectomy, was advocated by Jaretzki and others and involves a cervicomediastinal approach with both a cervical incision and median sternotomy. The extent of this procedure exceeds that of the extended thymectomy by including the cervical region, the aortopulmonary window, and the lateral region of the phrenic nerves. The pericardium is taken along with both pleural reflections. As might be expected, the incidence of complications following this procedure exceeds that reported for other procedures including phrenic and recurrent laryngeal nerve injuries as well as postoperative respiratory failure.

Despite the assumption made by advocates for the more extensive procedures, it seems likely that in a patient with multiple aberrant rests of thymus any procedure will remove all thymic tissue, especially since many of these areas are visible only microscopically. Indeed, results with a less invasive approach, transcervical thymectomy, are equivalent to those achieved by the "extended" approaches with significantly less morbidity and shorter hospital stay.

Our preferred operation for thymectomy is via the transcervical approach utilizing the technique popularized by Joel Cooper. This less invasive approach is contraindicated only when a large thymoma (>4 cm) is present or hyperextension of the neck is unable to be achieved. Otherwise, cervical thymectomy is the approach that we have now used in over 200 patients.

2 The patient is positioned supine with an inflatable bag behind the scapulae and with the neck hyperextended. A transverse skin incision is made just at the level of the sternal notch and deepened through the platysma. Superior and inferior subplatysmal flaps are raised so as to maximize the operative field and allow for the placement of skin retractors. Dissection is carried along the midline separating the right and left strap muscles, specifically the sternohyoid and sternothyroid muscles. The sternothyroid muscle is elevated, and the dissection proceeds along the posterior surface of the muscle.

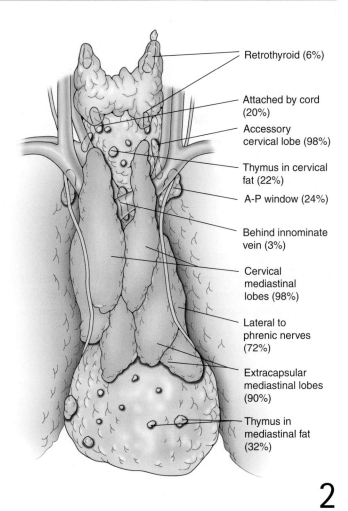

Retrothyroid (6%)

Attached by cord (20%)

Accessory cervical lobe (98%)

Thymus in cervical fat (22%)

A-P window (24%)

Behind innominate vein (3%)

Cervical mediastinal lobes (98%)

Lateral to phrenic nerves (72%)

Extracapsular mediastinal lobes (90%)

Thymus in mediastinal fat (32%)

2

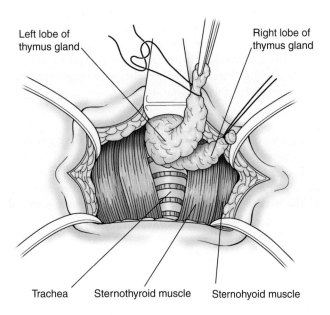

Left lobe of thymus gland

Right lobe of thymus gland

Trachea Sternothyroid muscle Sternohyoid muscle

3

3 The lobe of the thymus gland is identified anterior to the inferior thyroid vein. The gland can be distinguished from adjacent fat by its salmon pink color and by the presence of a capsule. Once the gland is identified it is freed up laterally and medially, and the dissection proceeds superiorly while applying downward retraction on the gland. This maneuver allows for complete dissection of the gland up to its origin where a small vein usually is found. The vein is clipped, and the gland is mobilized anteriorly and freed away from adjacent structures. A silk ligature is placed at the apex of the lobe of the gland to be used as a "handle" to facilitate the mobilization. Dissection then proceeds toward the mediastinum until the innominate vein is encountered. Both lobes of the gland are freed away from surrounding structures in a similar manner. Locating one lobe of the gland leads to the other lobe as the dissection proceeds in a caudad direction. The gland is always located anterior to the inferior thyroid veins, and the veins are dissected away from the gland and left intact.

4 Both lobes of the gland are lifted anteriorly, and using blunt dissection with peanut sponges, the gland is separated away from the innominate vein. As this maneuver proceeds, individual thymic venous branches come into view. These branches are individually ligated and divided. The number of branches varies, but usually at least two or three are identified and must be divided in order to mobilize the gland away from the vein. Care must be taken to avoid avulsing one of these venous branches since bleeding is difficult to control in the limited operative field. The gland usually courses anterior to the innominate vein, but in the occasional patient either a lobe or the entire gland may pass posterior to the vein. This anatomical variant needs to be recognized and dealt with appropriately so as not to leave any residual gland. Using ball sponges on a ring forceps, the gland is separated away from the sternum anteriorly.

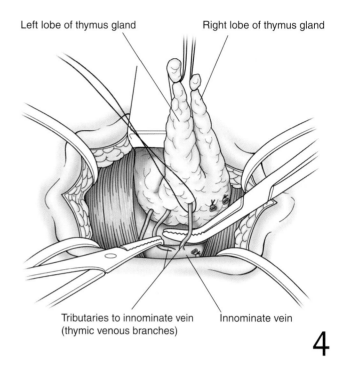

Left lobe of thymus gland   Right lobe of thymus gland

Tributaries to innominate vein
(thymic venous branches)   Innominate vein

4

Cooper thymectomy retractor

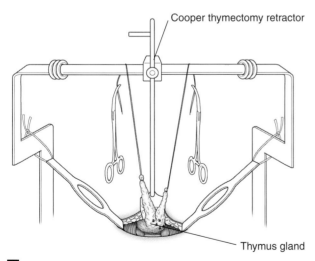

Thymus gland

5

5 The Cooper Thymectomy Retractor (Pilling-Weck Co., Ft. Washington, PA) is put in place to further define the operative field and allow for better visualization of the anterior mediastinum. This retractor attaches to the operating table, and the L-shaped blade is placed behind the sternal notch and lifted. The inflatable bag is deflated so that an optimal view of the mediastinum is provided. If the neck is able to be well extended, the entire thymus gland may be visualized, and the mediastinum is viewed down to the diaphragm with appropriate downward traction applied to the pericardium.

6 Once the retractor is in place, additional skin retraction is provided by an army-navy retractor placed on each side of the incision held in place by Penrose drains attached to the arms of the Cooper retractor. The gland is completely dissected away from the pericardium down to its inferior extent by blunt dissection with ball sponges. Likewise, the gland is completely separated from the sternum anteriorly. The gland is bluntly dissected away from the right pleural reflection and reflected from right to left. Care is taken to avoid entry into the pleural space; but if a rent is made in the pleura, the lung simply is re-expanded at the time of closure by placing a red rubber tube through the pleural rent while the anesthesiologist inflates the lungs. The gland is easily distinguished from pleural fat by the difference in appearance and texture. The gland readily separates from the pleural reflection with blunt dissection. Once the gland is freed off the right pleural reflection, the left lobe is likewise freed. Often, a tongue of gland tracks down into the aortopulmonary window, and this extension needs to be followed to its termination to assure complete removal of the gland. All of the dissection in this area is done bluntly, taking care to avoid any significant traction on the phrenic nerve. The gland is then reflected from inferiorly up into the neck sweeping off any residual pericardial attachments, some of which may need to be divided sharply. Following this maneuver the gland is delivered into the neck and removed. With the retractor still in place a thorough inspection is made to assure hemostasis as no drains are left. Both pleural reflections should be assessed for integrity. The retractor is then removed. The neck is closed in layers in the usual fashion, first reapproximating the strap muscles in the midline followed by a subcuticular skin closure.

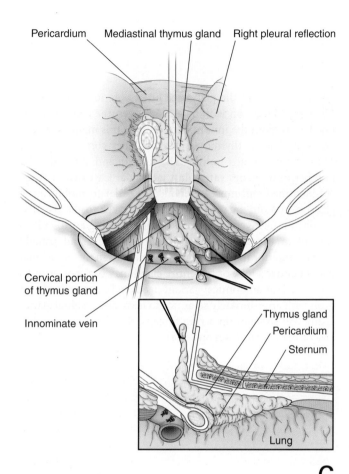

Pericardium Mediastinal thymus gland Right pleural reflection

Cervical portion of thymus gland

Innominate vein

Thymus gland
Pericardium
Sternum

Lung

6

POSTOPERATIVE CARE

With careful neuromuscular monitoring the patient should be easily awakened and extubated prior to transfer to the postanesthesia recovery area. A chest radiograph should be obtained to assure that both lungs are fully inflated in case any entry into the pleural space had been made. Preoperative medications are resumed as soon as the patient is fully awake and able to take fluids by mouth. Patients are watched for several hours in the recovery area prior to discharge. Routinely in our experience, patients are discharged home on the day of the procedure, though early in our experience they were discharged on the morning of the first postoperative day. Mild analgesics are prescribed for the postoperative discomfort, and patients usually return to full activity within 1 week.

OUTCOME

The goal of thymectomy in MG is the induction of remission or improvement of symptoms with less reliance on medication. Remission can be expected in 40–50% of patients undergoing thymectomy, but the time that it takes to achieve this rate may be somewhat prolonged. Patients may see continued improvement for up to 18 months following operation, and some patients may not go into remission until some time after that. Our data and that from Cooper's group suggest that results obtained following transcervical thymectomy do not differ from those obtained via the trans-sternal route, either the extended or the maximal approach.

FURTHER READING

Baraka A. Anesthesia and critical care of thymectomy for myasthenia gravis. *Chest Surgery Clinics of North America* 2001; **11**: 337–61.

Blalock A, McGehee HA, Ford FR, et al. The treatment of myasthenia gravis by removal of the thymus gland. *Journal of the American Medical Association* 1941; **117**: 1529.

Bril V, Kojic J, Ilse WK, et al. Long-term clinical outcome after transcervical thymectomy for myasthenia gravis. *Annals of Thoracic Surgery* 1998; **65**: 1520–2.

Jaretzki A III, Wolff M. Maximal thymectomy for myasthenia gravis: surgical anatomy and operative technique. *Journal of Thoracic and Cardiovascular Surgery* 1988; **96**: 711–6.

Masaoka A, Yamakawa Y, Niwa H, et al. Extended thymectomy for myasthenia gravis patients: a 20-year review. *Annals of Thoracic Surgery* 1996; **62**: 853–9.

Chylothorax

ROBERT J. CERFOLIO MD, FACS, FACCP
Associate Professor of Surgery, Chief of Section of Thoracic Surgery, University of Alabama at Birmingham; Department of Surgery, Division of Cardiothoracic Surgery, Birmingham, Alabama, USA

HISTORY

Munk and Rosenstein first described chylothorax in 1891. They noted that the clear pleural effluent from a patient's chest tube turned milky when the patient ate a fatty meal. Chylothorax is now defined as the presence of lymphatic fluid in the pleural space that results from a leak in the main thoracic duct or one of its branches. Chylothorax is suggested today, as Munk described over 100 years ago, by the presence of milky drainage from a tube that is in the chest, or the accumulation of this type of fluid in the pleural space. The diagnosis is confirmed by analysis of the effluent with measurement of a triglyceride concentration that is greater than 110 mg/dl. The diagnosis may also be established by the presence of fat and chylomicrons via microscopic examination of the effluent. Staining with Sudan-3 is another diagnostic test because it highlights fat globules. If the patient is not eating, the fluid may not be milky, and the diagnosis should be suspected by a persistently high, unexplained chest tube output in a patient with stable hemoglobin who does not have a subarachnoid–pleural fistula.

Thoracic duct fluid is a mixture of chyle, which contains cholesterol, protein, and lymphatic fluid, from the small intestine. The main cellular element is lymphocytes. In the past chylothorax had extremely high operative mortality because it used to lead to leukopenia and malnutrition mainly because of delayed treatment. However, because of a heightened awareness of this problem by surgeons, chylothorax is being more quickly diagnosed and treated.

Chylothorax is classified as congenital, traumatic, neoplastic, spontaneous, or miscellaneous. Operative chylothorax (an iatrogenic subset of the traumatic type) is the most common form that the surgeon needs to address operatively, and this type will be the main scope of this chapter. A 1996 report found chylothorax to be a very rare complication after a general thoracic surgical procedure. We found the incidence of chylothorax to be 0.26% after lobectomy and 0.37% after pneumonectomy. However, after esophagectomy, we found this complication to occur in 2.9% of patients. Because esophagectomy is by far the most common setting in which chylothorax requires operative intervention, we will focus on this operation in the remainder of this chapter.

PRINCIPLES AND JUSTIFICATION

The best way to manage chylothorax after esophagectomy is to prevent it. Prevention is best accomplished during an Ivor Lewis-type approach by carefully examining the posterior mediastinum prior to doing the esophageal–gastric anastomosis. The thoracic duct, if visualized, should be ligated. If it is not seen, sponges should be placed in the area and should be observed for 1 minute to ensure that clear fluid does not collect. Similarly, during a transhiatal approach, the posterior mediastinum at the hiatus should be examined prior to passing the conduit from the abdomen to the neck.

PREOPERATIVE ASSESSMENT AND PREPARATION

Once diagnosed postoperatively, chylothorax usually requires operative intervention. We have shown that if the chest output is consistently greater than 1000 ml per day for 4–5 days after esophageal resection, nonoperative management with total parenteral nutrition or medium chain triglycerides diet will probably fail. Because esophagectomy, coupled with a high output, suggests an injury to the main duct or to a major tributary, thoracic duct ligation is required. Delay can lead to serious morbidity. Lymphangiography prior to surgery can be helpful. This test may demonstrate a leak from a large collateral, and this information can help guide treatment. Moreover, 40% of patients have a thoracic duct that has an atypical course. Lymphangiography helps not only to identify the leak, but also to identify the course of the main thoracic duct that may help in ligation. A gastrografin swallow should be performed prior to reoperation to ensure no anastomotic leaks exist. If one is present, perhaps that can be addressed at the same time as the chylothorax. Usually, though, a small anastomotic leak is best left alone as it will heal on its own.

OPERATION

Once surgical intervention is decided, many surgical approaches are available. The options include both a right and left video-assisted thoracoscopy, laparoscopy, redo celiotomy, right or left thoracotomy, and even a neck approach. The site of drainage is the most important determinant as to the side and type of surgical approach chosen. However, if a patient has had an Ivor Lewis operation initially, we prefer a redo right thoracotomy, even if the drainage is mostly coming out of a left chest tube. The duct can be ligated from the right, and this approach saves the patient the morbidity of a left thoracotomy several days after having had a right.

The goal of operative therapy is to ligate the thoracic duct and to also perform a pleurodesis. We prefer a mechanical pleurodesis, but some use chemical pleurodesis. Others have used fibrin glue over the duct as well. Another option is to use a pleural shunt, which we believe does not address the problem, but merely reroutes it.

The best way to identify the chylous fistula at the time of surgery is to give the patient a fatty meal, either through the feeding tube (that many surgeons place at the time of esophageal resection), or though the nasogastric tube. Cream, milk, or olive oil can be given approximately 1 hour before the operation. This maneuver is done so the surgeon can see the duct actively spurting the milky discharge. Once identified, the duct can be clipped or ligated.

1 Probably the best and most commonly selected way to identify the duct is through a right thoracotomy. One may re-enter the chest over the same rib used initially (usually the fifth rib), or go over the eighth rib for easier access to the lower chest.

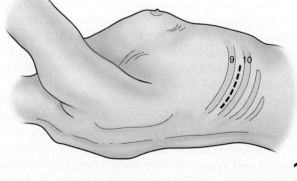

1

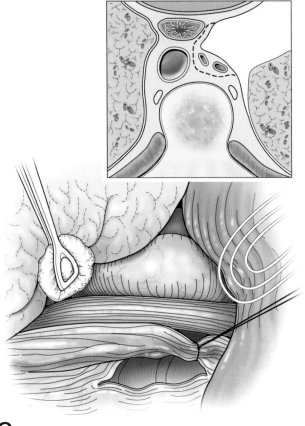

2

2 Since this reoperation is most commonly performed after an Ivor Lewis esophagogastrectomy, the gastric conduit lies on top of the main thoracic duct, and this is where most fistulas lie. One needs to mobilize the conduit carefully to avoid injuring the freshly formed anastomosis, which is usually only a few days old, and to avoid injuring the gastroepiploic artery. For this reason, we prefer placing a lap pad along the lesser curve (which always lies against the right chest), and retracting gently with a retractor to lift the conduit up slightly.

Once the duct is visualized with the milky discharge coming out of it, the surrounding tissue should be oversewn with Prolene suture buttressed by pledgets.

If the duct cannot be found, then mass ligation of all of the supradiaphragmatic tissue lying on top of the vertebral body should be performed. This maneuver is done just above the diaphragm on top of the vertebral body. Fibrin glue can then be placed over this area as well. Others have described the use of talc. Mechanical pleurodesis helps create pleural symphysis and helps prevent the re-accumulation of chyle. The system should be continuously challenged with a fatty meal prior to closure, to ensure that the fistula has been properly closed. The chest is closed with a right angle chest tube placed posterior-inferior and a straight chest tube placed apical-anterior.

POSTOPERATIVE CARE

Keys to good postoperative care include challenging the patient with a high fatty meal both via tube feeds initially and later by mouth, prior to removing any chest tubes. If mechanical and/or chemical pleurodesis has been performed, and if no air leaks exist, we prefer leaving the chest tubes on suction. The patient should have chest physical therapy, nebulizer treatments, frequent ambulation daily, incentive spirometry, and strict aspiration precautions.

OUTCOME

With quick diagnosis, careful intraoperative management and diligent custodial, postoperative care results are outstanding. Early intervention is crucial; and when performed, most patients have few to no sequelae. This complication may only add a few extra days to the usual 7-day postoperative course that most patients who undergo Ivor Lewis esophagogastrectomy currently have.

FURTHER READING

Cerfolio RJ, Allen MS. Postoperative chylothorax. *Journal of Thoracic and Cardiovascular Surgery* 1996; **112**:1361–6.

Miller JI. Anatomy of the thoracic duct and chylothorax. *General Thoracic Surgery* 2000; **LWW**: 747–56.

Munk I, Rosenstein A. Zur Lehre von Reporption in Darm nach Untersuchungen an einer. Lymph(chylus)fistel beim Menschen. *Virchow Archives of Pathology and Anatomy* 1891; **123**: 484.

Bronchoscopy

JOHN C. KUCHARCZUK MD
Assistant Professor of Surgery, Division of Cardiothoracic Surgery, Hospital of the University of Pennsylvania, Philadelphia, PA, USA

HISTORY

In the late 1890s, Gustav Killian used a rigid tube to remove an impacted piece of bone from the right mainstem bronchus of an awake 63-year-old man. Twenty years later, Chevalier Jackson popularized extensive examination and therapeutic interventions using rigid bronchoscopy. Jackson developed a rigid bronchoscope with a small light at its tip to illuminate the airways. His techniques were effective; however, they required specialized training, and only a few physicians obtained the skills required to safely perform the procedures. Awake rigid bronchoscopy is rarely practiced today. Nevertheless, rigid bronchoscopy under general anesthesia remains a valuable tool for the thoracic surgeon and is irreplaceable in certain circumstances. Bronchoscopy requires specialized skill and knowledge to safely intubate the airway, as well as the participation of an experienced anesthesiologist to manage ventilation via the rigid bronchoscope.

The advent of the flexible bronchoscope in the 1970s has revolutionized the field of bronchoscopy. Flexible bronchoscopy is easy to perform in the awake patient as well as the patient under general anesthesia. Bronchoscopy can be used for diagnostic as well as therapeutic interventions. Flexible bronchoscopes are available in a number of sizes and specialized configurations designed for particular applications. Working channels from 1.2 mm up to 3.2 mm allow for aspiration of secretions as well as deployment of a number of instruments into the airway under direct vision.

The modern thoracic surgeon must be an expert bronchoscopist comfortable with both flexible and rigid bronchoscopy. He must be able to choose the approach and instrument most appropriate to the airway for a given clinical situation.

PRINCIPLES AND JUSTIFICATION

Flexible bronchoscopy

Awake flexible bronchoscopy can be performed in the outpatient setting for a variety of diagnostic and therapeutic reasons (Table 7.1).

Table 7.1 *Indications for flexible bronchoscopy*

Examination of airway to the subsegmental level
Aspiration of secretions
Mucosal brushings
Biopsy of endobronchial lesions
Deployment of expandable airway stents
Removal of small foreign bodies
Transbronchial needle biopsy

1 Flexible bronchoscopy allows for examination down to the subsegmental level. Usually, these procedures are performed in a specially designed endoscopy suite. The suite should include a supplemental oxygen supply, pulse oximetry, cardiac monitoring and intubation equipment in the event of an airway emergency. In our practice most of the awake outpatient bronchoscopy is performed by the pulmonologists. The thoracic surgeon is usually involved in difficult cases or those in which an untoward event has occurred. On the other hand, all awake bronchoscopy performed in the postoperative period on our ward is done by the thoracic surgeon. The most common indication is atelectasis due to mucus plugging in the postoperative period. A well-timed therapeutic bronchoscopy in the postoperative patient with mucus plugging can avoid more serious complications such as pneumonia and reintubation.

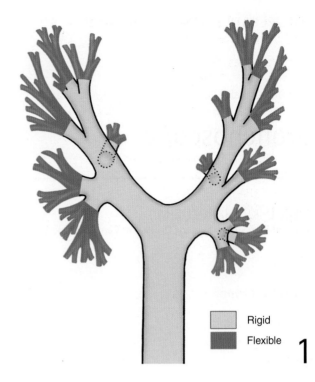

Rigid

Flexible

1

Flexible bronchoscopy under general anesthesia is performed in the operating room after the patient is anesthetized. If examination of the upper portions of the trachea is required, the patient can be mask ventilated initially and then intubated over the bronchoscope after the proximal airway has been examined. Following intubation, the patient can be ventilated through the endotracheal tube with use of a bronchoscopy adapter while the remainder of the distal airway examination is completed. Flexible bronchoscopy allows examination of the airways down to the subsegmental level.

Rigid bronchoscopy

Rigid bronchoscopy is performed in the operating room under general anesthesia. A number of specific applications exist for rigid bronchoscopy which are listed in Table 7.2.

Table 7.2 *Indications for rigid bronchoscopy*

Removal of foreign bodies
Evaluation of tracheal stenosis
Placement of nonexpandable stents
Control of massive hemoptysis
Evaluation of tracheobronchial mobility
Evaluating airway invasion or adherence by esophageal tumors
Palliation of airway obstruction by tumor ("coring out")

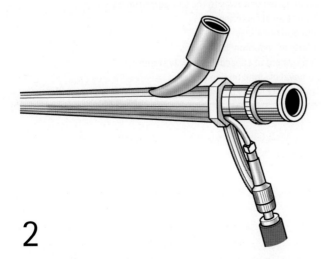

2 Ventilating rigid bronchoscopes have a side port adapter to allow for connection to the anesthesia circuit. A venturi apparatus should also be available to provide oxygen insufflation in the event that a nonventilating scope is used.

2

PREOPERATIVE ASSESSMENT AND PREPARATION

General considerations for bronchoscopy

The initial evaluation of the patient begins with a complete review of their medical and surgical history. Identification of medical issues which will alter the conduct of the procedure, such as bleeding dyscrasias or significant allergy to an anesthetic agent, is important. All recent radiographic studies should be reviewed and the appropriate method of bronchoscopy (rigid, flexible, or both) selected. Prior to performing any procedure, we have a detailed discussion with the patient and family concerning the risks and benefits of the procedure. Except in truly emergent situations, we always obtain a signed permit prior to the procedure.

Flexible bronchoscopy

We provide supplemental oxygen to all patients undergoing bronchoscopy. For awake bronchoscopy, oxygen is provided either via a nasal cannula or by a face mask with an opening to allow for the passage of the bronchoscope. Monitoring in the awake patient should include pulse oximetry and heart rate at a minimum. Most patients have an intravenous line in place; however, with properly administered topical anesthesia intravenous sedation is rarely required. We perform awake bronchoscopy on an outpatient basis in the bronchoscopy suite and on an inpatient basis on the general patient wards. On the inpatient ward, we maintain bronchoscopy carts in conjunction with the respiratory therapists. These carts are stocked with a flexible bronchoscope, a light source, suction tubing, bite blocks, oxygen masks, local anesthetics, pulse oximetry, and emergency airway equipment. These simple carts minimize the frustration encountered when performing a procedure on an awake patient without all the appropriate equipment available. We use a standard adult bronchoscope with an external diameter of 5.9 mm for these procedures.

Flexible bronchoscopy under general anesthesia is performed in the operating room in conjunction with an anesthesiologist. Monitoring includes pulse oximetry, noninvasive blood pressure monitoring, and three-lead electrocardiogram (ECG) monitoring. Following the induction of general anesthesia, direct laryngoscopy is performed and an endotracheal tube is placed. Tube position is confirmed by auscultation, observation of the chest, and end-tidal carbon dioxide monitoring. In the adult patient we like to place an 8.0 mm endotracheal tube. This tube size allows ventilation via a bronchoscopy adapter during use of a standard 5.9 mm outside diameter (OD) bronchoscope. We generally prefer the 5.9 mm OD bronchoscope because it has a working channel of 2.8 mm which is large enough to aspirate thick secretions without becoming clogged. Using smaller endotracheal tubes with smaller bronchoscopes is often frustrating, due to difficulty in clearing the secretions in order to obtain an adequate view. The "pediatric bronchoscope," for example, has an outside diameter of 3.5 mm and a working channel of only 1.2 mm. For specialized use such as laser bronchoscopy we use a 6.2 mm OD scope which has a 3.2 mm working channel. If possible, we place a 9.0 mm endotracheal tube in these situations.

Rigid bronchoscopy

The preoperative assessment of patients undergoing rigid bronchoscopy also includes examination of the neck and oral cavity. Severe cervical arthritis with a contracted, flexed neck may make rigid bronchoscopy difficult. Poor dentition should be noted; loose teeth are at risk during rigid bronchoscopy. Removable dental work such as bridges and dentures should be taken out prior to arrival in the operating room. The presence of a mature tracheostomy is not a contraindication to rigid bronchoscopy. The tracheostomy device can be removed and the patient intubated with the rigid scope from above, or in some circumstances intubated directly through the stoma with care taken to avoid injury to the membranous portion of the trachea posterioly. Likewise, rigid bronchoscopy can be performed through the tracheal stoma in a patient following total laryngectomy.

ANESTHESIA

Awake flexible bronchoscopy

Adequate topical anesthesia is paramount to the performance of awake flexible bronchoscopy. We begin the anesthetizing process with the administration of a lidocaine nebulizer treatment (5 ml of 1% lidocaine solution) by a respiratory therapist. Following this, the posterior pharynx, tonsilar pillars, and soft palate are sprayed with a 1% cetacaine spray. Next, 2–5 ml of a 2% lidocaine solution is injected transtracheally through the cricothyroid membrane with a 21 gauge needle. This maneuver causes the patient to cough but results in topical anesthesia of the airway. Finally, a bite block is placed in the mouth, and the bronchoscope is introduced through the mouth and advanced down to the level of the vocal cords. One milliliter of a 4% lidocaine is sprayed through the working channel of the bronchoscope onto each vocal cord under direct vision. The scope is removed, and the patient is encouraged to cough. At this point the local anesthesia is complete, and awake bronchoscopy can be easily performed with satisfactory patient comfort. Intravenous sedation can lead to hypoxemia, hypercarbia, and hypotension. With properly administered local anesthesia the patient remains comfortable throughout the procedure, and we rarely find it necessary to administer any intravenous sedation.

Flexible bronchoscopy under general anesthesia

Once appropriate monitoring has been established, the patient is preoxygenated, and general anesthesia is induced.

General anesthesia is usually accomplished with a combination of intravenous and inhalation agents. A muscle relaxant is administered, and direct laryngoscopy is performed. An endotracheal tube is placed under direct vision, and its position confirmed by the presence of end-tidal carbon dioxide. The endotracheal tube is connected to the ventilator circuit via a bronchoscopy adapter, and the patient is ready to undergo the procedure. Special anesthetic considerations include minimizing the inspiratory oxygen content to below 50% when using laser bronchoscopy to avoid an airway fire as well as increasing gas flow rates into the anesthetic circuit when vigorous and prolonged suctioning is required.

Rigid bronchoscopy under general anesthesia

The performance of rigid bronchoscopy under general anesthesia requires close coordination between the anesthesiologist and surgeon. While the anesthesiologist institutes the appropriate monitoring and intravenous access, the surgeon readies the rigid bronchoscope along with its light source and supporting hardware. During "routine" rigid bronchoscopy, general anesthesia is induced with a combination of intravenous and inhalation anesthetics. Secretions are aspirated from the posterior pharynx, and the patient is maskventilated. A muscle relaxant is administered to allow easier placement of the rigid bronchoscope. Patients with large mediastinal masses or near complete obstructing tracheal tumors represent a particularly challenging subset that require special anesthetic consideration. Placement of these patients in a supine position or administration of general anesthesia with a muscle relaxant can lead to complete airway obstruction and life-threatening hypoxemia. In this group the airway is topicalized with local anesthesia first. The patient remains in a somewhat upright position, and general anesthesia is slowly induced with intravenous agents. The anesthesiologist assists the patient's spontaneous ventilation, and the use of muscle relaxants is initially avoided until the airway is secured. The patient is quickly positioned and intubated with the rigid scope by the surgeon. Ventilation through the anesthesia circuit connected to the side port of the ventilating scope is begun. If a nonventilating scope is used, insufflation of oxygen via a Venturi apparatus can be used to maintain oxygenation.

OPERATION

Awake flexible bronchoscopy

The patient is placed in a bed or stretcher and the back is elevated to 60 degrees. Pulse oximetry and heart rate monitoring is begun. Supplemental oxygen is provided by a face mask with a hole cut in it to allow passage of the bronchoscope. Topical anesthesia is provided as described above in the anesthesia section. Once the oral pharynx, vocal cords, and airway have been completely anesthetized, a bite block is placed in the mouth, and the bronchoscope is introduced into the oral pharynx. If the topical anesthesia has been complete, the patient does not cough and remains comfortable throughout the procedure.

3 The right-handed surgeon should stand on the patient's right side The surgeon's left hand is used to introduce the scope while the right hand is used on the scope control and suction buttons. The scope is advanced to a position above the vocal cords, and the patient is asked to take a deep breath and vocalize. This maneuver allows direct visualization of the vocal cords in motion. It is important to rule out a paralyzed vocal cord in the postoperative patient who aspirates, especially if they have undergone mediastinoscopy or a left upper lobectomy. If a vocal cord is paralyzed but fixed in the midline, no further intervention is required. Lateralization of paralyzed vocal cord predisposes to aspiration and may require Teflon injection to medialize the cord.

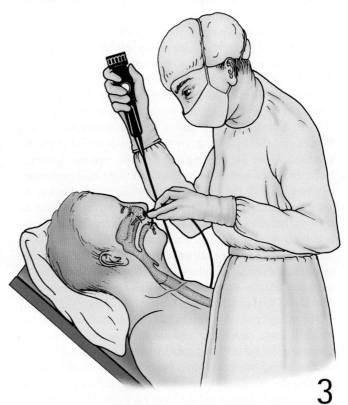

3

The patient is again asked to take a deep breath opening the vocal cords, and the bronchoscope is passed into the proximal trachea. The observer is oriented by noting the posterior longitudinal muscle along the membranous portion of the trachea. The carina is located, and a systematic examination of the airway is carried out down to the subsegmental level. Mucus plugs and thick secretions are aspirated out with the aide of saline lavage. A sample is usually obtained for gram stain as well as bacterial culture and antibiotic sensitivity.

Flexible bronchoscopy under general anesthesia

The patient is brought to the operating room, and general anesthesia is induced. Direct laryngoscopy is performed, and an 8.0 endotracheal tube is placed. The endotracheal tube is connected to the ventilator through a bronchoscopy adapter. The surgeon stands at the head of the table. Flexible bronchoscopy is carried out. Following this exam, the single lumen tube is removed, and a double lumen endotracheal tube is placed for isolated lung ventilation during the procedure.

We perform flexible bronchoscopy under general anesthesia on all patients undergoing a thoracic surgical procedure. Our examination is complete and includes inspection down to the subsegmental level on both sides. This step is especially important in those patients undergoing a pulmonary resection associated with an endobronchial lesion. Direct visualization of the lesion allows us to plan how we will handle division of the bronchus. If the endobronchial lesion is very distal at the segmental or subsegmental level, we will divide the lobar bronchus in our normal fashion with a linear stapling device. By contrast, if bronchoscopy raises the question of a positive or "close margin" we routinely take the bronchus open and obtain a frozen section. If the frozen section is negative, we proceed to close the bronchus with an interrupted, hand-sewn technique. On the other hand, if the margin is positive, we perform a sleeve resection if possible. It is unwise to rely on an "outside" preoperative bronchoscopy when performing a pulmonary resection, and the information gained is vital when contemplating the more complex bronchoplastic procedures.

Rigid bronchoscopy under general anesthesia

4 Once ready to introduce the rigid bronchoscope, the patient is positioned supine with the neck slightly flexed ("sniffing position"). The surgeon stands behind the patient's head, secretions are suctioned from the posterior pharynx, and mouth guards are placed. The surgeon's left hand is used to control the patient's head by gripping the maxilla with the middle and ring fingers. The index finger and thumb of the left hand are used to hold the scope in the manner in which one would hold a pool stick. The right hand grasps the scope at the level of the eyepiece.

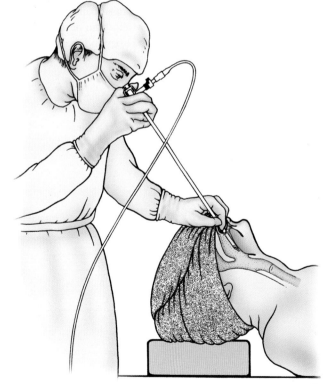

4

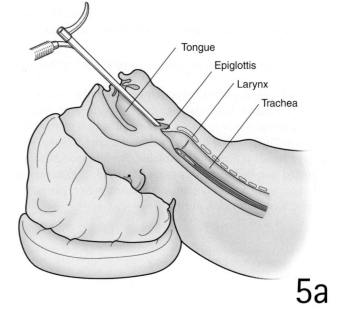

Tongue

Epiglottis

Larynx

Trachea

5a

5 The instrument is introduced with the bevel down and advanced until the epiglottis is visualized. The bronchoscope is placed just under the leading edge of the epiglottis which is gently elevated to reveal the vocal cords. Elevation is provided by the operator's left thumb. Use of the teeth or gums as a fulcrum to elevate the epiglottis results in damage to the teeth and must be avoided. The most common mistake made is advancing the scope further than 1 cm beyond the tip of the epiglottis thus placing the scope beyond the larynx.

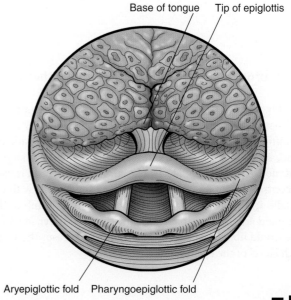

Base of tongue   Tip of epiglottis

Aryepiglottic fold   Pharyngoepiglottic fold

5b

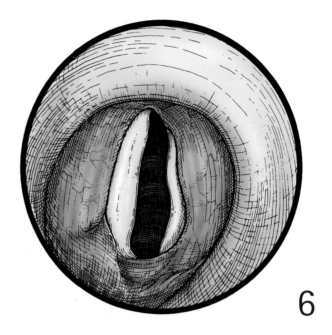

6 Once the vocal cords are visualized, the scope is rotated 90 degrees to the right and advanced into the trachea. When in the trachea, the scope is rotated back to its original position. The supporting pillow is removed from behind the head, and the table headboard is lowered to extend the neck. Ventilation is begun either through the side port with an eyepiece in place or via the Venturi apparatus with the nonventilating scope.

6

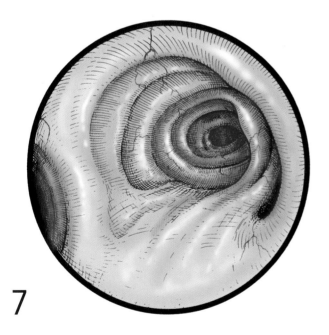

7

7 In order to manipulate the rigid scope, the patient's head is turned to the side opposite to that you wish to examine. To examine the right side the head is slightly turned to the left, and the scope is passed into the right mainstem.

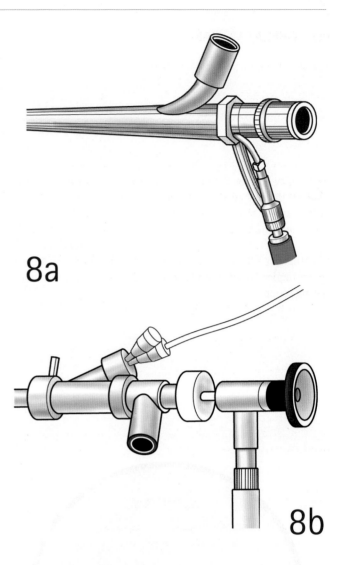

8 We usually suspend ventilation and remove the eyepiece when advancing the scope. If closer inspection of the airway is required, a Hopkins rod telescope is passed through an adapter on the main channel of the rigid scope. These telescopes provide magnification as well as a variety of angled views. If telescopes are not available, a flexible bronchoscope can also be passed through the rigid scope.

8a

8b

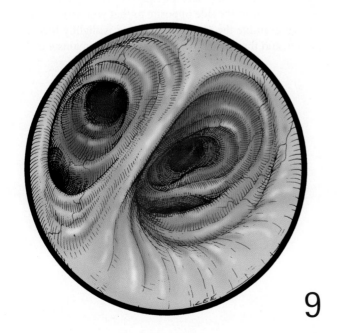

9

9 To examine the left side the head is rotated far to the right. This maneuver allows for easy introduction into the left mainstem bronchus.

POSTOPERATIVE CARE

Awake flexible bronchoscopy

Following awake flexible bronchoscopy with general anesthesia, we continue to monitor the patient's pulse oximetry for a short period to assure the patient's oxygenation is satisfactory. We generally obtain a chest X-ray to evaluate the results following a therapeutic bronchoscopy, such as removing a mucus plug in the postoperative period. Since the posterior pharynx and vocal cords have been locally anesthetized, we keep the patient NPO for 3–4 hours to avoid aspiration.

Flexible bronchoscopy or rigid bronchoscopy under general anesthesia

Following these procedures, the patients are allowed to recover from general anesthesia in a monitored recovery room setting. Since these procedures are often done in conjunction with another thoracic surgical procedure, the more invasive procedure, such as a pulmonary resection, dictates the postoperative care.

Patients undergoing laser ablation of an obstructing lesion or relief of airway obstruction by a "coring technique" utilizing the rigid bronchoscope are hospitalized and observed overnight to ensure an adequate airway.

OUTCOME

Complication rates for these procedures should be low. Bleeding dyscrasias should be addressed prior to the procedure, especially if a biopsy is planned. A high percentage of complications surrounding awake flexible bronchoscopy are related to preprocedural intravenous sedation. This issue can be avoided altogether with the proper application of local anesthesia and avoidance or minimal use of intravenous sedation. This principle is of particular importance in the frail and elderly. Significant hypoxemia must be avoided during these procedures. Some particularly tenuous patients are probably better off undergoing elective intubation followed by therapeutic bronchoscopy rather than struggling with awake bronchoscopy. Avoiding hypoxemia during rigid bronchoscopy requires teamwork and coordination between the anesthesiologist and surgeon.

Rigid and flexible bronchoscopy are invaluable tools for the thoracic surgeon. While flexible bronchoscopy has become the norm, situations arise which demand the use of rigid bronchoscopy necessitating training and confidence with this procedure.

FURTHER READING

Fulkerson WJ. Fiberoptic bronchoscopy. *New England Journal of Medicine* 1984; **311:** 511–5.

Lukomsky GI, Ovchinnikow AA, Bilal A. Complications of bronchoscopy: comparison of rigid bronchoscopy under general anesthesia and flexible fiberoptic bronchoscopy under topical anesthesia. *Chest* 1981; **79:** 316–21.

Miller JL. Rigid bronchoscopy. *Chest Surgery Clinics of North America* 1996; **6:** 161–7.

Miller MB, Kvale PA. Diagnostic bronchoscopy. *Chest Surgery Clinics of North America* 1992; **2:** 599.

8

Video-assisted thoracic surgery

LUIZ EDUARDO V. LEÃO MD, PHD
Professor and Chairman, Department of Surgery, Division of Thoracic Surgery, Escola Paulista de Medicina – Universidade Federal de São Paulo, São Paulo, Brazil

HISTORY

Thoracoscopy was used for exploration of the pleural space in the early twentieth century by Jacobeus, but only in the late 1980s and early 1990s with development of video technology and endoscopic instrumentation did this field expand to what is known today as video-assisted thoracic surgery (VATS). This approach follows the trend of less invasive techniques that have been developed for most surgical areas.

PRINCIPLES AND JUSTIFICATION

VATS is not an operation but an approach to performing operations. The same surgical principles should be applied as in an open procedure, although in some cases surgical technique and strategies may be different. VATS operations also include diagnostic and therapeutic procedures. Indication for operation should be the same as for the open procedure.

With this less invasive approach, most operations can be performed through two to four access ports with minimal muscle incision and no rib spreading. Thus, less operative pain, easier coughing, and preserved respiratory mechanics are to be expected in the immediate postoperative period. This less invasive procedure should result in a shorter hospitalization and, in most cases, in lower costs and earlier return to normal and productive life.

The initial enthusiasm for and expansion of the technique also have raised some concern regarding which procedures *can* be performed by VATS and which procedures *should* be performed by VATS. After more than 10 years of use, VATS has now withstood the test of time, and several VATS techniques now have a definite role in the diagnosis and treatment of certain thoracic conditions. Of course, the skill and judgment of the surgeon are fundamental; most importantly, every surgeon performing VATS operations should have surgical training, and operative setup facilities should be available to allow immediate conversion to an open procedure, if necessary.

PREOPERATIVE ASSESSMENT AND PREPARATION

Because VATS is an approach, rather than an operation, preoperative evaluation may be very different, depending on the underlying disease and the planned surgery. Although VATS potentially carries less morbidity and is less invasive than thoracotomy, certain principles must be adhered to in the preoperative evaluation of the patient for thoracoscopic surgery. Surgical indications for each situation should be the same as those for the open procedure.

The presence of adhesions and previous pleurodesis, thoracic surgery, chest trauma, and chest tube insertions should be carefully assessed from patient data, and computed tomographic (CT) evaluation may be included. The presence of dense adhesions generally precludes use of a VATS procedure.

As does the patient undergoing thoracotomy, the patient undergoing thoracoscopic surgery requires a general anesthetic. In addition, one-lung ventilation is a prerequisite for this surgical procedure. One must also realize that any thoracoscopic procedure may have to be converted to an open thoracotomy due either to the inability to complete the planned procedure thoracoscopically or to technical complications such as vascular injury and hemorrhage. Thus, although thoracoscopic surgery may be planned, the patient must not present a prohibitive risk for thoracotomy. The preoperative evaluation of the patient undergoing thoracoscopic surgery should be no less rigorous than that of the patient undergoing thoracotomy.

A preoperative consultation with the anesthesiologist is very important. In a young, otherwise healthy patient undergoing thoracoscopy for spontaneous pneumothorax or sympathectomy, preanesthetic evaluation can occur the day before or the morning of surgery. Older patients, however, and patients with complex medical problems should be seen in advance of the planned procedure.

ANESTHESIA

With few exceptions, VATS operations are performed with the patient in the lateral position, under general anesthesia, and with single-lung ventilation. Most patients are managed with a double-lumen tube to allow collapse of the ipsilateral lung. As the first access port is opened to the atmosphere, air enters the chest, and the lung is deflated. In most thoracic procedures, no CO_2 insufflation is required, and a valved port is not necessary. In children and adults too small to allow placement of a double-lumen tube, a tube with a bronchial blocker may be used.

The anesthesia team should be familiar with open thoracic procedures and be prepared for a rapid conversion to an open thoracotomy should complications arise or difficulties develop in performing the thoracoscopic operation. One possible exception to this anesthesia setup is the thoracic bilateral sympathectomy, in which the patient may be placed in a sitting position with a regular single-lumen tracheal tube. In this operation, a skilled surgeon can perform each side of the procedure under a few minutes of apnea.

In most simple operations, an arterial line is not used, but anesthetic monitoring with non invasive blood pressure measurement, pulse oximetry, and end-tidal CO_2 measurement are standard monitoring. In advanced procedures, as well as in compromised patients, an arterial line is placed for hemodynamic monitoring.

OPERATION

Basic operative setting and general principles

1 The patient is placed in a full lateral position. A roll or sandbag is placed in the axilla. One or two monitors may be used. The surgeon must have a direct view of the monitor across the operative field.

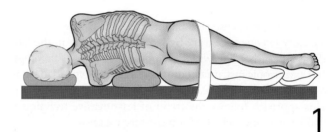

1

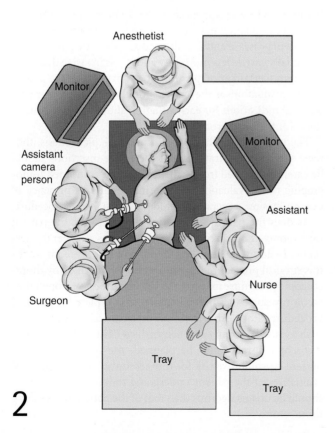

2

2 The surgeon, camera, and instruments should be in the same direction with regard to the pathology. This principle avoids an awkward handling of the instruments due to the 'mirror imaging' effect that results when instruments are pointed toward the camera. Triangulation of the scope and the accessory instruments prevents the interference of one instrument with the others during the operation. Before the trocars are inserted, the lung should be deflated. Because collapse of the alveoli takes some time, a useful practice is to request lung deflation as soon as the patient is positioned.

3,4 The first access port should be planned for visualization of the lesion from a distance and exploration of the hemithorax. After the skin and soft tissue incision, digital exploration can be very helpful in feeling a chest free of adhesions or in separating adhesions. The presence of firm and extensive pleural symphysis requires conversion of the procedure to an open thoracotomy.

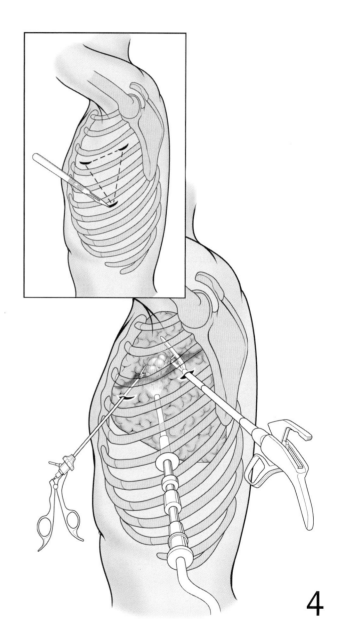

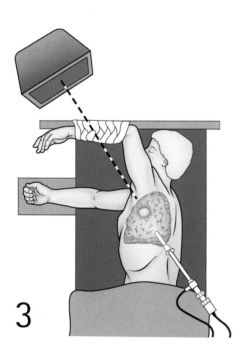

3

4

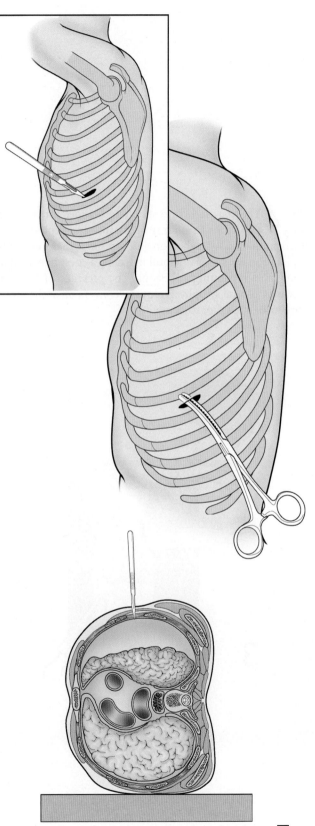

5a–c Most operations are performed using three ports in an inverted triangle position. The two working ports are placed under direct vision from inside the chest; they are planned after initial evaluation of the whole hemithorax and placed according to the position of the lesion and handling of the instruments. Some form of thoracoscopic port always should be used for passage of the scope. Direct passage of instruments through the chest wall is an acceptable technique, however, particularly when standard thoracic instruments are being used. One or two additional ports may be necessary for retraction.

Most of the procedures are performed with a 10-mm 0-degree scope. Some surgeons often use a 30-degree scope in several situations. Periodic warming of the thoracoscope is essential to prevent fogging of the lens due to the temperature difference between the thorax and operating room air. Disposable as well as reusable endoscopic instruments are used. In most VATS operations, regular surgical instruments – such as ring forceps – may be used that also may be placed inside the chest without use of the trocar port.

One important issue arises in VATS procedures in which malignant or infected specimens are removed from the thoracic cavity. Implants of malignant tissue in the port site have been reported. As a rule, all of these specimens should be removed inside a plastic bag to prevent the spread of disease at the port site. In most operations, a chest tube (generally a 24–28 Fr thoracic catheter) is placed in the lower access port. The other access sites are closed with subcutaneous and subcuticular absorbable stitches. The lung is re-expanded, and the tube is connected to suction. The chest tube is removed when all air leaks are sealed and drainage is less than 100 mL per day.

5a

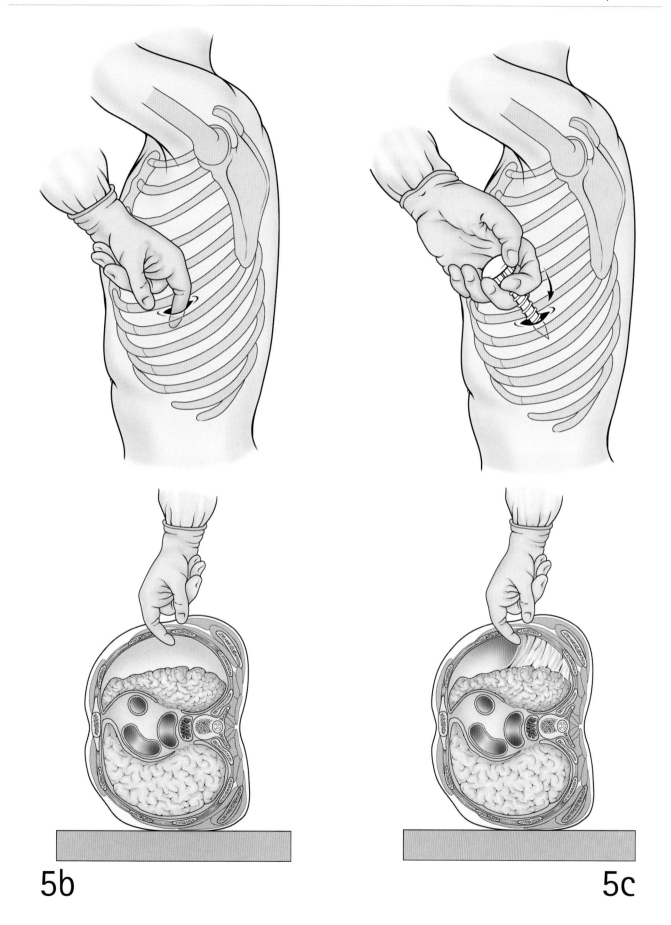

5b

5c

Procedures

As stated earlier, a large number of thoracic procedures can be performed successfully through a VATS approach. This chapter, however, describes only some procedures that have been widely accepted by most thoracic surgeons as straight-forward operations to perform using the videothoracoscopic approach.

Several advanced procedures performed on VATS, as pulmonary lobectomy, thymectomy, esophagectomy, resection of first rib for thoracic outlet syndrome, thoracoscopic approach to spinal surgery and other complex procedures will be discussed in the respective chapters.

Pleural biopsy

6a,b The patient is positioned in a lateral decubitus position, and a pneumothorax is created by collapsing the side of highest yield predicted by preoperative radiographical evaluation. Usually, a standard three- or two-entry port technique is directed at the lower half of the thoracic cavity to maximize the biopsy yield. Identified masses are incised with an endoscopic scissors, knife, or biopsy forceps. Care should be taken not to excise tissue deeply on the diaphragm or apex to avoid vascular injury or phrenic perforation. Multiple biopsy specimens are obtained to ensure that enough tissue is available. Consultation with a surgical pathologist with or without frozen section diagnosis may be useful to ensure that a proper amount of tissue is obtained for appropriate histological and histochemical staining procedures.

When a 10-mm telescope with a 5-mm working channel is available, the operation can be performed through this single 10-mm incision. Thus, several pleural procedures – including treatment of most pleural effusions – can be performed via a single port access site. Use of a spoon-shaped biting forceps usually allows removal of adequate pleural specimens for diagnosis and histochemical studies without producing crushing artifacts.

For diagnosis of a malignant pleural effusion, a therapeutic procedure such as the surgical creation of pleural symphysis is often undertaken. The preferred sclerosing agent in malignant cases has been talc. Effective pleurodesis can be achieved by insufflation of 4–5 g of sterile talc. Under direct vision, talc powder is insufflated over the lung and parietal surfaces through the working channel of the thoracoscope or through the other working port. A chest tube is placed through the lower port site and left in place until the volume of drainage is approximately 100 mL daily.

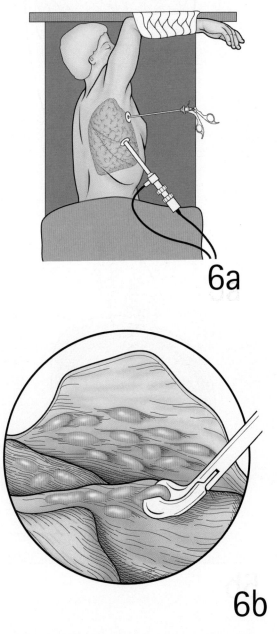

6a

6b

Lung biopsy – wedge resection of the lung

A common procedure performed is lung biopsy for diagnosis of diffuse lung disease or for a detailed histological evaluation of pulmonary interstitial disease. The videothoracoscopic procedure allows a complete evaluation of the chest cavity, and lung tissue can be resected from any area of the lung.

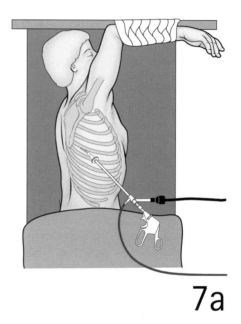

7a

7a,b With the operated lung collapsed by one-lung ventilation, the thoracoscope is introduced through an initial port site placed in the fifth to seventh intercostal spaces in the mid to posterior axillary line. After a thorough exploratory thoracoscopy, the accessory access sites for lung biopsy are selected, aimed at the areas of interest under direct visual control. Two additional access sites are typically required. They should be placed at least 10 cm apart in the anterior axillary line and the posterior axillary to midscapular line. The target area is determined by CT studies, and at least two specimens are resected. The usual inverted triangle is used for placing the port access sites, with special attention given to locating them far enough from the target area to allow opening of the endostapling device. The target area is grasped with a lung clamp or a ring forceps. Stapling can be performed from the same port site, or the first and second staplings may alternate between grasper port and stapler port sites.

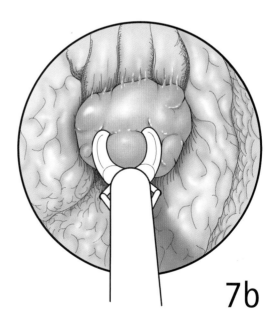

7b

8a,b The lung is grasped in the area of interest for the application of the stapler. Specially designed endoscopic lung clamps may be used. Alternatively, one can introduce the traditional thoracotomy instruments (ring forceps, lung forceps) through the access site without using the thoracoscopic port. The endoscopic stapler is introduced through another access site for pulmonary biopsy. Usually, the procedure can be completed with two or three staplings. The resected specimen can be pulled out from one of the access sites and is sent for pathological and microbiological studies. Air leakage can be checked by instillation of saline on the suture line. Adequate homeostasis is essential. A chest tube is inserted into the pleural cavity through the lowest access site for underwater sealed drainage. The incisions are closed in layers.

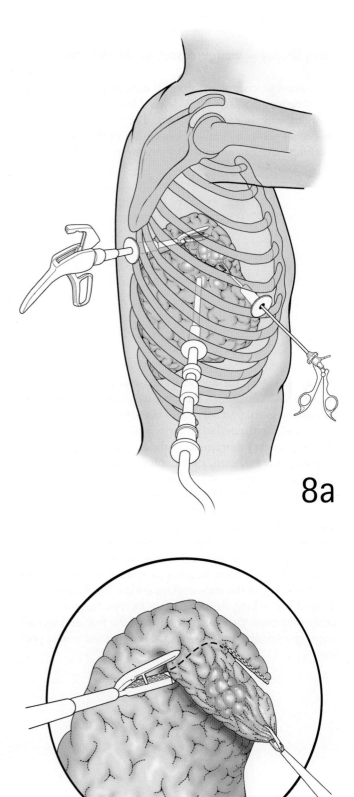

8a

8b

Pulmonary solitary nodules

Solitary pulmonary nodules up to 2.5–3 cm in diameter and peripherally located are easily treated by VATS techniques. The surgical strategy is similar to that of wedge resection of the lung for biopsy.

With the operated lung collapsed by one-lung anesthesia, the thoracoscope is introduced through the initial port site. After a thorough exploratory thoracoscopy, the accessory access sites for lung resection are selected, aimed at the areas of interest under direct visual control. The wise course is to keep all but one trocar site away from the nodule to allow plenty of room to move the instruments inside the chest and to provide adequate distance for stapling devices to open.

One trocar site may preferentially be placed near the suspected location of the nodule (as noted from the CT scan). This strategy allows the index finger to be introduced into the chest for palpation. Grasping the lung and moving it over the index finger has proven to be very sensitive in detecting even small nodules.

The first step is to identify the pulmonary nodule. The nodule can be identified by inspection, by instrumental palpation, or by digital examination. The trocar site near the nodule allows the index finger to be introduced into the chest for palpation. Grasping the lung and moving it over the index finger has proven to be very sensitive in identifying even small nodules. Sometimes palpation with inflation of the lung also may be useful.

9 Once located, the nodule is grasped and resected with stapling techniques. The port sites of the stapler and the grasper are switched to complete the wedge resection. Stapling should be planned so as to resect the lesion with generous margins.

Usually, the whole procedure can be completed with two or three staplings. The resected specimen can be extracted from one of the access sites. Before removal, the specimen should be placed in a specially designed plastic bag or a surgical glove. The specimen is sent for frozen section. If the result is inconclusive, thoracotomy may be required. After hemostasis is ensured, a chest tube is inserted into the pleural cavity through the lowest access site and connected to an underwater sealed drain. The other incisions are closed in layers.

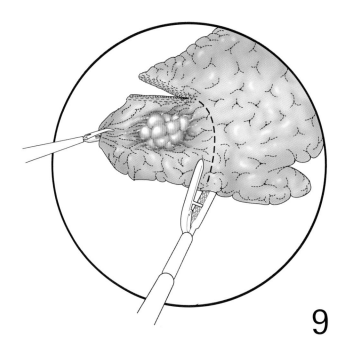

9

Primary spontaneous pneumothorax

The operation for pneumothorax is directed both to treatment of the current episode and prevention of recurrent episodes. The thoracoscopic operation allows an excellent evaluation of the lung surface and obliteration and resection of the blebs, and also allows an efficient method of pleural symphysis.

Most patients operated on are those experiencing a second episode of spontaneous pneumothorax or a first episode with persistent bronchopleural fistula or bilateral disease. Currently, for patients in whom a chest tube was initially

placed and in whom an air leak persists for more than 3–4 days, a thoracoscopic operation is advised.

Working ports are usually placed posteriorly and anteriorly, near the anterior axillary line. The lung is inspected for blebs, usually with two lung forceps placed through the working ports. Most of the blebs are located in the apical area, but fissures, the mediastinal aspect of the superior lobe, and the superior segment of the lower lobe also are carefully inspected.

Although most of the blebs are easily identified, sometimes asking the anesthesiologist for a partial inflation of the lung, placing the patient in the Trendelenburg position, and keeping the target area under saline may be useful.

10 The blebs are resected together with a good portion of the lung apex. Usually, the bleb resection can be completed with two or three firings of the stapler. The target should be approached from different directions by switching the position of the grasper and the stapler. When no blebs are found, we recommend that the apex be resected with the endostapler and a more radical pleurectomy be performed.

After resection of the blebs, pleurodesis should also be performed to decrease the probability of recurrent pneumothorax. A mechanical abrasion with gauze or a piece of Marlex mesh rubbed vigorously against parietal pleura allows a very effective abrasion. Alternatively, the parietal pleura may be excised. The dissection plane is created, and blunt dissection is performed. This approach is more aggressive, and bleeding points should be carefully coagulated.

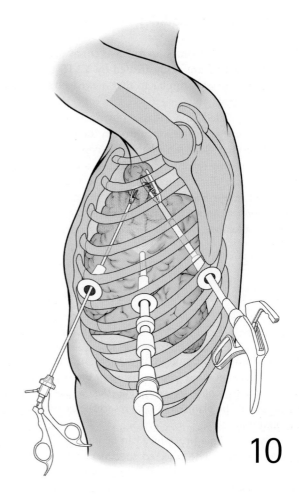

10

11

Mediastinal cysts and tumors

11 To reach the posterior mediastinum, the first access incision is made at the fifth intercostal space in the anterior axillary line for introduction of the thoracoscope. Another incision is made at the fourth intercostal space, also in the anterior axillary line, for introduction of the lung retractor. The lung is retracted anteriorly with a fan retractor. For upper and middle posterior mediastinal tumors, the working ports should be made at the anterior to middle axillary lines between the second to fourth intercostal spaces. On the other hand, for lower posterior mediastinal tumors, the working access sites should be made at the midaxillary line between the fifth and seventh intercostal spaces. A slight tilting of the operative table to the ventral side of the patient allows the lung to shift anteriorly and improves the endoscopic visual fields.

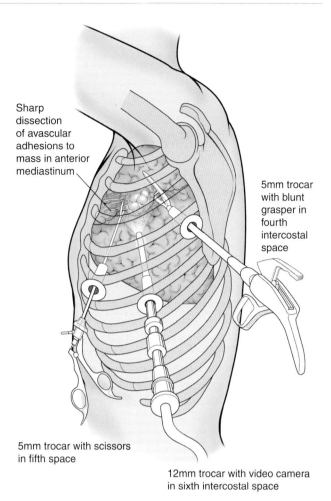

Sharp dissection of avascular adhesions to mass in anterior mediastinum

5mm trocar with blunt grasper in fourth intercostal space

5mm trocar with scissors in fifth space

12mm trocar with video camera in sixth intercostal space

12a

12a,b When anterior mediastinal tumors are approached, the initial trocar for the camera is placed within the mid to posterior axillary line in the fifth intercostal space. The other ports for instruments are placed in the fifth intercostal space in the anterior axillary line and the third intercostal space in the posterior axillary line. This trocar positioning properly triangulates the instrumentation and enables one to add more ports if necessary. The initial recognition of the pathology is begun inferiorly and laterally and extended medially, with meticulous clipping and coagulation of all bleeders, especially branches of the innominate vein.

Cysts can be treated using the same principles as in an open operation. The cyst usually can be carefully dissected with sharp and blunt dissection. When rupture occurs, the remaining cyst content is suctioned, and the cyst walls are dissected and resected as completely as possible. When the procedure is completed and the surgeon is assured that no bleeding is occurring from the port sites, a chest tube is inserted through one of the port sites and connected to the underwater suction.

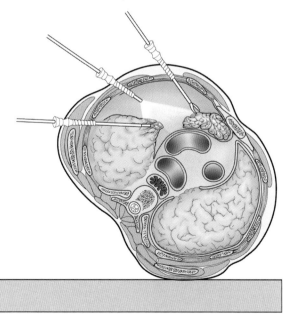

12b

Thoracoscopic sympathectomy

Thoracoscopic sympathectomy has been the treatment of choice for palmar hyperhidrosis, and also for facial and axillary hyperhidrosis. Other indications are Raynaud's disease and reflex causalgia. Unlike the classical open operation, in which section of stellate ganglion or brachial plexus was a common complication, the thoracoscopic approach allows a very simple operation without major risks.

Thoracic sympathectomy has become one of the straightforward procedures to be approached through VATS.

An adequate sympathetic denervation of the upper limb can be achieved through an operation with an upper level at the T2 ganglia. Operations as simple as a section of the sympathetic trunk over the second rib had been widely employed with good results achieving a dry hand, but with an important side-effect, with a high incidence of severe compensatory sweating that could adversely affect quality of life of patients.

This uncomfortable result led to several technical modifications of the operation in order to decrease compensatory sweating (also called reflex hyperhidrosis). Soon it become clear for most surgeons that a sympathectomy or sympathicotomy performed at T2 level can be associated with severe compensatory sweating and should be avoided when possible.

Therefore, our technique aims to spare the T2 ganglion in all cases of palmar and axillary hyperhidrosis. At the same time, it is very important to remember that sympathetic innervation to the axilla is provided not only by fibers that reach the axilla through brachial plexus, but also those sympathetic fibers that reach the axillary region from intercostal nerves, though rami communicantes. In our current technique we perform a true sympathectomy (with resection) using an ultrasonic scalpel. We adopt a T3-T4 resection for palmar hyperhidrosis and a T3-T5 sympathectomy for axillary hyperhidrosis.

Under special conditions where a T2 section is mandatory (craniofacial hyperhidrosis or facial blushing) the procedure can be performed through a section of the sympathetic chain over the second rib (sympathicotomy). Alternatively, this procedure can be performed with clipping of the sympathetic chain over the second rib.

Most of the operation is performed with a double-lumen tube and one-lung ventilation, although in some cases a tracheal tube and apnea during the sympathectomy can be used.

Some surgeons may prefer to routinely use a single lumen tracheal tube, under CO_2 insufflation through a Veress needle.

13 Patients are placed in a semisitting position with both arms abducted about 60°. Adequate positioning of patient on the operative table is important to avoid any chance of brachial plexus injury.

Two 5-mm access ports are used, one for the telescope and camera. The 4- or 5-mm telescope is usually placed in the third or fourth intercostal space in the line of the anterior iliac spine. The second port is placed in the midaxillary line, generally one intercostal space above.

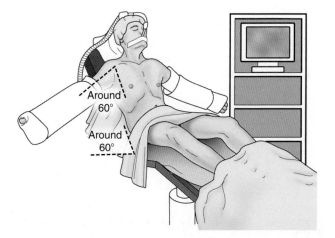

13

14 After the anesthesiologist deflates the right lung, the sympathetic chain is identified, and ribs and ganglia are identified. The first rib runs in a completely different plane and the second rib is usually easily identified.

A careful identification of all anatomic points before any surgical manipulation is essential. One must identify correctly the sympathetic trunk, ganglia and ribs. A very important point to remember is that anatomical variations are very common, and a mistake may result in an asymmetric result or failure of the procedure.

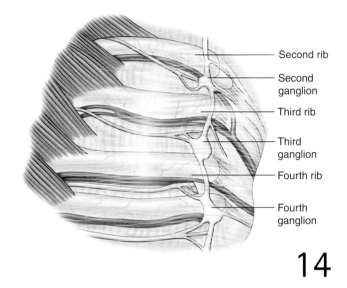

Second rib
Second ganglion
Third rib
Third ganglion
Fourth rib
Fourth ganglion

14

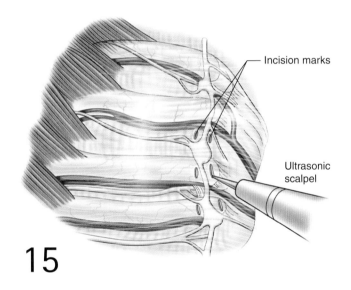

Incision marks

Ultrasonic scalpel

15

15 We begin the procedure performing small incisions at each side of the sympathetic chain, usually next to each ganglion.

16 When all the ganglia to be resected are identified, we begin slowly cutting each side of the chain, medially and laterally.

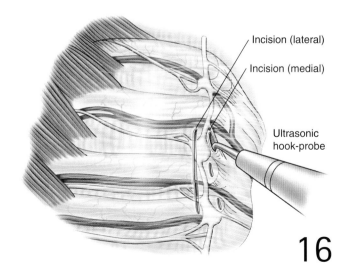

Incision (lateral)

Incision (medial)

Ultrasonic hook-probe

16

17 The hook probe of the ultrasonic scalpel is useful to retract and dissect the sympathetic chain at each side. If necessary, a nerve hook can be placed along the sympathetic chain, to be sure that no loose attachments are present. The cranial and caudal ends of nerves to be resected are sectioned. Usually, the lateral side of the rami communicantes are easily identified and sectioned.

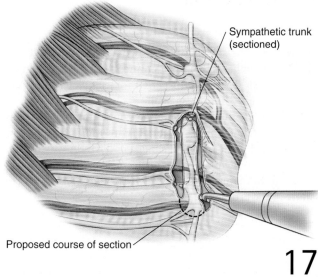

Sympathetic trunk (sectioned)

Proposed course of section

17

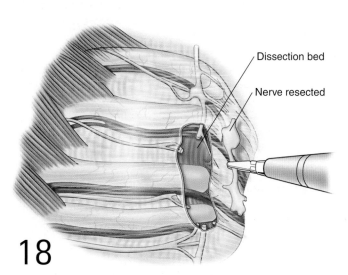

Dissection bed

Nerve resected

18

18 The portion of the sympathetic nerve specimen is grasped with a dissector and resected. Careful hemostasis is performed in dissected bed.

19 The left side operation is essentially the same, but again it is very important to identify the anatomic landmarks and identify subclavian artery, esophagus, descending aorta and the phrenic nerve. Any imprecise maneuver may lead to disaster. On the left side the exposure of the caudal end of the sympathetic trunk is usually more easily achieved. If necessary for downward retraction of the lung or laterally descending aorta, a third 3 to 5 mm port may be necessary and endo-peanuts may be used to apply gentle retraction.

Air is evacuated from the thoracic cavity through a 14F catheter placed through one of the ports. Lung expansion is achieved with gentle positive pressure delivered by the anesthesiologist and aspiration of the catheter in the operative field; final check is made by placing the end of this catheter in a water seal system over the operating table. Once bubbling disappears, the catheter is withdrawn, and the skin is closed with a subcuticular suture or surgical skin glue. The same procedure is performed on the left side. A radiograph is taken in the recovery room, and the patient usually can leave the hospital after 12–24 hours.

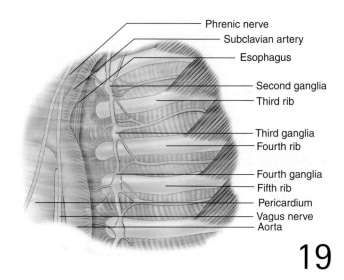

Phrenic nerve
Subclavian artery
Esophagus
Second ganglia
Third rib
Third ganglia
Fourth rib
Fourth ganglia
Fifth rib
Pericardium
Vagus nerve
Aorta

19

POSTOPERATIVE CARE

Postoperative care is significantly simplified in most patients undergoing the VATS procedure. Most patients can return to the general thoracic ward after a short stay in the recovery room. Rarely, admission to the intensive care unit is required.

In general, the VATS procedure is performed with a minimal disarrangement of chest architecture. No rib spreading and no muscle section are necessary. Thus, at least in theory, one should expect less pain and no compromise in respiratory function, because the patient has kept the ability to breathe deeply and cough. This procedure should also result in a short hospital stay and rapid return to work.

Unfortunately, these potential advantages have not always been realized. Some pain is experienced after VATS operations, and the improvement in respiratory function is not as great as one could expect from a merely theoretical viewpoint. In fact, most patients undergoing a VATS operation have pain, which is usually well controlled with oral analgesics. Also, the discomfort caused by the chest tube seems to be the main reason for the postoperative pain. In several VATS operations we have successfully abandoned the use of a chest tube. If it is necessary, use of a smaller tube and a faster withdrawal makes the postoperative period easier, and patients are able to go home earlier.

Most patients receive extra analgesia by intercostal nerve block or direct infiltration of port sites with bupivacaine hydrochloride 0.25%. We also usually give these patients a nonsteroidal anti-inflammatory drug. This strategy is usually enough to control pain and help patients to tolerate early physiotherapy (incentive spirometry) and mobilization.

When malignancies are diagnosed and treated, keeping in mind the common oncologic principles is essential. If the standard operation for lung cancer is a lobectomy with lymph node dissection, the surgeon should use a VATS procedure only if the same operation can be done with VATS. The possibility of seeding of the tumor in trocar ports should always be kept in mind when malignancies are considered. In these situations, all specimens should be removed from the chest cavity protected by a plastic bag or a glove.

OUTCOME

Because VATS is an approach, not an operation itself, the outcome for the given disease and/or the performed procedure should be considered. Complications can occur with any surgical procedure. Due to the less invasive nature of VATS, the number and severity of complications are expected to be decreased. Of course, as with all thoracic operations, open or closed, the potential for complications exists. Although incisions are small, VATS is a major operation, and patients deserve all the care normally given to patients undergoing thoracotomy.

Air leaks can be a significant problem after a VATS procedure. Air leaks are less of a problem after VATS procedures than after standard open operations, however, possibly because of better visualization of the cut surface of the lung and the secure staple line placed by modern endoscopic instruments.

The usual post-thoracotomy pain has not been completely eliminated in VATS operations. This kind of pain can be minimized by avoiding instrument levering and using small-diameter trocar sites to lessen pressure on intercostal nerves.

Careful, judicious integration of VATS access for thoracic procedures in the thoracic surgical practice will serve as a valuable addition to the thoracic surgeon's armamentarium. One should take care not to become overly enthusiastic regarding this less-invasive approach and not to compromise accepted thoracic surgical and oncologic principles in using the VATS technique.

FURTHER READING

Daniel TM. A proposed diagnostic approach to the patient with the subcentimeter pulmonary nodule: techniques that facilitate video-assisted thoracic surgery excision. *Seminars In Thoracacic and Cardiovascular Surgery* 2005; **17(2):** 115–22.

de Hoyos A, Litle VR, Luketich JD. Minimally invasive esophagectomy. *Surgical Clinics of North America* 2005; **85(3):** 631–47.

Leao LEV, Almeida R, Oliveira R, Cameron AEP, Franco M. Sympathectomy (resectional) sparing T2 with ultrasonic scalpel – an excellent operative technique for ETS. *Clinical Autonomic Research* 2005; **15(2):** 136.

Manlulu A, Lee TW, Wan I, Law CY, Chang C, Garzon JC, Yim A. Video-assisted thoracic surgery thymectomy for nonthymomatous myasthenia gravis. *Chest* 2005; **128(5):** 3454–60.

McKenna RJ Jr, Houck W, Fuller CB. Video-assisted thoracic surgery lobectomy: experience with 1,100 cases. *Annals of Thoracic Surgery* 2006; **81(2):** 421–5; discussion 425–6.

Reisfeld R. Video-assisted thoracic surgery sympathectomy for hyperhidrosis. *Archives of Surgery* 2004; **139(6):** 586–9; discussion 589.

Video-assisted thorascopic sympathectomy

M. BLAIR MARSHALL, MD
Chief, Division of Thoracic Surgery, Georgetown University Medical Center, Washington DC, USA

HISTORY

Dorsal sympathectomies have been performed since the first part of the twentieth century. Initially, they were used to treat a variety of ailments unrelated to the sympathetic nervous system. Before the invention of endotracheal intubation, upper thoracic sympathectomies were performed via a posterior or supraclavicular approach. Once the ability to operate safely within the thoracic cavity was established, the intrathoracic approach was widely adopted. Over the past few decades, the thoracoscopic approach has been most widely utilized. The majority of these procedures are performed for primary hyperhidrosis with a smaller fraction of patients having a thoracoscopic sympathectomy for upper extremity ischemia. Currently, we use a bilateral video-assisted technique with a 2 mm 0 degree rigid thoracoscope. This procedure is performed as an outpatient.

PRINCIPLES AND JUSTIFICATION

No long-term effective therapies exist for the treatment of hyperhidrosis other than sympathectomy. Although not life threatening, this problem can be psychologically traumatic and socially disabling. Topical creams and lotions do not work well, and the side effects are usually intolerable for most. Iontophoresis, electrical water baths, can be effective; however they require frequent use to maintain their effect. Patients may be placed on beta-blockers or antidepressants by some physicians, but these therapies are generally ineffective. The only oral preparation we have found to be effective is Robinul (glycopyrrolate), a synthetic anticholinergic. Recently, botulinum toxin has demonstrated to be an effective alternative therapy. However, the effects are temporary, and the treatments are expensive. Also, for those with palmar symptoms, the injections are painful and not always effective. Occasionally, one can see decreased strength of the intrinsic muscles of the hand with this treatment.

Besides palmar and axillary hyperhidrosis, thoracic sympathectomies are performed to treat severe facial blushing and ischemic distal upper extremities due to small vessel disease of varying etiology.

PREOPERATIVE ASSESSMENT AND PREPARATION

Because the majority of patients presenting for a sympathectomy are young and healthy, we do not routinely perform any preoperative testing other than a complete history and physical. If there is any history of endocrine disorders, these should be completely evaluated before performing surgery. For those patients with co-morbidities, one should follow the standard preoperative guidelines for general endotracheal anesthesia.

ANESTHESIA

1 Our current technique uses a 2 mm thoracoscope and two Veress needle ports. The procedure is performed under general anesthesia with a single-lumen endotracheal tube. The patient is positioned supine with the arms extended to 90 degrees at the shoulder and the elbows flexed. Pay special attention to positioning of the arms to avoid an inadvertent brachial plexus injury.

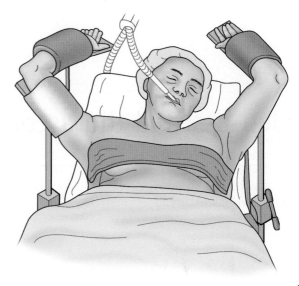

1

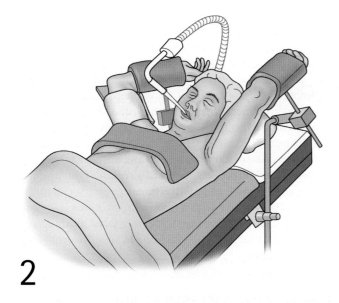

2

2 After draping, the table is flexed to bring the patient's head up approximately 45 degrees. This maneuver allows gravity to assist in visualizing the apex of the chest. Bilateral temperature probes are placed on the distal upper extremities, and baseline temperatures are recorded for each hand.

OPERATION

3 The table is rotated away from the operative side. Two intercostal spaces along the anterior axillary line are marked for the placement of trocars. The superior one is located in the inferior margin of the axillary hair line, in approximately the second or third intercostal space just posterior to the border of the pectoralis.

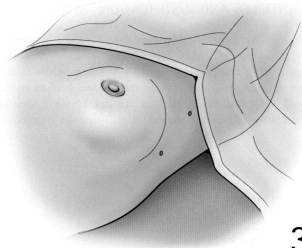

3

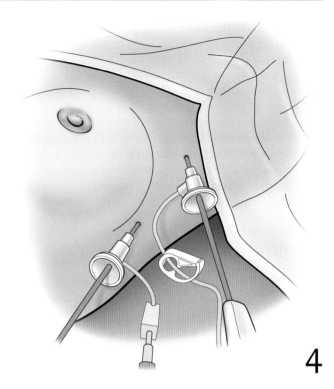

4 The second trocar is placed in the fifth intercostal space in the midaxillary line. The first trocar is placed through the inferior site while ventilation is being held. Carbon dioxide insufflation is used to compress the lung. One must insure that the pressure gauge on the CO_2 is set below 10 mmHg to avoid hemodynamic compromise.

4

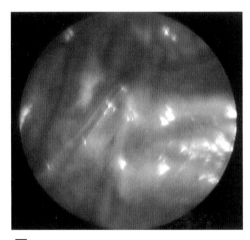

5a

5a–c Once the apex of the lung is sufficiently away from the apical chest wall, the second trocar is placed under direct vision. The sympathetic chain is identified, and the ribs are counted by initially identifying the first rib, the majority of which is mostly hidden. Cautery is used to divide the pleura and then the sympathetic chain overlying the rib head. For facial and palmar symptoms, we divide the chain at the level of T2. We continue this incision out laterally for 3 cm to include the Kuntz fibers. For axillary symptoms, we divide the chain at both T3 and T4. Once an increase in temperature has been observed, the CO_2 is evacuated, and the lung is allowed to re-expand. The identical procedure is performed on the opposite side. No skin sutures are needed, and dressings are placed.

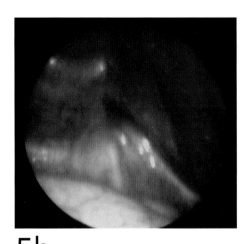

5b

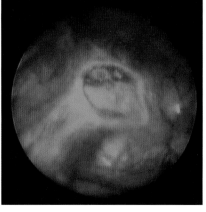

5c

POSTOPERATIVE CARE

In recovery, a chest X-ray is performed. It is not uncommon to have one or even bilateral small apical pneumothoraces from residual CO_2 left in the pleural space. We usually place the patients on nasal cannula oxygen to expedite reabsorption while they are in the postoperative recovery area. If any question of a parenchymal injury exists, we repeat a chest X-ray 2 hours following the initial one. For those with an increasing pneumothorax, a small pleural catheter is placed. The leak usually seals in less than 24 hours. The majority of patients are discharged home on the same day.

OUTCOME

For those patients undergoing sympathectomy for hyperhidrosis, the results are immediate. Most patients are very satisfied with the result. The reported success of the procedure ranges from 85-98% for palmar hyperhidrosis and is approximately 70% for axillary hyperhidrosis. Although the sympathetic innervation of the feet should not be affected with this approach, 50% of patients will report improvement in pedal symptoms. In those patients who fail or develop a recurrence, we have performed repeat sympathectomies with this approach. In this circumstance, we usually cut the pleura and underlying tissue out along the rib head to potentially divide any aberrant nerves.

The majority of morbidity with this procedure is compensatory hyperhidrosis. This problem occurs in approximately 30–80% of patients. For most, the issue of compensatory sweating is insignificant; however, in a small fraction of patients, the compensatory sweating is worse than their presenting complaints. Reversal of a sympathectomy has been reported but is not commonly performed.

Additional complications include gustatory sweating in approximately 35% of patients. Other complications include Horner's syndrome, parenchymal injury, bleeding, and prolonged pain. These problems are rare (1%).

FURTHER READING

Goh PM, Cheah WK, De Costa M, Sim EK. Needlescopic thoracic sympathectomy: treatment for palmar hyperhidrosis. *Annals of Thoracic Surgery* 2000; **70**: 240–2.

Herbst EG, Plas R, Fugger, Fritsch A. Endoscopic thoracic sympathectomy for primary hyperhidrosis of the upper limbs: a critical analysis and long-term results of 480 operations. *Annals of Surgery* 1994; **220**: 86–90.

Lee DY, Yoon YH, Shin HK, Kim HK, Hong YJ. Needle thoracic sympathectomy for essential hyperhidrosis: intermediate-term follow-up. *Annals of Thoracic Surgery* 2000; **69**: 251–3.

10

Mediastinoscopy

MAHER DEEB
Fellow, Hospital of the University of Pennsylvania, Philadelphia, Pennsylvania, USA
Shaare Zedek Medical Center, Jerusalem, Israel

HISTORY

Mediastinoscopy was first described by Carlins in 1959; since then, few major changes have occurred from the technical aspect.

PRINCIPLES AND JUSTIFICATION

Mediastinoscopy is mainly used for lung cancer staging and for tissue diagnosis in patients with mediastinal lymphadenopathy. Even with the great improvement in thoracic imaging, mediastinoscopy remains the gold standard. For preoperative mediastinal node involvement computerized tomography (CT) has a sensitivity of 87%, and a specifity of 82%.

PREOPERATIVE ASSESSMENT AND PREPARATION

Aneurysm of the aortic arch and innominate artery are considered a contraindication for the procedure; however, a few circumstances may justify more precautions during the procedure such as superior vena cava (SVC) syndrome, cerebrovascular disease, and atherosclerosis of the carotid system (mainly on the right side).

The procedure is simple and can be performed as an outpatient procedure. Hammoud et al., summarizing the Washington University experience with 2137 mediastinoscopy cases, reported four cases with perioperative mortality (only one case directly related to the procedure) and 12 cases with complications.

Equipment

A cautery, insulated cautery, mediastinoscope, cupped mediastinoscopy forceps, insulated suction, and long aspiration needle with syringe are all that is required.

ANESTHESIA

General anesthesia is performed with single-lumen tube intubation with the endobronchial tube fixed to the same side of the anesthesia apparatus to avoid the path of the mediastinoscope. Bronchoscopy usually is performed by the surgeon immediately before the mediastinoscopy, and in some cases can make mediastinoscopy unnecessary.

OPERATION

1 An inflatable bag is positioned behind the shoulders, with the head resting on a donut, in order to maximize cervical extension. The neck and anterior chest down to the xiphoid are prepared and draped.

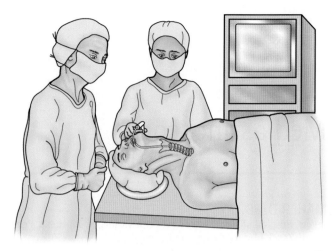

1

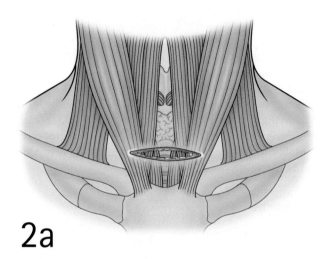

2a

2 A transverse 3 cm incision between the anterior borders of the sternocleidomastoid muscle is made 1 cm above the suprasternal notch. The dissection is taken through the platysma down to the strap muscles (the sternohyoid and the deeper sternothyroid), the midline is identified, and the straps are separated. If any significant bleeding is encountered, this situation indicates that the dissection is off the midline. To become reoriented, it is always helpful to have a feel of the trachea below. After dissecting the straps, the pretracheal fascia is elevated and opened, and the tracheal rings should be clearly visualized.

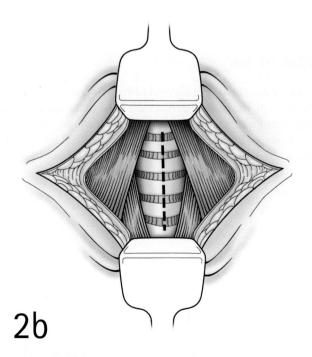

2b

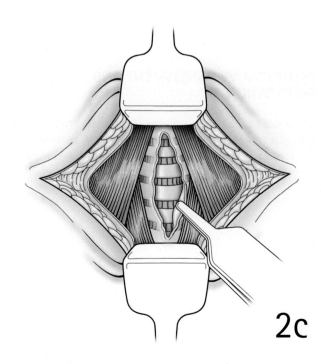

2c

3 Blunt dissection with the index finger is performed. The innominate artery is felt anteriorly and the trachea posteriorly. This maneuver is extremely important in delineating the planes of dissection. Further blunt dissection is performed in order to break the pretracheal fascia on the right and on the left of the trachea.

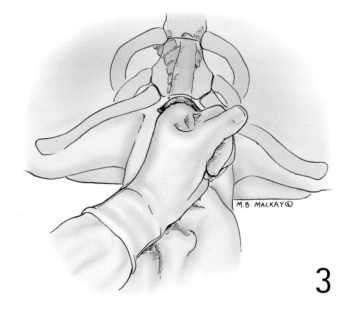

3

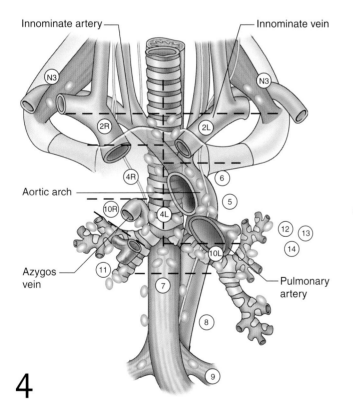

4 This illustration demonstrates the mediastinal lymph node distribution.

4

5a An excellent knowledge of the anatomy of the mediastinal structures is mandatory for the safety of the procedure. This cadaver dissection demonstrates the brachiocephalic trunk crossing the trachea from left to right.

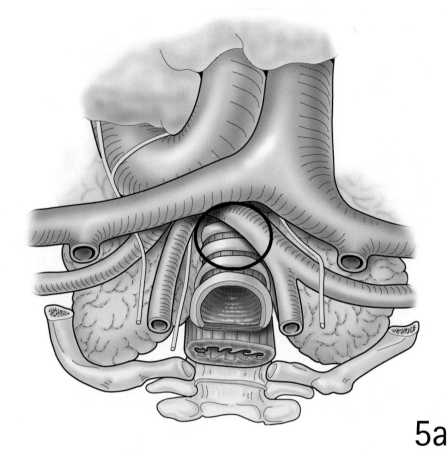

5a

5b In this illustration the brachiocephalic trunk was dissected out. Notice the relationship of the azygos vein to the right border of the trachea. Notice also the relationship between the right pulmonary artery and the right main bronchus, and the proximity of the left recurrent laryngeal nerve to the left border of the trachea.

5b

The mediastinoscope is inserted below the pretracheal fascia and introduced gently. The suction tip is used for dissection purposes. Any suspicious structure should be punctured with the aspiration needle first after ascertaining that the structure is not a blood vessel and that it is a lymph node. A cupped biopsy forceps may be used for the biopsy. It is preferable not to use the electrocautery on the left side due to the left recurrent laryngeal nerve.

If the procedure is being performed for lung cancer staging, some surgeons will start sampling the lymph nodes on the contralateral side of the lung lesion. If these nodes are positive for malignancy, then the patient will be staged as N3 disease and will not be a surgical candidate. The pathology of the ipsilateral lymph nodes will not change the final decision.

OUTCOME

Due to the proximity of the mediastinal lymph nodes to major blood vessels and bronchial circulation, bleeding can be a major problem. Major bleeding that necessitates thoracotomy or mediasternotomy for control is reported in 0.2–0.5% of patients. Minor bleeding that can be controlled with local pressure or coagulation is reported in 1.5% of patients. In cases of major bleeding that is not controlled with local pressure the surgical approach should be adjusted to each patient separately depending on the source of the bleeding and the location of the tumor. Resection is peformed at the time of the exploration.

Tracheal rupture is reported in patients with significant fibrosis of the mediastinum, and this problem is treated with local covering of the laceration with oxidized adhesive. Recurrent nerve paralysis, mainly on the left side, pneumothorax and lung injury, and wound infection are also potential complications. Sporadic cases of stroke have been reported in patients with atherosclerosis. Finally, tumor seeding may occur in the pathway of the scope.

FURTHER READING

Carlens EL. Mediastinoscopy: a method for inspection and tissue biopsy in the superior mediastinum. *Diseases of the Chest* 1959; **36:** 343–52.

Hammoud TZ, Anderson CR, Meyers FB, Guthrie JT, Roper LC, Cooper DJ, Patterson GA. The current role of mediastinoscopy in the evaluation of thoracic disease. *Journal of Thoracic and Cardiovascular Surgery* 1999; **118:** 894–9.

Patterson GA, Ginsberg RJ, Poon JD, et al. A prospective evaluation of magnetic resonance, computer tomography and mediastinoscopy in the preoperative assessment of mediastinal node status of bronchogenic carcinoma. *Journal of Thoracic and Cardiovascular Surgery* 1987; **94:** 679–84.

11

Mediastinotomy

JOSEPH S. FRIEDBERG MD, FACS
Associate Professor of Surgery, Division of Thoracic Surgery, Penn–Presbyterian Medical Center, Philadelphia, Pennsylvania, USA

HISTORY

Mediastinotomy, also commonly referred to as anterior mediastinoscopy or the 'Chamberlain procedure', was reported in 1966 as a technique for assessing the resectability of lung cancers in the left upper lobe. Since that time, the operation has changed little, but the indications have broadened to establish the procedure as an excellent operative approach for acquiring macroscopic tissue samples from tumors in the anterosuperior mediastinum on either side of the sternum. Although some proponents of video-assisted thoracic surgery (VATS) have challenged mediastinotomy as an outdated procedure, mediastinotomy has endured as a 'minimally invasive' surgical procedure in its own right and one that all thoracic surgeons should have in their armamentarium.

PRINCIPLES AND JUSTIFICATION

The role of mediastinotomy should be viewed separately with respect to its place in staging lung cancer and its role as a diagnostic procedure for anterosuperior mediastinal masses. For anterosuperior mediastinal masses, the indication is to obtain a tissue diagnosis when other modalities have failed or are inadequate. One of the most common indications for this procedure at our institution is to obtain a sufficiently large tissue sample of suspected lymphoma such that the specimen is adequate for routine and special-stain pathological examinations as well as flow cytometry. Generally, a presumptive diagnosis of thymoma is viewed as a contraindication to mediastinotomy for biopsy. Partial excision of an encapsulated thymoma can result in tumor dissemination; and therefore, many thoracic surgeons proceed directly to en bloc resection of the mass if thymoma is the leading diagnosis.

The use of mediastinotomy for staging of lung cancers is essentially limited to cancers involving the left upper lobe. This lobe drains preferentially to the aortopulmonary window (level 5) and the anterior mediastinal station (level 6). This lobe also drains to the nodal stations accessible via standard (cervical) mediastinoscopy. The staging rendered by the presence of metastatic disease in the lymph nodes accessed via cervical mediastinoscopy equals or exceeds the staging generated by the presence of metastatic disease in the lymph nodes accessed via left anterior mediastinotomy. Many thoracic oncologists will treat patients with known N2 disease (stage IIIa) with neoadjuvant therapy (preoperative chemotherapy with or without radiation) before surgical resection. Level 5 and 6 lymph nodes are categorized as N2 lymph nodes in compliance with the TNM staging system for lung cancer. Strong evidence exists, however, that lymph nodes at these stations are more likely to impart the prognosis rendered by positive N1 lymph nodes, especially if they are resected at the time of surgery. As a result, positive level 5 or 6 lymph nodes that are resectable do not serve as a contraindication to proceeding with a left upper lobectomy in a patient who is otherwise a surgical candidate. Unless the mediastinotomy is being carried out to confirm unresectable malignant involvement of the aortopulmonary window (as suggested by left vocal cord paralysis), the decision whether or not to perform a biopsy of those lymph nodes preoperatively is determined by the surgeon's commitment to neoadjuvant therapy. Many thoracic surgeons, even those who routinely perform cervical mediastinoscopy, have adopted a selective approach to left anterior mediastinotomy.

When mediastinotomy is performed for staging lung cancer, this procedure should be preceded by cervical mediastinoscopy. The recovery of any malignant lymph nodes from the mediastinoscopy obviates the need to proceed with mediastinotomy. If the lymph node biopsy specimens from the paratracheal stations are negative, however, then the cervical incision should be left open while the mediastinotomy is performed. This maneuver allows the surgeon to introduce an index finger through each incision to allow bimanual palpation of the aortopulmonary window and para-aortic region.

An alternative procedure to mediastinotomy is VATS. Whether to proceed with VATS instead of mediastinotomy is determined by the goal of the operation. If biopsy of an accessible mass or sampling of the level 5 and 6 lymph nodes is the goal, then mediastinotomy should be performed. If additional information is required, such as concomitant evaluation of the pleura, lung, or other mediastinal structures, then VATS is a better choice. A VATS procedure can provide more information, but it requires single-lung ventilation, is not an outpatient procedure, and requires some type of drainage tube in the chest postoperatively. Mediastinotomy is generally a less painful procedure for the patient than VATS.

The same risk factors that make a patient a poor surgical candidate for other operations apply to mediastinotomy as well. Specific contraindications are few and are essentially limited to previous mediastinotomy or a history of heart surgery in which a mammary graft was harvested. Previous mediastinotomy is a relative contraindication, and performing a reoperative mediastinotomy could be considered to obtain more tissue from a mediastinal mass that had been previously biopsied uneventfully, but failed to yield sufficient diagnostic material. The author would consider the presence of a patent internal mammary graft to the heart as an absolute contraindication to mediastinotomy because of the potential risk of a fatal complication resulting from inadvertent damage to the vessel.

The potential morbidities of the operation include bleeding from injury to major vascular structures, injury to the recurrent laryngeal nerve or phrenic nerve, pneumothorax, incisional tumor implantation, and chylothorax. The author was unable to identify any published reports of mortality associated with this operation but is aware of one anecdotal case in which death resulted from injury to the pulmonary artery. Postoperative discomfort is variable: some patients require no narcotic analgesia and return to work in several days whereas others need narcotic pain medication for more than a month. In the vast majority of patients, the procedure is very well tolerated. Cosmetically, a thin patient can expect to have a visible indentation on the chest if the costal cartilage was resected.

PREOPERATIVE ASSESSMENT AND PREPARATION

No procedure-specific preparations are made for patients undergoing a mediastinotomy beyond the standard preoperative preparations for other thoracic surgical procedures.

All patients should have a computed tomographic (CT) scan to guide the surgeon; and when the mediastinotomy is being performed to stage lung cancer, it should be carried out after cervical mediastinoscopy but during the same operation.

ANESTHESIA

Standard general anesthesia without single-lung ventilation is most commonly used for mediastinotomy. The procedure can be performed under local anesthesia. If the goal is to biopsy a mass abutting the chest wall, if deemed safe, general anesthesia is preferred and standard.

OPERATION

A single dose of preoperative antibiotic is given, and the usual deep venous thrombosis preventive measures are taken (pneumatic compression stockings and/or subcutaneous heparin sodium). The patient is positioned supine with the arms tucked at the sides. If the procedure is being performed to stage a lung cancer, then the patient is positioned for a cervical mediastinoscopy with the head at the very end of the operating table and a rolled towel or inflatable thyroid bag under the shoulders to maximally extend the neck. If the procedure is being performed to obtain tissue from a mediastinal mass, then elevation of the shoulders is optional. If the operation is being performed to stage lung cancer, then the cervical mediastinoscopy is performed first, and a left mediastinotomy is performed only if the frozen section pathological examination indicates no metastatic tumor in any of the superior mediastinal lymph nodes from which tissue was taken. In either case, a wide preparation is used so that any incision can be performed in an emergency should an untoward event occur.

Incision

If the operation is being performed to biopsy a mediastinal mass, then the incision is made over the appropriate site as dictated by the CT scan. A useful way to estimate the best location for the incision is to identify the CT cut with the most anteriorly accessible area of the mass and to estimate its distance, based on the number and thickness of the intervening slices, to the CT cut in which the manubrium is first visualized. The top of the manubrium can then be used as the landmark to estimate the correct position to place the incision. If the operation is being performed for staging a left upper lobe lung cancer, then the incision is placed over the second costal cartilage on the left side, with the sternomanubrial junction used as the landmark.

1 Once the appropriate site has been determined, a 3–6 cm incision is created in a transverse manner starting approximately 1 cm lateral to the sternal border. In the absence of any contraindications, I inject the operative site preemptively with a generous amount of 0.25% bupivacaine hydrochloride (Marcaine) before making the incision. After the skin is divided, the pectoralis muscle is exposed, and the fascia is incised along the length of the incision with electro-cautery. The underlying muscle fibers are then split along their axis. This step can usually be accomplished with blunt digital dissection. Once the costal cartilage is exposed, placing a self-retaining retractor in the incision to pull back the skin and muscle is useful. Even through a small skin incision, the retractor can be moved medially and laterally to expose an additional 1–4 cm of the cartilage.

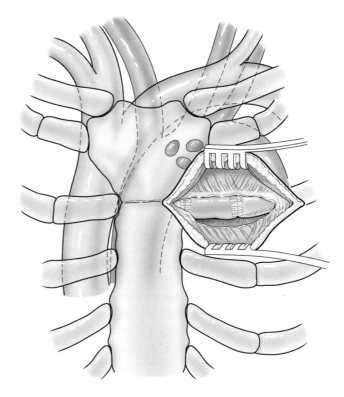

1

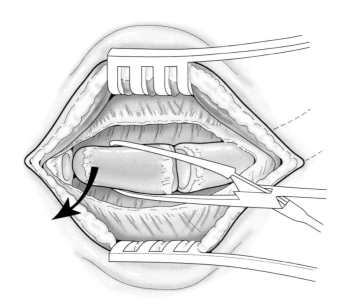

2

Approach

2 If the mass is abutting the undersurface of the chest wall, or if the interspace is very large, then the intercostal mus-cle can be divided along the superior surface of the under-lying rib. Otherwise, the perichondrium is incised with electrocautery along its length and a rib instrument or periosteal elevator is used to liberate the cartilage from the investing perichondrium. This portion of the procedure should be performed without violating the pleural space. The cartilage can be distinguished from the attached bony skeletal elements by both appearance and feel. Frequently, one can incise the margins of the costal cartilage with a scalpel and, by grasping the cartilage with a stout instrument such as a Kocher clamp, pop it free. If this technique is not successful, the cartilage can be divided with a standard rib-cutting instrument.

Mammary vessels

3 At this point the surgeon is looking at the posterior perichondrium, which is divided sharply along its length. The structures in jeopardy for the next portion of the procedure are the internal mammary vessels. The intrusiveness of these vessels is variable. The majority of the time, the vessels can be bluntly mobilized and retracted medially out of harm's way. Great care must be taken with the mammary vessels as they are very fragile, and although bleeding from a torn artery is generally not life threatening, it can be difficult to control due to retraction out of the immediate field. If the mammary bundle cannot be retracted, it should be pre-emptively ligated and divided.

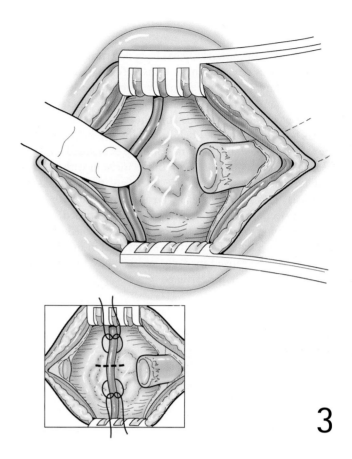

3

4

Biopsy

4 With the mammary vessels cleared from the field, the mediastinal pleura is then swept laterally, which exposes the mediastinum without violating the pleural envelope. This maneuver is best performed with digital dissection, although it can also be performed under direct vision using a small peanut dissector. If the procedure is being performed for biopsy of a mediastinal mass, then the mass should be visible at this point, and tissue can be removed. Sounding the mass with a 25- or 22-gauge needle before taking any biopsies is always prudent if the surgeon has any doubt as to what is visualized, what lies beyond the mass, and how the mass will behave once it is incised. The options for performing the biopsy include dissecting with a scalpel to carve out a specimen, taking bites with a standard mediastinoscopy forceps, or using a device designed for obtaining core needle biopsies. The vascularity of the mass, its firmness, its size, and the experience of the surgeon will dictate the best approach.

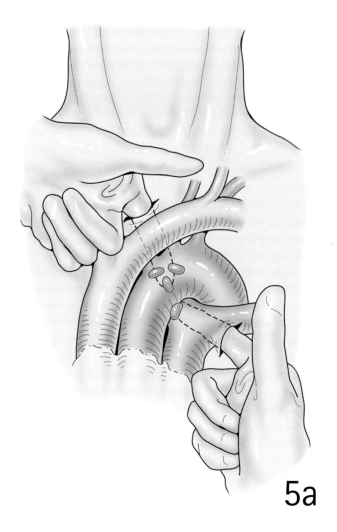

5a

Tumor assessment

5a,b If the procedure is being performed for staging of a left upper lobe lung cancer, then digital palpation is the next step after exposing the mediastinum. At this point a helpful approach is for the surgeon to place one index finger in the cervical incision and the other index finger in the mediastinotomy incision. This maneuver allows the surgeon to develop a mental 'road map' of the aortopulmonary region and to assess the degree of involvement of the lymph nodes with the mediastinal structures. The arch of the aorta is the most obvious and useful landmark to help the surgeon gain bearings.

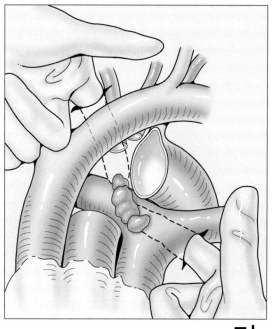

5b

Mediastinoscopy

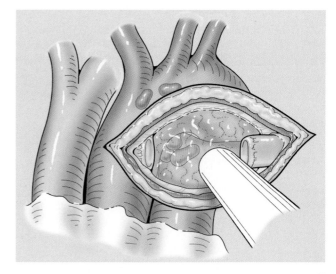

6

6 Mediastinal fat usually fills this space, so that a mediastinoscope must be introduced to adequately visualize the aortopulmonary region for safe lymph node biopsy. The scope is introduced and directed as dictated by the mental image of the mediastinum that the surgeon has established from tactile cues. Again, the surgeon should not hesitate to probe and aspirate the area of interest with a thin-gauge spinal needle if any question exists about the safety of performing the biopsy. The biopsy is performed using the same technique and guidelines as those used for cervical mediastinoscopy. In addition to the major arteries, the recurrent laryngeal nerve is the structure at greatest risk during this portion of the operation.

The pleural envelope can be disrupted to allow the surgeon to introduce the mediastinoscope into the left pleural space. Through the mediastinoscope some limited information can be obtained regarding the status of the parietal pleura and lung. If evaluation of the lung and pleural space is the principal goal of the operation, however, then VATS is likely to be a better operative approach.

Closure

7a,b Intentional or unintentional transgression of the pleura during mediastinotomy will result in a pneumothorax. If an air leak is present, then a small-bore chest tube should be placed. If any question exists as to whether an air leak is present, it is a simple matter to have the anesthesiologist deliver and hold a large breath while the incision is flooded with saline. An air leak will result in a persistent stream of bubbles. If no air leak from inadvertent lung injury is present, this complication can be treated without a chest tube. At the time of closure, the rent in the pleura is identified, and a 12- or 14-Fr red rubber catheter is passed into the pleural space. The incision is then closed in layers

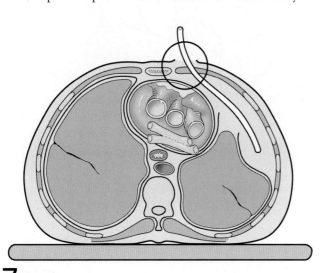

7a

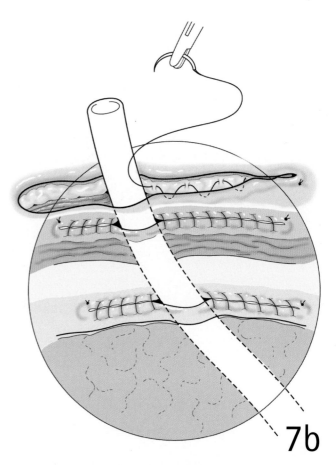

7b

with absorbable sutures. Each successive layer is closed around the red rubber catheter so that it describes an oblique course as it exits from the chest. The goal is to have the catheter exit through a tissue 'flap valve' that will collapse and form an airtight seal when the catheter is removed. The skin is closed with a running subcuticular absorbable stitch until the catheter is encountered. At this point, the catheter is occupying the last several millimeters of the skin incision that remain to be closed. The anesthesiologist is then asked to give the patient several large breaths while suction is applied to the catheter. The catheter is gradually withdrawn as the breaths are given. As the last several centimeters of the catheter are approached, a large breath is held to produce constant positive pressure to keep the lung fully expanded while suction is maintained on the catheter and it is slowly withdrawn. The remaining corner of the skin incision is then completed, Steri-Strips are applied, and the area occupied by the Steri-Strips is then covered with a sterile gauze to prevent the Steri-Strips from being dislodged when the outer dressing is removed. A waterproof clear bandage, such as a Tegaderm, is then placed over the gauze. The patient is then extubated and recovered.

POSTOPERATIVE CARE

In the recovery room, an upright chest film, to rule out pneumothorax or hemothorax, and any other routine studies requested by the surgeon are obtained. The usual postoperative check should also make note of the quality of the patient's voice to assure that recurrent laryngeal nerve injury has not occurred. If the operation proceeded without incident and no issues of concern arise in the recovery room, the patient may be discharged home with the appropriate precautions, pain medication and follow-up instructions. The patient is instructed to leave the waterproof dressing in place for 2 days and then remove it, leaving only the Steri-Strips. The patient may shower on the day of discharge with the waterproof dressing in place. Any postoperative issues, particularly suspicion of bleeding, are an indication for hospital admission and close observation along with performance of the indicated tests and studies.

OUTCOME

Mediastinotomy shares the same high sensitivity and specificity as cervical mediastinoscopy. Mediastinotomy is a small procedure that can yield diagnostic information for mediastinal tumors or dramatically alter the staging and subsequent approach to treatment of a patient with lung cancer. Reported complications are rare, mortalities are exceedingly rare and the procedure can generally be performed on an outpatient basis.

FURTHER READING

McNeill TM, Chamberlain JM. Diagnostic anterior mediastinotomy. *Annals of Thoracic Surgery* 1966; **2**(4): 532–9.

Olak J. Parasternal mediastinotomy (Chamberlain procedure). *Chest Surgery Clinics of North America* 1996; **6**(1): 31–40.

Okada M, Tsubota N, Yoshimura M, Miyamoto Y, Matsuoka H. Prognosis of completely resected pN2 non-small cell lung carcinomas: what is the significant node that affects survival? *Journal of Thoracic and Cardiovascular Surgery* 1999; **118**(2): 270–5.

Patterson GA, Piazza D, Pearson FG, *et al.* Significance of metastatic disease in subaortic lymph nodes. *Annals of Thoracic Surgery* 1987; **43**(2): 155–9.

Ponn RB, Federico JA. Mediastinoscopy and staging. In: Kaiser LR, Kron IL, Spray TL eds. *Mastery of cardiothoracic surgery*. Philadelphia: Lippincott–Raven, 1998: 11–27.

Watanabe M, Takagi K, Aoki T, *et al.* A comparison of biopsy through a parasternal anterior mediastinotomy under local anesthesia and percutaneous needle biopsy for malignant anterior mediastinal tumors. *Surgery Today* 1998; **28**(10): 1022–6.

12

Intercostal drainage

NORIAKI TSUBOTA MD, PHD

Clinical Professor, Department of Thoracic and Cardiovascular Surgery, Kobe University School of Medicine, Kobe, Hyogo, Japan; Vice President, Department of General Thoracic Surgery, Hyogo Medical Center, Akashi, Hyogo, Japan

PRINCIPLES AND JUSTIFICATION

The rather simple but important procedure of intercostal drainage must be correctly taught to young surgeons. Indications for insertion, size of the tubes, site of placement, number of tubes, use or nonuse of suction, grade of negative pressure, and timing of removal should be carefully specified. If these are poorly judged, the patient may face a more complicated and even dangerous situation.

PREOPERATIVE ASSESSMENT AND PREPARATION

Spontaneous pneumothorax

Spontaneous pneumothorax is one of the most common indications for intercostal drainage. Rapid re-expansion of the lung may produce pain, coughing, and even serious re-expansion pulmonary edema, which must be kept in mind especially when the lung has been completely collapsed for a few days. The equipment and drugs for an emergency should be kept ready in the room. To avoid these complications, the vacuum system is not used initially; the chest tube is just left in the water seal bottle for a while and then suction may be slowly added.

Tension pneumothorax is an emergency and usually results from rupture of a bulla in patients with emphysema. Urgent insertion of a chest tube with suction may relieve a patient's acute dyspnea. The lung fistula is frequently large.

Post-traumatic drainage

Pneumo- or hemothorax is a common acute condition encountered after thoracic injury. If the condition is accompanied by tension and is associated with injury in the contralateral side, the patient will surely be in a very precarious state. A proper diagnosis must be made, and procedures should be started immediately. If the emergency chest radiograph shows an opaque appearance and deviation of the mediastinum, the attending doctor should consider the possibility of performing thoracentesis, which is described earlier. Other injuries, such as ruptured bronchus and esophagus or damage to other vital organs, must be considered if the condition is serious.

Postoperative drainage

After lung resection, two tubes with a moderate negative pressure of approximately 10–20 cm H_2O have traditionally been recommended for proper drainage, one tube for air and the other for fluid. Now, in the thoracoscopic era, however, if the endoscopic procedure is not complicated, a single tube might be sufficient, even for postlobectomy drainage. In such instances, postoperative drainage is routinely provided by using the scope port. Usually, the opening is larger than needed by the tube, so that an additional skin stitch around the tube is required to prevent leakage of fluid and air.

When air leakage is not massive, some thoracic surgeons prefer not to suction the air and just leave in the tube connected to a water seal. In general, one should wait until absolutely no air leakage remains to remove the tube. However, in a very limited number of cases with minor leakage, the tube can be removed without any problem.

Postpneumonectomy drainage

Postpneumonectomy drainage differs somewhat from that described earlier. Neither fluid nor air is suctioned out. Some surgeons may not even leave a chest tube in the postpneumonectomy space. In my opinion, however, use of a chest tube sealed with water for 1–3 days after the operation is helpful in recognizing postoperative bleeding. Sudden discharge of a bloody content, which often surprises the attending doctor, may be caused by posture change and may be followed by chest pain or even faintness. Proper management easily resolves these symptoms.

Postpneumonectomy air leakage is a very serious condition. Two types are seen: one that develops early in the acute recovery phase and another that develops late after discharge. When a patient begins to expectorate sanguineous sputum and an accompanying decrease of fluid is seen on the chest radiograph, prevention of aspiration to the contralateral lung is mandatory. Immediate bronchoscopy may disclose an opening at the stump. If this occurs early after the operation and it is still in the nonempyema stage, reopening the thorax and reclosing the bronchus may be successful. If it develops at a late stage, open-window thoracostomy should be chosen as a temporary procedure.

Postresection drainage

Air leakage after lung resection usually ceases within several days. Sometimes, when a large free space remains, such as in the case of middle and lower lobectomy or left upper lobectomy, it may be prolonged, especially if the patient has an emphysematous lung.

The first attempt is to reduce the chest tube pressure to a level low enough to preserve lung expansion. Then, the tube may be withdrawn 2 or 3 cm in a second attempt to allow the air leak spot on the lung touched by the tube to change to native tissue. By appositioning the parietal pleura, one may facilitate healing of the leakage spot. Repeated trials of withdrawing the tube while watching the side hole position, lowering the suction pressure, and even instituting a water seal trial are sometimes very helpful. In fact, in the era when operation for tuberculosis was common, suction was not a standard practice.

Changing the tube for a smaller one with a Heimlich-valve bottle is another option and is very attractive, as the patient is kept ambulatory. Sclerotherapeutic agents such as tetracycline hydrochloride, OK-432, and asbestos-free talc may serve to stop both air leakage and effusion. They may be ineffective, however, if the space is relatively large. Otherwise the discharge will become turbid, and the patient will develop empyema. At this stage, thoracoscopic closure of the lung fistula using a sealant or stitches is easily tried with minimal invasion and is effective, so that one should not hesitate to choose this procedure.

Empyema

Parapneumonic empyema may be recognized when the discharge changes from serous to fibrinous or turbid during the course of pneumonia with chest tube care. Rupture of a severely infected lung or tumor produces pyopneumothorax with multiple air-fluid level.

When the patient presents with these symptoms, closed-tube drainage is no longer effective, and the discharge soon becomes purulent. If the chest tube is not properly managed at this stage, the patient easily enters the purulent phase with a multi-loculated space, which can no longer be managed by conservative methods and requires operative procedures such as rib resection drainage and even the Eloesser procedure.

The reasons for failure during treatment of the parapneumonic space are as follows. Nondependent drainage is most often a cause for chronicity. Tube size may not be large enough to drain thick and large amounts of fluid, the tube may be inserted late after the formation of a thick peel or bronchopleural fistula, or drainage may be choked up with coagula or foreign bodies.

Video-assisted thoracoscopy is another alternative for treatment of this condition. Debridement and compact decortication at the beginning of the organizing phase may be achieved by this maneuver. Fibrin and loculations are swept under endoscopic vision, and the peel is dissected from the parietal and visceral surfaces of the pleura.

Acute exacerbation of a silent tuberculous empyema may be encountered in a patient known to have a silent empyema who is thin and has been in relatively good condition despite having restricted lung function. To prevent pneumonia due to aspiration to the opposite side through a bronchopleural fistula, open thoracostomy drainage with a large window is the first choice rather than closed tube drainage and must be performed immediately after admission.

Malignant effusion

The tube insertion technique for malignant effusion does not differ from the basic one; however, some points should be remembered. Generally, patients with this condition are undernourished, chronically ill, and even cachectic. Drainage must be started slowly without suction. The attending doctor should remain watchful for 20–30 minutes until the patient becomes stable. If the patient develops any acute distress, such as dyspnea, chest pain, or collapse, drainage should be ceased immediately, and a chest radiograph should be taken. If the chest radiograph discloses major mediastinal shift, this may be corrected by the entrance of air, accompanied by measures to alleviate the acute symptoms.

Although massive bloody, wine-like effusion is a typical sign of malignant disease, such as lung cancer or diffuse mesothelioma, negative results of cytological examination for malignant cells and thin serous yellow fluid do not mean the absence of malignancy. One should not make a quick diagnosis of tuberculosis and should not prescribe a long course of antitubercular drugs without performing thoracoscopy. Biopsy of the pleura must be carried out at this stage using this technique.

Instillation of an anticancer drug into the thoracic cavity is often indicated for this condition after complete evacuation of fluid and good re-expansion of the lung is achieved. Effusion may be temporarily stopped with this procedure.

ANESTHESIA

Local anesthesia is started with a sufficient amount of intradermally injected anesthetic followed by subcutaneous infiltration and anesthesia of the muscles. Intercostal vessels run beneath the ribs at the posterior and lateral thorax. After feeling the rib with the tip of the needle, one slides it upward along the upper edge of the rib to avoid an injury to the vessels. Because the pleura is very sensitive, an adequate amount of anesthetic must be infiltrated around it. A lower intercostal space must not be entered. One must be aware that when a pathological condition develops, such as post-traumatic or parapneumonic pleuritis, the diaphragm is usually at a higher than normal position.

OPERATION

Basic technique of thoracentesis and chest tube insertion

1 Thoracentesis is one of the most common procedures and may be carried out very easily. One must remember, however, that it can be more dangerous than tube insertion. Use of the wrong site for introduction of a sharp needle and repeated trials may produce unnecessary complications such as bleeding and iatrogenic pneumothorax, liver injury, and even cardiac injury.

The surgeon waits several minutes until analgesia develops well. The needle is introduced slowly, following the route of the local anesthesia infiltrated. As soon as fluid is observed, the needle is fixed using a hemostat. The hemostat is attached along the skin to make sure that the tip of the needle remains within the thoracic cavity at the same depth. Once the content is determined, the content is slowly and carefully withdrawn. When the patient begins to complain of dyspnea or chest pain, the procedure is halted, and the needle is replaced with a chest tube if necessary.

The chest tube is inserted through a 2-cm skin incision over the second intercostal space in the midclavicular line or fourth space in the anterior axillary line after ascertaining that sufficient anesthesia has been attained. This site is adequate for air drainage. A lower site, that is, the fifth or sixth intercostal space in the posterior axillary line, is chosen for fluid drainage. A free pleural space is recognized through direct vision of the pleural cavity. Some adhesion between the parietal and visceral pleura may be opened by finger dissection. A

No. 24–28 tube held with a large curved hemostat is introduced into the affected space. This support is helpful to guide the tube to the place where it is needed.

A tube containing a rigid stent may be quickly introduced into the chest cavity through a smaller skin incision and with little exploring. This technique should be used only in a patient with a completely collapsed lung. Using this type of tube is not recommended, however, because it requires force when inserted. This technique may result in a serious injury to the lung or other structures.

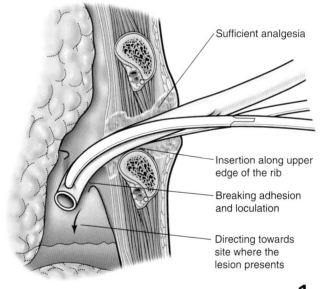

Sufficient analgesia

Insertion along upper edge of the rib

Breaking adhesion and loculation

Directing towards site where the lesion presents

1

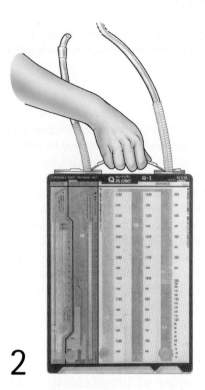

2

Drainage device

2, 3 The traditional three-bottle drainage system, which includes a collection bottle, a water seal bottle, and a suction-regulating bottle, is now available as a plastic unit with molded compartments. This unit, which is provided with a large No. 28 chest tube, adequately manages relatively large volumes of air leak and discharge in the acute postoperative period. In the chronic stage, however, when little air leakage and small amounts of discharge are present, it might be replaced by simpler systems of drainage with smaller No. 20–24 tubes, which allow the patient to walk around. One of these is a collecting bottle equipped with a one-way Heimlich valve; the other is the smallest unit, an aspiration kit, which can inform the patient by a piping sound when an air leak persists. The No. 8–10 tube of this unit is easily inserted into the space with little discomfort. The patient can even be sent home with the simpler unit. If the attending doctor can manage three different types of drainage devices according to the patient's condition, the patient can enjoy freedom from a chain of drainage tubes. Needless to say, early ambulation is one of the most important factors promoting recovery.

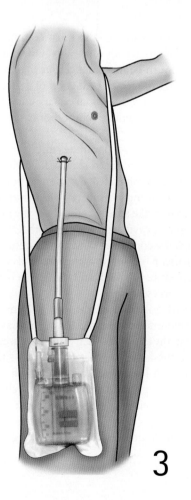

3

POSTOPERATIVE CARE

The whole route of the chest tube, from the site of insertion to the bottle, must be inspected. Every day one must check for smooth and moderate swinging of the fluid in the tube synchronized with the breathing cycle (tidaling) and for adequate water level in the sealed column, as well as noting both the character and amount of the air leakage and the discharge. Large swinging in the chest tube, as is usually observed after pneumonectomy, indicates poor reaeration of the underlying lung. Aggressive transbronchial suctioning or bronchoscopy might be required to prevent the affected lung from developing microatelectasis. Sudden cessation of the discharge might be a sign of tube trouble, especially if the content is bloody. Massive development of subcutaneous emphysema, which is seldom life threatening although it greatly worries the patient, indicates a need to increase the suction flow by adding another tube, or kinking of the tube behind the patient's back.

FURTHER READING

Cerfolio RJ, Tummala RP, Holman WL, et al. A prospective algorithm for the management of air leaks after pulmonary resection. Annals of Thoracic Surgery 1998; 66: 1726–31.

Kirsh MM, Rotman H, Behrent DM, Orringer MB, Sloan H. Complications of pulmonary resection. Annals of Thoracic Surgery 1975; 20: 215–36.

Okada M, Tsubota N, Yoshimura M, Miyamoto Y, Yamagishi H, Satake S. Surgical treatment for chronic pleural empyema. Surgery Today 2000; 30: 506–10.

Ponn RB, Silverman HJ, Dederico JA. Outpatient chest tube management. Annals of Thoracic Surgery 1997; 64: 1437–40.

Schfers SJ, Dresler CM. Update on talc, bleomycin, and the tetracyclines in the treatment of malignant pleural effusions. Pharmacotherapy 1995; 15: 228–35.

Weissberg D, Refaely Y. Pleural empyema: 24-year experience. Annals of Thoracic Surgery 1996; 62: 1026–9.

13

Tracheostomy

RANDAL S. WEBER, MD, FACS
Hubert L. and Oliver Stringer Distinguished Professor of Cancer Research, Chairman Department of Head and Neck Surgery, University of Texas MD Anderson Cancer Center, Houston, Texas, USA

ARA A. CHALIAN, MD, FACS
Specialist Associate Professor, Director Head and Neck Reconstructive Surgery Service, Department of Otorhinolaryngology–Head and Neck Surgery, University of Pennsylvania Health System, Philadelphia, PA, USA

SARAH H. KAGAN, PHD, RN
Associate Professor of Gerontological Nursing; School of Nursing, Gerontology Clinical Nurse Specialist, Hospital of the University of Pennsylvania; Secondary Faculty, Department of Otorhinolaryngology–Head and Neck Surgery, University of Pennsylvania, Philadelphia, PA, USA

HISTORY

The creation of an opening into the trachea for establishment or maintenance of the airway dates back to antiquity. In the early 1800s the procedure was performed by a few pioneering surgeons for patients in danger of asphyxiation. In the latter half of the nineteenth century and the early portion of the twentieth century, tracheostomy has evolved into a lifesaving procedure safely performed for patients with airway obstruction.

PRINCIPLES AND JUSTIFICATION

Elective tracheostomy is performed for various indications but most commonly for respiratory failure and ventilator dependency. Other indications include acute airway obstruction, congenital or acquired stenosis of the larynx, subglottis or trachea, and the presence of copious secretions that cannot be cleared by the patient. Surgical procedures on the upper aerodigestive tract, which have the potential to produce swelling of the base of tongue, larynx, or pharynx, are managed by elective tracheostomy.

PREOPERATIVE ASSESSMENT AND PREPARATION

For elective tracheostomy under general anesthesia, the airway is first controlled by endotracheal intubation. When the patient has some degree of airway obstruction and endotracheal intubation is considered hazardous, the tracheostomy is performed with the patient awake and breathing spontaneously while monitored by the anesthesiologist.

OPERATION

The patient is supine, a transverse roll is placed beneath the shoulders, and the neck is extended. This position hyperextends the neck, elevates the cricoid, and allows identification of the laryngeal skeleton. The anesthesiologist has access to the patient's airway and remains in control of the endotracheal tube during the course of the tracheostomy. Among patients with airway distress who are unable to lie flat on the operating table, the procedure is performed in the semi-Fowler position with the head elevated. Hyperextension of the neck, which may result in further airway embarrassment, should be avoided. Administration of intravenous sedation is avoided in this setting to prevent suppression of respiratory drive, which could produce apnea, and loss of the airway.

The two key surgical principles necessary to perform a rapid, efficient, and safe tracheostomy are: (1) maintaining orientation in the midline without deviation to the side of the trachea and (2) meticulous hemostasis. The patient's neck and upper chest are prepped with an antiseptic solution, and sterile drapes are placed appropriately for adequate exposure of the surgical field.

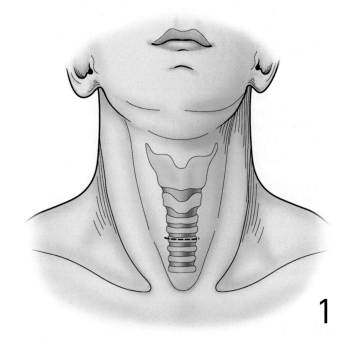

1 The incision is marked 2 cm above the sternal notch, or halfway between the cricoid cartilage and the sternal notch. A 2–4 cm horizontal incision is routinely used for elective tracheostomy, while a vertical incision is preferred by some for emergency airway access. When performed under local anesthesia, the incision and deeper tissues are infiltrated with 1% lidocaine with 1:100 000 epinephrine.

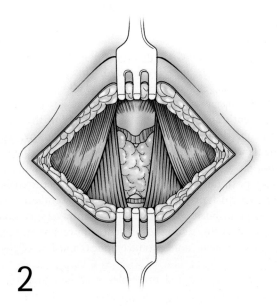

2 The incision is deepened in a horizontal orientation through the subcutaneous tissue. Once the fascia overlying the strap muscles is encountered, the plane of dissection shifts from horizontal to vertical. Using Army-Navy retractors, the subcutaneous fat is retracted laterally, exposing the midline fascia overlying the strap muscles. The midline fascial decussation is incised, and the superficial strap muscles (sternohyoid) are retracted laterally. The thinner sternothyroid muscles are encountered next, separated vertically and are retracted laterally.

By gently elevating the muscles off the trachea with a hemostat, the Army-Navy retractors can be used to retract both strap muscles laterally, exposing the thyroid isthmus, pretracheal fascia, and inferior thyroid veins.

3 The veins overlying the trachea may be retracted later-ally; or if large and arborizing, they are ligated. Following retraction or ligation of these veins, the pretracheal fascia is incised vertically and swept off of the anterior trachea to expose the tracheal rings. The isthmus of the thyroid may vary from 5 mm to several centimeters in vertical dimension. If the isthmus is not excessively bulky, it may be elevated from the anterior tracheal wall and retracted superiorly.

However, when the isthmus is large and prevents exposure of tracheal rings 2–4, it should be divided. Using a curved mosquito hemostat, the isthmus is elevated off of the under-lying tracheal cartilages. This maneuver frequently requires dissection from both the superior and inferior aspect of the isthmus. Care is taken not to perform lateral dissection in order to avoid injury to the recurrent laryngeal nerves and the inferior thyroid veins. Once the isthmus is mobilized, clamps are placed on either side, and it is divided in the midline. The cut edges of the isthmus are oversewn with a running 3-0 chromic suture.

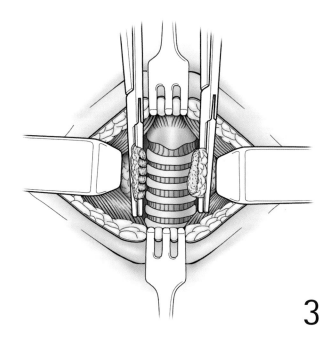

3

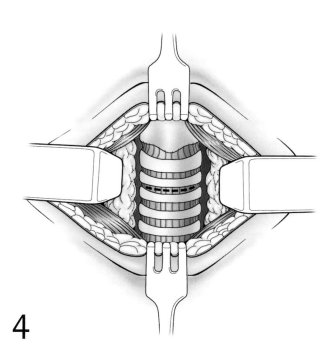

4

4 Following division of the isthmus, the thyroid is easily retracted laterally to expose the upper tracheal rings. To insure proper placement of the tracheostomy opening, the tracheal rings should be counted at least down to tracheal ring 4. The trachea is entered most often between the second and third tracheal rings or occasionally between rings 3 and 4. Tracheostomy between rings 1 and 2 should be avoided due to the concern for granulation tissue formation and subse-quent subglottic stenosis. Conversely, a low tracheostomy (inferior to ring 4) should be avoided whenever possible due to the potential for erosion of the innominate artery. The ves-sel crosses the anterior tracheal wall and the anterior curve of the tip of the tracheostomy tube may erode the walls of the trachea and innominate artery creating a tracheo-innominate fistula. Exsanguination is almost immediate, should this complication occur.

Various types of tracheal incisions and flaps have been advocated for the tracheotomy site. Some authors use an inferiorly based Bjork flap. This flap is fashioned by dividing tracheal rings 2 and 3 lateral to the midline. The inferiorly based flap is then sutured to the inferior aspect of the neck incision. In obese patients this flap when sutured to the lower neck skin may facilitate replacement of the tracheostomy tube should inadvertent decannulation occur. Potential problems with the Bjork flap include weakening and telescop-ing of the anterior tracheal wall, granulation tissue formation, and tracheal stenosis.

In most patients, a horizontal incision at the muscular interspace between tracheal rings 2 and 3 will permit easy access to the tracheal lumen and will avoid problems occa-sionally encountered with the Bjork flap.

Before opening the airway, a cricoid hook is placed beneath the lower edge of the cricoid, and upward traction elevates the trachea into the surgical field as well as maintaining stability of the trachea during insertion of the tracheostomy tube.

Selection of the appropriate tracheostomy tube should be made prior to opening the trachea. In general, adult males will require a larger tube than females due to the larger size of their trachea. A cuffed tracheostomy tube is placed when ventilatory support is required, and the scrub nurse inflates the tracheostomy tube cuff to insure its integrity prior to insertion. The anesthesiologist deflates the endotracheal tube cuff before the airway is incised to prevent premature puncture of the endotracheal tube balloon.

The tracheal incision is made with a knife blade rather than with electrocautery. In the oxygen-rich environment, incising the trachea with the electrocautery may ignite the drapes or the endotracheal tube. Once the trachea is opened, the endotracheal tube cuff is reinflated while all material is made ready for insertion of the tracheostomy tube. In some patients with a thick neck and a deep tracheostomy wound, it is advisable to place a stay suture from the inferior tracheostomy skin incision around the third tracheal ring. The ends of the sutures are tied with an air knot, left long, and taped to the chest wall. Traction on this suture will permit replacement of the tracheostomy tube in the event of a premature decannulation. All remaining air is removed from the tracheostomy tube cuff, and the inner cannula is removed and replaced by the obturator within the lumen of the tube.

5 After the horizontal tracheal incision is made, the opening is enlarged with a tracheostomy dilator or a hemostat. Prior to inserting the tracheostomy tube, the anesthesiologist removes the tape from the endotracheal tube, and the tip of the tube is retracted to just above the tracheostomy site. When the opening in the trachea is adequate, the previously lubricated tracheostomy tube is inserted with gentle pressure until the lumen is entered.

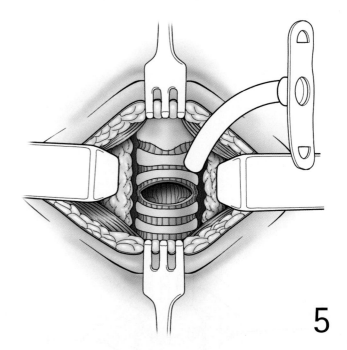

5

Once the tube is inserted, the anesthesia circuit is completed, the patient is ventilated and the CO_2 monitor confirms the patient is being ventilated. The tracheal hook and the Army-Navy retractors are removed, once ventilation is confirmed. The tracheostomy tube flange is then secured to the anterior neck skin with either 2-0 silk or 2-0 prolene stay sutures. Tracheostomy ties may also be placed circumferentially around the neck; however, sutures provide added security against premature decannulation. The incision is not closed, and packing or dressings are unnecessary.

POSTOPERATIVE CARE

Humidified oxygen or room air is administered to prevent dryness and crusting of secretions within the tracheostomy tube lumen which could lead to airway obstruction. The inner cannula is removed and frequently cleaned of secretions and dried mucus. Tracheostomy care also includes cleaning the wound with dilute hydrogen peroxide every 8 hours for the first 5 days to remove secretions and reduce encrustation.

The initial tracheostomy tube change occurs on postoperative day 4 or 5. The wound tract is well formed by this time, and creation of a false passage is unlikely. The new tracheostomy tube is secured by cotton twill tape placed circumferentially around the neck and tied securely to the flange of the tracheostomy tube.

OUTCOME

Local infections following tracheostomy are generally uncommon and prophylactic antibiotics are unnecessary. In obese patients who have a thick subcutaneous adipose layer, fat necrosis can occur which predisposes to wound infection. Also patients with an active pulmonary infection are at increased risk for infection. Redness of the surrounding skin or purulence in the tracheostomy site may indicate infection. Cultures are obtained, and therapeutic antibiotics administered. Other rare complications of tracheostomy include intra- or postoperative hemorrhage, which is usually due to bleeding from the thyroid isthmus or the pretracheal veins. Packing the wound with oxidized cellulose will often control postoperative bleeding; however, wound re-exploration may be necessary for significant bleeding. Even rarer is life-threatening hemorrhage from the innominate artery. This complication occurs when the tracheostomy site is low and the patient is mechanically ventilated. Excursion of the tip of the tracheostomy tube erodes the anterior tracheal wall and the wall of the artery producing massive hemorrhage. Avoidance of a low tracheostomy has greatly reduced the incidence of this complication. Finally, overinflation of the tracheostomy tube cuff may result in ischemic necrosis of a circumferential segment of the tracheal wall. The use of a tracheostomy tube with a high-volume low-pressure cuff and avoiding overinflation will prevent this significant complication.

FURTHER READING

Goldenberg D, Ari EG, Golz A, Danino J, Netzer A, Joachims HZ. Tracheotomy complications: a retrospective study of 1130 cases. *Otolaryngology – Head & Neck Surgery* 2000; **123**: 495–500.

Gysin C, Dulguerov P, Guyot JP, Perneger TV, Abajo B, Chevrolet JC. Percutaneous versus surgical tracheostomy: a double-blind randomized trial. *Annals of Surgery* 1999; **230**: 708–14.

Pryor JP, Reilly PM, Shapiro MB. Surgical airway management in the intensive care unit. *Critical Care Clinics* 2000; **16**: 473–88.

Walts PA, Murthy SC, DeCamp MM. Techniques of surgical tracheostomy. *Clinics in Chest Medicine* 2003; **24**: 413–22.

Right-sided pulmonary resections

RYOSUKE TSUCHIYA, MD
Chief, Division of Thoracic Surgery, National Cancer Center Hospital, Tokyo, Japan

HISTORY

Graham performed the first successful pneumonectomy for lung cancer in 1933. Pulmonary resection was also applied to patients with tuberculosis before effective drugs were developed. Lobectomy became the standard procedure as a radical resection for lung cancer in the 1950s. Cahan described procedures of mediastinal and hilar lymph node dissection for pneumonectomy and lobectomy in 1951 and 1960. Bronchoplasty and vasculoplasty were introduced to lung cancer surgery in the 1970s. Techniques for locally advanced lung cancer invading great vessels and/or the heart were described in the 1960s and were applied as clinical practice in the 1980s. Limited resection, that is segmentectomy or partial resection of the lung, were examined as potential operations for lung cancer. However, the results of a randomized controlled trial revealed that local and/or regional recurrence occurred more frequently in the limited resection group than in the conventional lobectomy group and this translated into a survival difference. VATS (video-assisted thoracic surgery) lobectomy has been introduced as an option for early stage lung cancer in recent years.

PRINCIPLES AND JUSTIFICATION

Right-sided pulmonary resections consist of pneumonectomy, lobectomy, segmentectomy, and partial (wedge) resection with or without broncho-vasculoplastic procedures. These procedures are applied to lung malignancies, inflammatory lesions, and congenital anomalies. Most of the inflammatory diseases can be controlled by medicine, and lung cancer has become the most common disease for pul-monary resection. Tracheal and bronchial plastic surgery is applied to the right lung much more frequently than to the left lung because of asymmetric anatomy of the tracheo-bronchial tree and the pulmonary artery. Combined resection of the superior vena cava is one of the characteristics of right lung resection.

PREOPERATIVE ASSESSMENT AND PREPARATION

Extent of the lesion is the most important factor in deciding what procedure to choose. Computerized tomography (CT) provides good information concerning the extent of the lesion, especially in the case of lung cancer. Lung cancer staging is defined by the primary tumor, nodal involvement, and distant metastasis. Thoracic CT defines the primary tumor, nodal involvement, intrapulmonary metastases, and pleural involvement with or without effusion or pleural dissemination. Malignant effusion and intrapulmonary metastases prohibit curative resection of lung cancer. Those lesions should be confirmed histologically or cytologically by a thoracoscopic approach. Upper mediastinal lymph node metastases can be diagnosed histologically by mediastinoscopy when thoracic CT shows increased size of those lymph nodes.

Upper airway obstruction causes obstructive pneumonia or air trapping of the lung and disturbs intratracheal intubation. Therefore, obstruction of the airway should be released by bronchoscopy before undertaking an intrathoracic procedure.

Smoking should be ceased at least 4 weeks before surgery to decrease bronchial secretion and to reduce postoperative pulmonary complications.

ANESTHESIA

In cases of inflammation or lung cancer with airway obstruction, secretions from the lesion and/or obstructed bronchi must be controlled during the operation. The face-down position prevents secretions from flowing into the opposite healthy lung. However, the face-down position limits the operative procedure. Recently, surgery has been performed in the lateral position under anesthesia, with a separate ventilation tube to suck up secretions during surgery.

Inhalation anesthesia stimulates the bronchial glands and increases secretion. Instead of inhalation anesthesia, intravenous anesthesia with epidural anesthesia is used in wet cases. Epidural anesthesia is usually continued until extraction of the chest tube after the operation.

OPERATION

Incision and exploration

Pneumonectomy and lobectomy may be performed through a standard posterolateral thoracotomy. However, with recent advances including the introduction of video-assisted thoracic surgery and the development of surgical instruments, skin incisions have become shorter than those by conventional standard thoracotomy. Although some doctors recommend VATS lobectomy even for cases of lung cancer, open thoracotomy is the most common procedure to perform radical resection with systematic nodal dissection for lung cancer.

Exposure of the hilum

1a,b Exposure of the hilum of the lung is the first step of pulmonary resection. The reflection of the mediastinal pleura is opened from front to back beyond the right main bronchus. The vagal nerve is taped to prevent injury, but taping of the phrenic nerve is not always necessary. In the case of lung cancer located in the hilum, intrapericardial ligature of pulmonary vessels is required, and the phrenic nerve should be taped to be preserved.

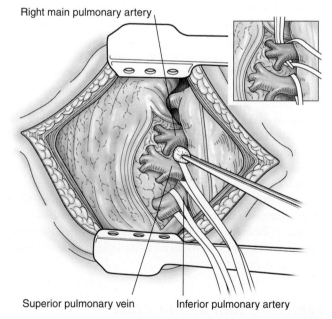

Right main pulmonary artery

Superior pulmonary vein

Inferior pulmonary artery

1

Pneumonectomy

In cases of lung cancer involving the main bronchus, right pulmonary artery, pulmonary veins, or left atrium, pneumonectomy would be chosen as a curative resection. Bronchoplasty and/or vasculoplasty should be discussed before a decision is made to perform a pneumonectomy.

DISSECTION OF THE PULMONARY LIGAMENT

2 In cases of lung cancer located in the lower or middle lobe, lower mediastinal lymph node dissection is required. After opening the pleura along with pulmonary ligament at the reflection, fatty tissue including lymph nodes is divided from the esophagus and the vagus nerve until exposing the lower border of the inferior pulmonary vein. Pulling the lower lobe and pushing the diaphragm are important techniques for exposure.

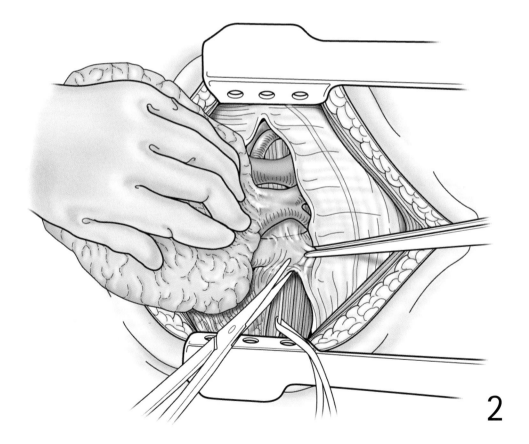

2

SUBCARINAL LYMPH NODE DISSECTION

3 The subcarinal lymph node space is triangle-shaped and connects with both hilar lymph nodes. Those lymph nodes make a boomerang-shaped mass located to the back of the right pulmonary artery, left atrium, and both pulmonary veins. Therefore, early dissection of the subcarinal lymph node improves the exposure and ligature of the inferior pulmonary vein.

Reflecting the esophagus from the subcarinal lymph nodes is the first step. Retraction of the vagal nerve with a tape makes finding the bronchial artery along the branch of the vagal nerve easy. At the lateral thoracotomy, a branch of the vagal nerve covers the bronchial artery because of the outside location of the vagal nerve against the bronchial artery. After cutting the branches of the vagal nerve and the bronchial artery, the left hilar lymph nodes located along the left main bronchus are dissected from the esophagus, vertebra, and thoracic aorta. The common wrapper covering the hilar nodes and left main bronchus should be penetrated along the border of lymph nodes and the bronchus. This procedure of penetration between the main bronchus and the lymph nodes should be done carefully because the bronchial artery runs along the bronchus. The left hilar lymph nodes are grasped and pulled by Allis forceps, and are dissected from the pericardium until the tracheal bifurcation. Next, the right hilar lymph nodes are divided from the right intermediate and right main bronchus and pericardium in a similar way to the left side. At the bifurcation, the bronchial artery is ligated, and subcarinal lymph node dissection is finished. The fibrous membrane dividing the subcarinal region and the upper mediastinal region can be observed after this dissection.

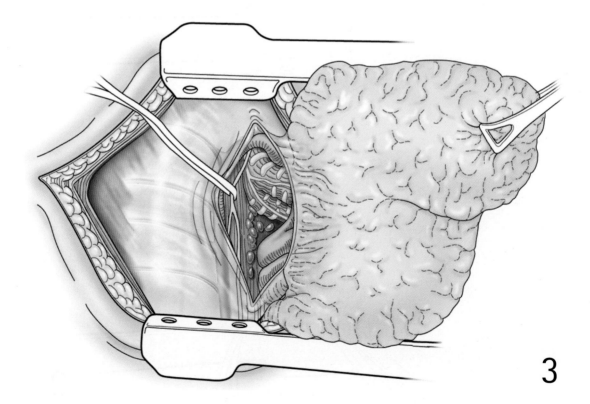

3

4

DIVISION OF THE INFERIOR PULMONARY VEIN

4 The inferior pulmonary vein is exposed after the inferior mediastinal and subcarinal lymph node dissection. Because of the short neck of the inferior pulmonary vein, further dissection of the vein is needed towards the inside of the lower lobe of the lung. Adventitia of the vein should be exposed to perform complete lymph node dissection and to confirm the reflection of the pericardium around the vein. The vein will be divided by a stapler or after double ligation with a transfixed suture.

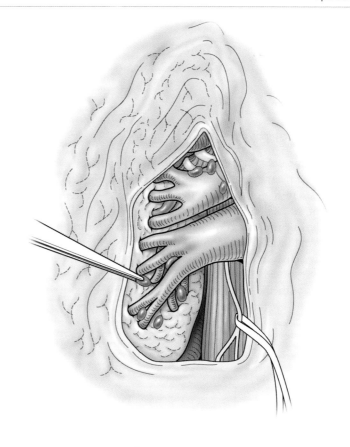

5 If the incision line crosses the pericardium, an intrapericardial procedure should be applied.

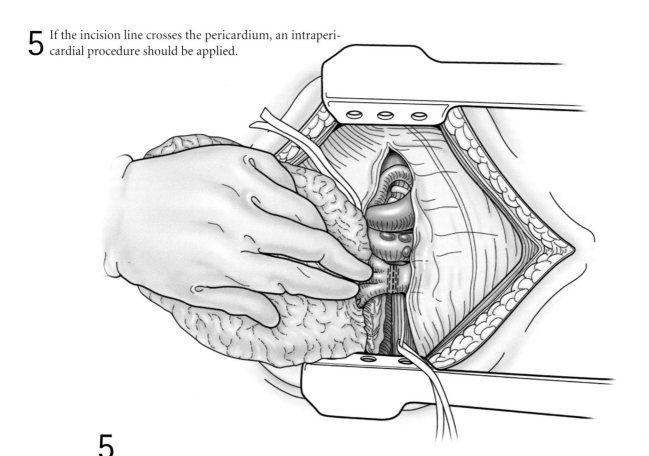

5

DIVISION OF THE SUPERIOR PULMONARY VEIN

6 The superior pulmonary vein will be easily exposed by incising the pleura. The lower border is free from other major organs. On the other hand, the upper border of the vein adjacent to the mediastinum crosses the right pulmonary artery. Before dissecting the upper border, the soft tissue and lymph nodes located in front of the superior vein should be dissected until the anterior adventitia of the vein is completely exposed. If the dissection of the vein is performed along with the adventitia, no damage to the pulmonary artery on the hilar lymph nodes will occur.

Recently, the superior pulmonary vein has almost always been divided with a stapler. However, in the case of a tumor invading or located in the hilum, a conventional suture and/or ligature are needed. Before ligation of the superior vein, each branch should be tied independently. This step is required to avoid the peripheral branches, when tied together, covering the right pulmonary artery and obscure the peripheral dissection of the superior branch of the pulmonary artery. This cautionary procedure is much more important when performing a lobectomy than in that of pneumonectomy.

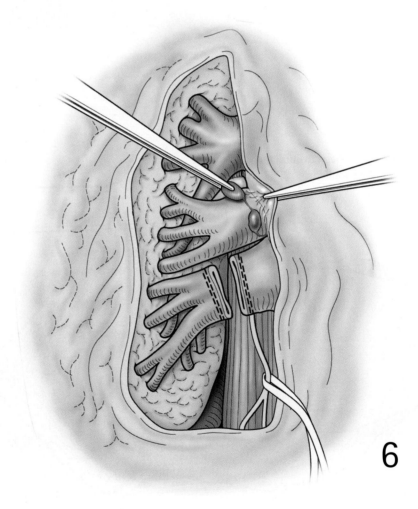

6

DIVISION OF THE RIGHT PULMONARY ARTERY

7 The right pulmonary artery and superior vena cava are connected by a fibrous membrane at the bifurcation of the upper and lower branches of the pulmonary artery. This membrane is a part of the pericardium. Division of this membrane makes central dissection of the front of the right pulmonary artery easy. Because the posterior wall of the right pulmonary artery is covered by a fibrous portion of the pericardium attaching the trachea and both main bronchi, this fibrous portion should be divided from the bronchus to expose the artery completely. This dissection totally around the artery is very important to prevent the ligature from slipping off from the stump of the artery. When the stapler to divide the pulmonary artery is used, misfiring should be avoided. Therefore, a vascular clamp should be placed on the pulmonary artery before it is divided. After the artery is cut, the central stump should be dissected from neighboring structures until the stump is free from tension to avoid slipping of the ligature or tearing near the staples.

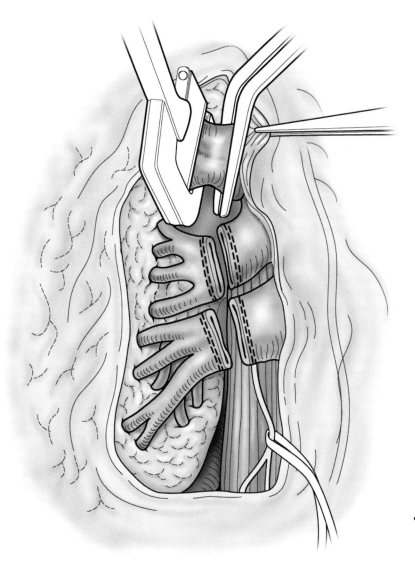

7

DISSECTION OF THE UPPER MEDIASTINUM

8 To expose the upper mediastinum, the mediastinal pleura is opened longitudinally from the azygos vein to the apex of the thorax as described by Cahan. The mediastinal pleura will be cut horizontally at the apex. The azygos vein should be divided when the upper mediastinal lymph nodes are swollen. To preserve the recurrent nerve, the vagal nerve should be taped and pulled toward the front at the border of the azygos and be stripped naked upward. The recurrent nerve is easily detected when the vagal nerve is pulled anteriorly. After the recurrent nerve is stripped, the right brachiocephalic artery is exposed toward the ascending aorta. Then, the superior vena cava is exposed from the upper mediastinal fat tissue including the lymph nodes at the azygos vein to both brachiocephalic veins. A mediastinal venous branch draining into the superior vena cava should be carefully ligated. When the bifurcation of both brachiocephalic veins is exposed, the inferior thyroid vein should be identified. Next, exposure of the tracheal wall should be started near the recurrent nerve and ended at the fibrous membrane detaching the tracheal carina and covering the pulmonary artery. After grasping the superior mediastinal lymph nodes with Allis or Babcok forceps and pulling them anteriorly, the upper mediastinal fat tissue including the lymph nodes will be detached from the pericardium covering the ascending aorta to the right pulmonary artery. The upper mediastinal lymph nodes will then be dissected as a compartment.

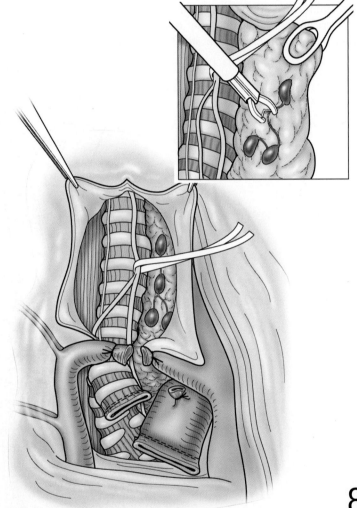

8

DIVISION OF THE RIGHT MAIN BRONCHUS

9 If there is enough length between the surgical margin of the bronchus and the tumor margin, mechanical closure with a stapler will be applied as described by Sweet. In the case of a short neck of the right main bronchus, the Overholt method will be applied with a stapler or with a manual pro-

cedure. Covering of the stump of the bronchus with a pericardial fat pad or with an intercostal muscle should be applied in cases of preoperative chemotherapy and/or radiotherapy. In the case of intense chemoradiotherapy, omentopexy should be applied.

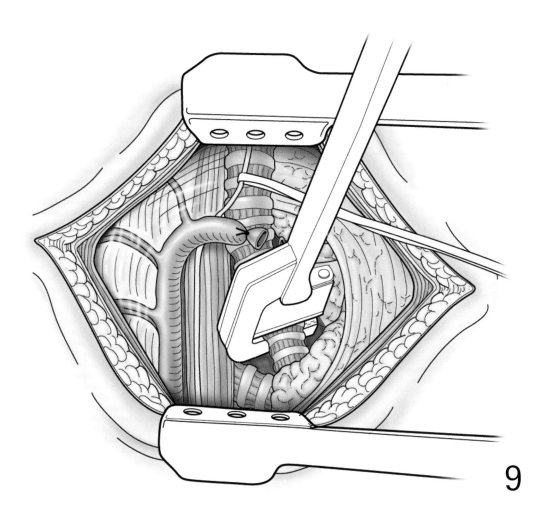

9

Upper lobectomy

A lung cancer located at the right upper lobe is the most common, although the reason is not clear. Therefore, right upper lobectomy with systematic nodal dissection is the most typical procedure for lung cancer surgery.

DIVISION OF THE SUPERIOR PULMONARY VEIN

10a,b The upper lobe of the right lung should be pulled posteriorly to expose the anterior hilum of the lung. After opening of the pleura of the hilum, the superior pulmonary vein is stripped, and the upper lobe vein will be ligated or stapled. When the vein is ligated, the branches of the vein should be ligated at the peripheral cut end to develop the surface of the upper pulmonary artery for safe management. When the stapler is applied, the stapler compresses the vein and separates the branches of vein. Therefore, stapler management of the pulmonary vein is safe.

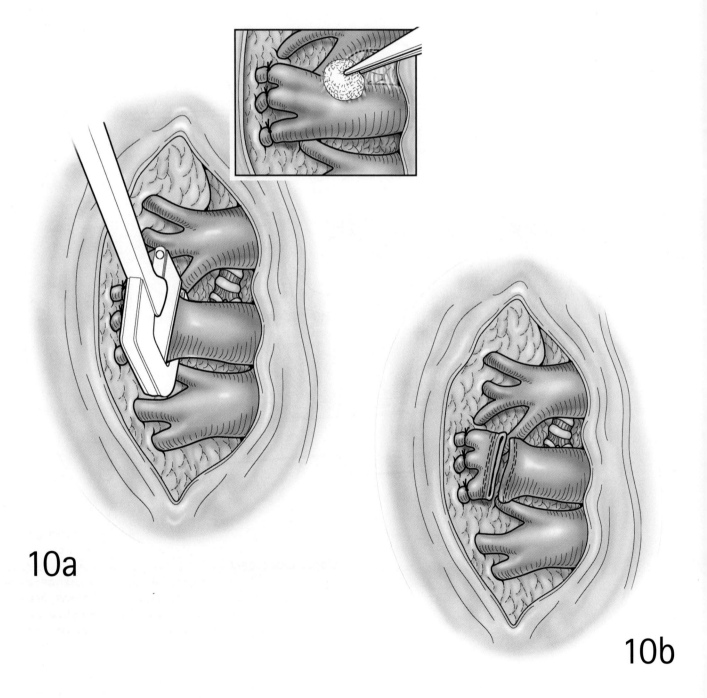

10a

10b

DIVISION OF THE SUPERIOR PULMONARY ARTERY

11 To strip the pulmonary artery, the fibrous membrane connecting the pulmonary artery to the superior vena cava should be divided with an electronic cautery or scissor. After division of this membrane, the right main pulmonary artery can be easily stripped peripherally, and the lymph nodes located. The bifurcation of the superior and intermediate pulmonary arteries is also dissected from the pulmonary artery. The superior pulmonary artery will be stapled and then the intermediate pulmonary artery will be stripped toward the periphery to detect the ascending artery or arteries. In most of the cases, the ascending arteries will be divided at this point. However, in cases with large hilar or intrapulmonary nodes, the ascending arteries will be cut after incomplete separation of the upper and middle lobes. After division of the right upper lobe pulmonary artery branch, the front wall of the right main, upper lobe and intermediate bronchi should be stripped, and bronchial arteries should be ligated.

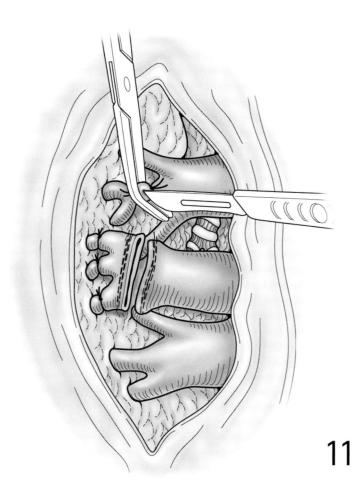

11

DISSECTION OF THE UPPER MEDIASTINUM

The upper mediastinal nodal dissection should be performed in a similar way to the description in the section on pneumonectomy above. After the upper mediastinal dissection, the back wall of the right main, upper lobe and intermediate bronchi should be stripped, and the bronchial arteries ligated. The lung parenchyma around the upper lobe bronchus should be dissected from the upper lobe bronchus and the lymph nodes located at the second carina. After those lymph nodes are carefully stripped, the posterior wall of the intermediate pulmonary artery can be exposed.

DIVISION OF THE INTERLOBAR SPACE

12 The major fissure separates the upper and middle lobes and the lower lobe, which are well separated from each other. However, separation of the minor fissure between the upper and middle lobes is incomplete in most cases. Therefore, even in cases of upper lobectomy, separation of the major fissure should be performed first at the point of crossing of both fissures. Separation of the major fissure will continue to expose the intermediate pulmonary artery or the lymph node attaching to the artery. The tunnels extend from the interlobar space to the posterior and anterior hilum beside the pulmonary artery. Staplers should be applied to divide the interlobar incomplete separation. Incomplete separation between the upper and lower lobes usually is thin; therefore, a stapler can be easily applied to separate the lobes. On the other hand, when the tissue is a thick division between the upper and middle lobes, staplers should be applied in multiple dissections.

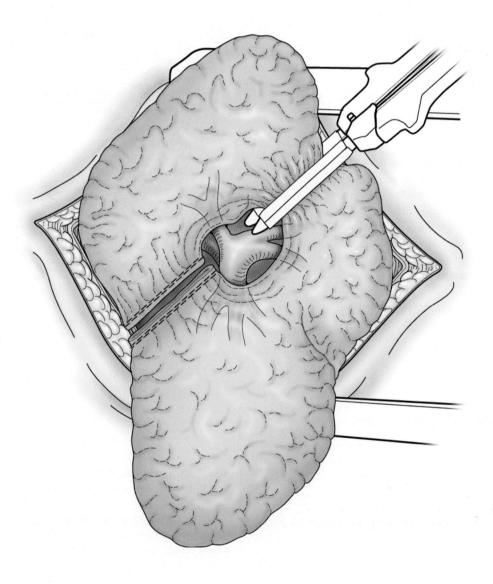

DISSECTION OF THE INTERLOBAR LYMPH NODES

13 After dividing the interlobar space, the interlobar lymph nodes will be exposed and should be dissected from the intermediate bronchus.

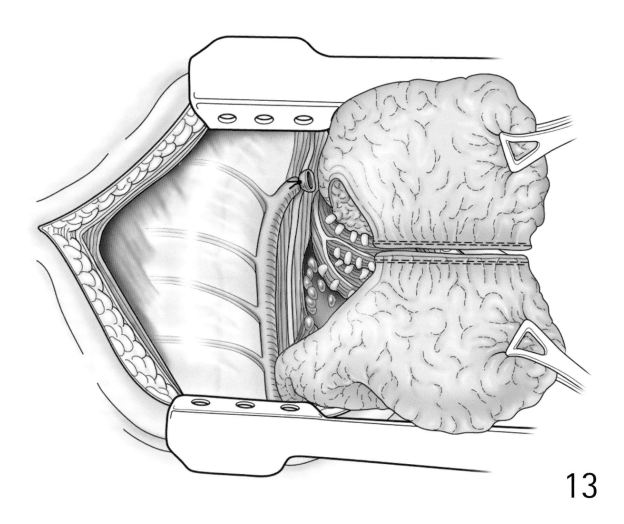

13

DIVISION OF THE UPPER LOBE BRONCHUS

The entrance of the upper lobe bronchus is extrapulmonary. Therefore, the upper lobe bronchus has a cartilaginous portion and a membranous portion. Two major procedures exist to close the bronchial stump, the Sweet procedure and the Overholt procedure. The Sweet procedure should not be applied in cases of a short neck of the bronchus, because a deformity of the residual main and intermediate bronchi will be made. The Overholt procedure is a good method to close a short neck of the upper lobe bronchial stump.

Lower lobectomy

The lower mediastinal and subcarinal lymph node dissection and ligature of the inferior pulmonary vein should be per-

formed in a similar manner to a pneumonectomy. After those procedures, most of the division of the interlobar space, division of the pulmonary artery, dissection of the interlobar lymph nodes, and division of the lower lobe bronchus are carried out through the interlobar space. Lymphatic flow from the lower lobe drains to the interlobar and hilar lymph nodes around the middle lobe, the upper lobe, the intermediate and main bronchi, and finally to the upper mediastinal lymph nodes. Therefore, those lymph nodes should be dissected completely as an *en bloc* dissection.

DIVISION OF THE INTERLOBAR SPACE

Most patients will have almost a complete separation between the middle and lower lobes. However, the interlobar space between the upper and lower lobes is separated incompletely.

Therefore, the interlobar space between the middle and lower lobes should be divided first by using electric cautery. In cases with incomplete separation, the interlobar space should be dissected near the crossing of three lobes until the lymph nodes located beside the pulmonary artery are exposed. A tunnel is thus establised from the interlobar space to the anterior hilum near the root of both pulmonary veins. A stapler should be used through the tunnel to divide the space. A similar tunnel should be made from the interlobar space to the posterior hilum between the upper and intermediate bronchi.

DIVISION OF THE PULMONARY ARTERY

14 The lymph nodes beside the pulmonary artery should be dissected from the pulmonary artery toward the lower lobe. The adventitia of the pulmonary artery should be cleared by using a scissor or electric cautery. The superior segmental artery is divided separately from the other basal arteries. The basal segmental artery is divided with a stapler. When the basal artery is ligated, the existence of a branch of the middle lobe artery from the anterior segmental artery of the lower lobe should be visualized. This branch of the anterior segmental artery should be ligated at the periphery.

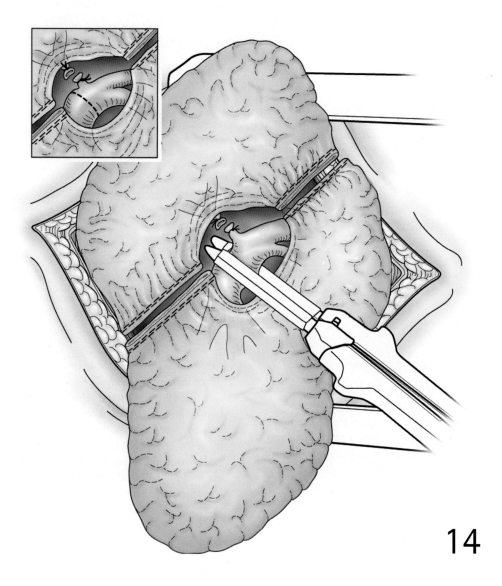

14

DISSECTION OF THE INTERLOBAR LYMPH NODES

Lymph nodes located around the lower lobe bronchus, the interbronchi between the lower lobe and the middle lobe bronchi, and the interbronchi between the intermediate and the upper lobe bronchi should be dissected toward the lower lobe. In cases with metastases of these lymph nodes, the intrapulmonary lymph nodes in the middle and upper lobes should be dissected completely, or bilobectomy should be performed.

An upper mediastinal lymph node dissection should be performed routinely even though the possibility of cure for patients with lower lobe lung cancer metastasizing to the upper mediastinum is extremely rare. Therefore, hilar and interlobar lymph node dissection is much more important than upper mediastinal dissection.

DIVISION OF THE LOWER LOBE BRONCHUS

15 Because the origin of the superior segmental bronchus is almost at the same level as the origin of the middle lobe bronchus, the resection line of the lower lobe bronchus should be set diagonally. Attention should be paid to prevent stricture of the middle lobe bronchus by closure of the bronchial stump. Therefore, in the case of a short surgical margin from the edge of the cancer, conversion to a bilobectomy of the middle and lower lobes should be done to obtain an adequate surgical margin.

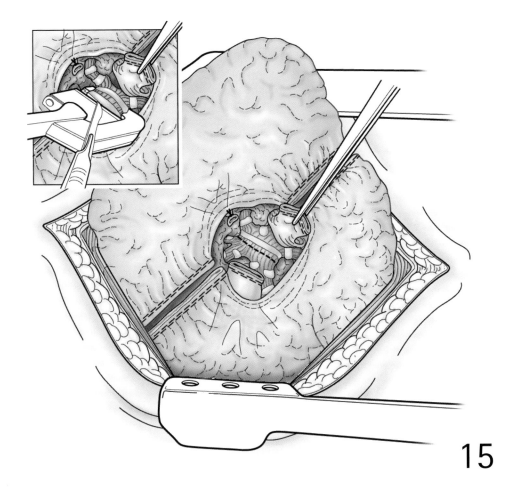

15

COVERING WITH THE PERICARDIAL FAT PAD

The stump of the upper lobe bronchus will be covered with residual lung, and dead space after upper lobectomy will vanish completely. On the other hand, dead space after lower lobectomy or bilobectomy of the middle and lower lobes will remain for a long time after surgery. As the bronchial stump is bare of covering, the frequency of bronchopleural fistula is higher in cases of lower lobectomy or bilobectomy of the middle and lower lobes than in cases of upper lobectomy. Therefore, the stump of bronchus after lower lobectomy and bilobectomy of the middle and lower lobes should be covered with the pericardial fat pad or an intercostal muscle to prevent bronchopleural fistula. A major part of the pericardial fat pad is located on the diaphragm; therefore, development of the pericardiophrenic angle is very important for providing enough of the pericardial fat pad.

Middle lobectomy

Middle lobectomy is applied only to cases of early stage lung cancer and carcinoid tumors because it is difficult to perform a systematic lymph node dissection.

16 The middle lobe pulmonary vein is ligated immediately after opening the pleura at the anterior hilum. Next, division of the interlobar space between the middle and lower lobes is performed, and the intermediate trunk of the pulmonary artery is dissected. A tunnel is then made from the interlobar space next to the pulmonary artery to the anterior hilum adjacent to the confluence of the upper and middle pulmonary veins. The stapler is used for separation of the upper and middle lobes. In most cases, lobulation between the upper and middle lobes is incomplete, and both lobes are connected to each other widely. Therefore, staples should be applied from three dimensions, anterior, lateral and aslant front-lateral to the tunnel. Because small veins from the medial segment of the middle lobe drain to the upper lobe vein, those veins should be ligated or stapled before or during the separation of an incomplete lobulation.

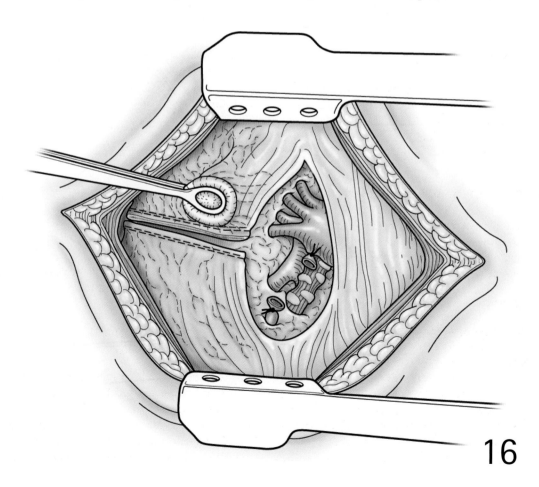

16

17 Finally , the middle lobe bronchus will be cut.

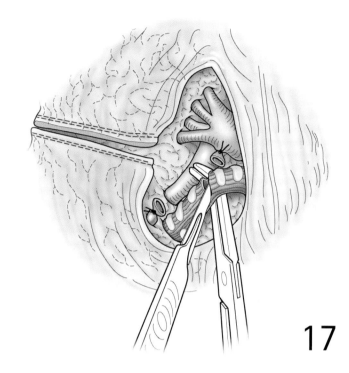

17

Middle and lower lobectomy

Middle and lower lobectomy is a standard procedure for cases of lung cancer located in either the middle or lower lobe because hilar and intrapulmonary lymph node dissection can be performed completely. Most of the procedures are similar to those described in the cases of middle or lower lobectomy.

Combined resection of superior vena cava

A right lung cancer located in the hilum and/or with mediastinal lymph node metastases is a good indication for sleeve pneumonectomy, and these tumors also frequently invade the superior vena cava.

BYPASS TECHNIQUES

In cases of severe invasion of the superior vena cava, a temporary or permanent bypass should be made to cut or to repair the superior vena cava during cross clamp. An internal bypass technique is not recommended because the tumor invading the superior vena cava is frequently exposed in the lumen. An external shunt from the left brachiocephalic to the right auricle is the most common type of shunt. Because it is difficult to maintain blood flow in this shunt, an additional permanent shunt from the right brachiocephalic vein to the root of the

superior vena cava is placed to maintain venous return from the upper half of the body.

ARTIFICIAL VESSEL

A Gore-Tex graft with a ring is frequently used for replacement of the superior vena cava.

PATCH GRAFT

A pericardial patch graft is used to cover the defect of the superior vena cava.

DIRECT SUTURE

In the case of a limited defect of the vena cava, repair of the cava is performed by direct suture.

POSTOPERATIVE CARE

Lung resection not only changes ventilation but also changes the circulatory condition of the patient because of a decrease of the pulmonary vascular bed. Two major issues exist during the postoperative care of patients with a pulmonary resection. First, the patient is adapting to the change of ventilation and circulation. The second issue is prevention of postoperative complications. The management of bronchial toilet and limiting fluids to avoid overload are important for a good recovery.

Early rehabilitation

Just after anesthesia, the patient should be sitting up in bed and drinking water to expectorate sputum. On the first postoperative day, the patient should sit on a chair beside the bed and take a meal. The patient should also walk around the ward with or without oxygen, depending on his or her condition.

Bronchial toilet

Oxygen and inhalation drugs used during the operation increase the secretion of sputum after surgery. Expectoration of sputum is the best method to clean the bronchial tree. However, some patients have difficulty in expectorating sputum, which may lead to a pneumonia. In such a case, a flexible bronchoscope is used to suck the sputum or a mini-tracheostomy is applied.

Limiting fluids

Fluids should be limited after surgery because lung resection decreases the pulmonary vascular bed. Overhydration will cause pulmonary edema. Therefore, a negative fluid balance should be maintained during the first postoperative week.

Chest tube management

The purposes of a chest tube are evacuation of air leakage and drainage of a pleural effusion, bleeding, and/or lymph fluid. Massive bleeding and lymph fluid usually require a reoperation. Prolonged air leakage will also require reopening of the thorax. The chest tube should be removed when the air leak has stopped and the daily amount of pleural effusion is less than 4–5 ml/day per kg body weight.

OUTCOME

The prognosis of a patient with a lung cancer depends on its postoperative pathological stage and whether a complete resection for cure was performed. Pathological stage IA lung cancer has a 5-year survival rate of greater than 80%. Stages IB, IIA, and IIB have over 59% 5-year survival rates, but advanced stages have less than a 50% 5-year survival rate. Early detection and early operation are needed to cure patients with lung cancer. Induction therapy followed by surgery may be indicated in selected patients to improve the results of lung cancer surgery.

Left-sided pulmonary resections

JEAN DESLAURIERS MD, FRCS(C)
Professor of Surgery at Laval University, Sainte-Foy, Quebec, Canada

REZA MEHRAN MD, FRCS(C)
Assistant Professor of Surgery, University of Ottawa, Ottawa, Ontario, Canada

PRINCIPLES AND JUSTIFICATION

The most common indication for left-sided pulmonary resection is lung cancer. Surgery may also be indicated for the management of less common malignancies affecting the lung or for benign diseases such as bronchiectasis.

The main objective of any type of resection done for lung cancer is the complete removal of both the tumor and involved nodes. Indeed, the main difference between resecting lung for carcinoma and resecting lung for benign diseases is the need in cancer procedures to include draining nodes and sometimes adjacent tissues such as the chest wall which may be directly invaded by the neoplasm. Limited resections such as wedge resections or segmentectomies are therefore only used under special circumstances. In general, incomplete or "debulking" procedures play no role in the management of lung cancer.

For most patients with early stage lung cancer, lobectomy is the procedure of choice. Whether each of these patients should also have a complete mediastinal lymphadenectomy remains controversial, especially in individuals with T1N0 and T2N0 tumors. If the tumor cannot be completely resected by lobectomy, pneumonectomy must be done. Left sleeve resections are done infrequently not only because no bronchus intermedius exists on that side but also because left pneumonectomy is better tolerated than right pneumonectomy. Pulmonary arterioplasties also have become standard procedures in some centers. For those who express concern about sleeve resection or arterioplasties for lung cancer treatment, adequacy of the resection is the major issue. On the other hand, those who are advocates of these techniques point out that negative frozen sections insure complete resection of the neoplasm. When the tumor involves either directly or through adjacent nodes, the hilum of the lung, the pulmonary vascular pedicle, or the aortopulmonary window,

mobilization and ligation of blood vessels may have to be done from within the pericardium.

PREOPERATIVE ASSESSMENT AND PREPARATION

Evaluation of physiological status

The evaluation of patients prior to left-sided pulmonary resection is somewhat different if the indication for surgery is lung cancer or if it is a benign process. Regardless of the underlying pathology, proper evaluation of cardiopulmonary function and of other risk factors for morbidity must be carried out. All of these patients should have a thorough history and physical examination. Of particular interest to the surgeon are the smoking history, possible occupational exposure, grade of dyspnea, weight loss, and associated comorbidities.

The evaluation of pulmonary function should be complemented by spirometric studies and analysis of arterial blood gases. If the patient has clinical or physiological evidence of impaired pulmonary function ($FEV_1 < 2.0$ L), additional information must be obtained especially when a strong possibility of pneumonectomy exists. This information is best obtained through exercise testing with measurements of O_2 saturation, arterial blood gases, and maximal O_2 consumption (VO_{2max}). A VO_{2max} lower than 15 ml/kg/min is a warning that pulmonary complications are likely to occur. Prediction of postoperative function through the use of isotopic scanning also can be useful. Very often, however, numbers only tell part of the story and experience as well as clinical judgement are just as important when deciding if a given individual has enough pulmonary reserve to withstand lung resection. Adjustment of pulmonary medication, stoppage of smoking, and a short period of rehabilitation will often improve the patient's endurance and reduce the likelihood of complications. Oral corticosteroids must be avoided as much as possible.

In addition, time and effort also must be spent to evaluate cardiac function if the patient has a history of coronary heart disease or an abnormal ECG. For most, an exercise test is all that will be required. If the test is positive either clinically or electrocardiographically, a thallium isotope scan should be done, and we recommend that all these patients are seen preoperatively by a cardiologist. One area that is frequently overlooked is the carotid arterial system, and in cases of possible compromised circulation, complementary investigation must be done. Similarly, all other comorbidities such as diabetes mellitus should be looked at carefully and their treatment optimized prior to operation.

In several cases, the actual planning of surgery is done at the time of bronchoscopic examination. Indeed, no patient should undergo any kind of pulmonary resection without prior bronchoscopy. Whether the examination should be done by the surgeon or by an experienced "medical" bronchoscopist remains controversial and may vary from center to center.

Resectability of the tumor

In addition to deciding whether the patient needs surgery and if he or she can withstand pulmonary resection, determination of whether the tumor is technically resectable is necessary. Anatomically, the extent of disease and therefore the type of resection likely to be required are best determined through the interpretation of CT images and bronchoscopy findings.

1a With specificity in the range of 70–80%, CT scan can accurately predict the need for chest wall resection. CT scanning also is useful to assess the status of mediastinal nodes. Obviously, bronchoscopic examination is of paramount importance to determine the feasibility of standard lobectomy, sleeve resection, and pneumonectomy.

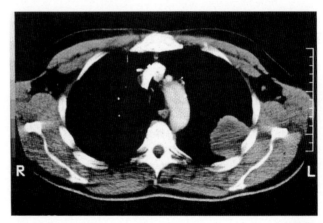

1a

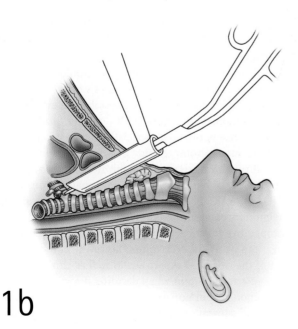

1b

1b Due to an overall CT diagnostic accuracy of less than 80% to assess lymph node status, many surgeons almost routinely perform a cervical mediastinoscopy before resecting a lung cancer. This examination allows for palpation, inspection, and biopsy of mediastinal nodes and is more sensitive and specific than either CT or MRI to detect metastatic nodes.

Accurate pretreatment staging of the mediastinum has now become an important priority because most patients with clinical N2 disease will undergo induction therapies. On the left side, upper lobe tumors can metastasize to the aortopulmonary or anterior mediastinal nodes in up to one third of cases. Since these nodes are not accessible by cervical mediastinoscopy, an anterior second space exploration (Chamberlain procedure) or an extended cervical mediastinoscopy is often added to standard mediastinoscopy.

A newer imaging technique that may be helpful in pretreatment staging of lung cancer patients is positron emission tomography (PET) scanning. This examination is a "one stop" test that can detect positive lymph nodes as well as distant metastases. This examination also can be combined with CT scanning to more accurately localize a lesion.

Another issue that must be considered is the need for a tissue diagnosis. Many surgeons feel that if CT scan and bronchoscopy demonstrate a potentially resectable tumor in a fit patient, preoperative biopsy is not indicated because the results of the biopsy are unlikely to alter the decision to operate. On the other hand, those who are advocates of preoperative biopsy (often done by fine needle aspiration) point out that having a diagnosis before operation can help streamline the investigation as well as avoid reliance on frozen section analysis at the time of surgery. Indeed, transthoracic needle biopsy (TTNB) can be done with very low morbidity, and in most series it has a very high diagnostic accuracy (90–95%). The concern that TTNB may spread tumor cells and adversely affect outcome is not substantiated.

Preparation for surgery

One of the most important steps in the preparation for surgery is the need to have a clear discussion with the patient and the relatives not only of what will happen during or after the operation but also of the risks involved, most common complications, and chances of prolonged survival. Ideally, patients should be off cigarette smoking, but this goal is difficult to achieve because of time constraints and the possible rise in patient stress towards the upcoming operation.

As previously alluded to, a 6-week period of rehabilitation has been shown to decrease morbidity in high-risk patients undergoing lung resection for carcinoma. During that time, medication and nutrition are optimized, and the patient's endurance is improved as evidenced by increased distances during the 6-minute walking test. Unfortunately, most centers do not favor this approach because they do not have the infrastructure to implement and supervise such programs.

The surgeon's preparation is also important, and he or she must be able to perform bronchoplasties instead of pneumonectomies in selected cases. The surgeon must also be able to deal with invasive tumors that may require intrapericardial ligation of blood vessels or concomitant chest wall resection for their complete removal.

ANESTHESIA

All patients are seen preoperatively by an anesthesiologist, and most are admitted on the day of surgery. Since it is common practice to use epidural analgesia during the postoperative period, the catheter is inserted before operation (awake patient) so that continuous analgesia can be delivered throughout the operation. All patients have an arterial line (radial artery) for monitoring, a central venous line which can be used for massive fluid infusion, and a Foley catheter.

All procedures require a general anesthetic, most often given through the use of a disposable double-lumen tube. These tubes come in right-sided and left-sided models, and their position is verified with a pediatric flexible bronchoscope. If any problems occur during the operation, the tube can easily be repositioned with the bronchoscope. Single lung ventilation also can be achieved with the use of a Fogarty catheter advanced and inflated in the mainstem bronchus of the operated side.

Our policy is to give the first dose of antibiotics as well as 5000 units of heparin (subcutaneously) prior to incising the skin.

OPERATION

Position, incision, and exploration

2a The posterolateral incision is used by most surgeons because it provides considerable exposure to the entire pleural space. This incision is versatile and allows the surgeon the possibility of modifying the operative strategy, if required. The patient is in the lateral decubitus position with the arm extended anteriorly and superiorly, gliding the scapula away from the fifth interspace. The head of the patient is supported, and a roll is inserted in the axilla to spread the intercostal spaces at the site of the incision. The table is broken at the lumbar area to push the pelvis away from the incision and spread the ribs even further. The legs are supported with pillows, and the patient is immobilized in a bean bag.

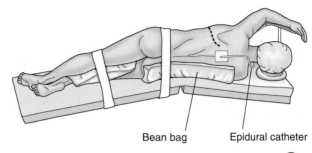

Bean bag   Epidural catheter

2a

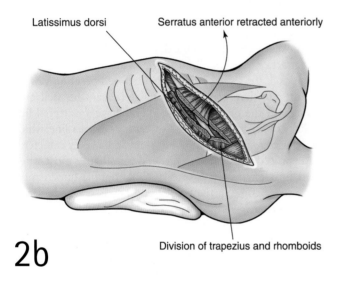

Latissimus dorsi   Serratus anterior retracted anteriorly

2b   Division of trapezius and rhomboids

2b A posterolateral thoracotomy which follows initially the posterior and inferior edges of the scapula is then performed. The incision is carried down to the latissimus dorsi which is incised with the cautery. The serratus anterior is preserved because it is a functional cough muscle as well as a potential source for a transposition flap in the future. The muscle is retracted anteriorly. The ribs and intercostal spaces are counted; and for most cases, the pleural space is entered in the fifth intercostal space. We almost never remove a rib and neither do we divide the lower rib to increase mobility as advocated by some surgeons.

The first stages of the operation involve the freeing of the lung if there are any adhesions and a thorough exploration of the lung itself, entire surfaces of the pleura, and mediastinum. Any suspicious lesion should be biopsied, and in lung cancer operations, routine sampling of nodes located in predetermined areas should be carried out. On the left side, biopsy of hilar nodes (level 10), aortopulmonary nodes (level 5), and subcarinal nodes (level 7) should be done prior to deciding which procedure must be carried out. Careful inspection and palpation of the tumor itself also can help in deciding the extent of resection that will be needed.

Sometimes, the resectability of large central tumors can only be determined by opening the pericardium and palpating the pulmonary artery and veins from within. In some cases, the decision to undertake resection requires considerable experience and judgment because once one is committed to resection, it may not be possible to abort the procedure.

General techniques of dissection and division of lung structures

Although the pulmonary artery and/or its branches are usually taken first, followed by the pulmonary veins and bronchus, anatomical and pathological considerations can bring about variations in the order of mobilization and division of lung structures. Some surgeons believe that the pulmonary veins must be ligated first in order to avoid potential spillage of tumor cells, but this concept has never been validated. One possible disadvantage of dividing the pulmonary vein first is that it may bring some degree of hypertension not only in the pulmonary arterial system but also in the bronchial arteries which, in turn, may increase blood loss throughout the operation. Depending on the type of lesion being dealt with and its location, the operator must be able to conceive and execute the most appropriate strategy. Often in difficult cases, for instance, it is easier to divide the bronchus first followed by ligation and division of the vascular pedicle.

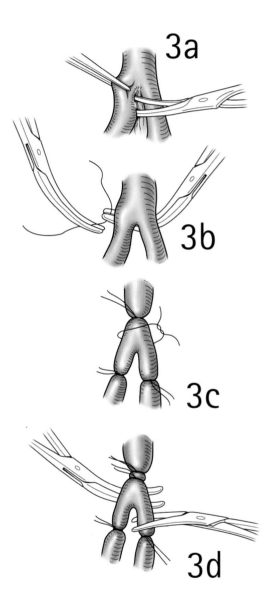

3a–d The main elements of the left lung pedicle are located underneath the mediastinal pleura which must be opened to reach them. Within the interlobar fissure, each branch of the pulmonary artery can be found after opening the deep recess of the visceral pleura. The mobilization of the main pulmonary artery (PA) or of any of its branches involves the opening of the adventitia of the blood vessel, dissection of its lateral borders, and use of a Lahey clamp to complete the mobilization posteriorly. The main PA is usually controlled with a vascular stapler while the individual branches are doubly ligated with 2-0 silk ties and divided against a clamp applied as far back as possible within the parenchyma. When one is using ligatures, it is important to leave a long enough stump as to prevent "dislocation" of the ties. These incidents can be dramatic and are always inelegant. In cases where dissection appears to be hazardous, it is always wise to get proximal control of the left main PA in case an injury occurs. In cases of pneumonectomy, one may have to enter the pericardium in order to get such control. Pulmonary veins are handled in the same general way as the pulmonary artery.

If an arterial injury should occur, it is important to digitally control the site of the tear and apply a vascular clamp more proximally. We have seen many cases where a small tear became a large one because clamps were put blindly, hurriedly, and with great panic. Once the hemorrhage is controlled, the operative field must be properly exposed so that the vascular wound can be adequately and safely repaired.

Currently, most surgeons use a stapling device to close the bronchus. These have been shown to be safe and indeed are very convenient for inexperienced surgeons. Sound surgical principles to avoid bronchial dehiscences include careful dissection trying to preserve the bronchial vascular supply, parallel stapling, or simple interrupted suture closure using reabsorbable sutures and covering of the suture line with autologous tissue in cases where the bronchus appears to be at risk of dehiscence.

Lobectomy

UPPER LOBECTOMY

4a–c With the apex of the lung gently retracted inferiorly, the mediastinal pleura is incised over the pulmonary artery, and the incision is extended around the left upper lobe (LUL) bronchus and into the fissure. Often dividing the posterior part of the fissure at this stage will help by opening up the space between the two lobes and providing better exposure to arterial branches to both lower and upper lobes. Each arterial branch to the upper lobe is then identified, ligated, and divided. We prefer to ligate and divide the most distal branch (lingula) first and then move proximally, because in this fashion it is easier to gain access to the apical dorsal branch (most proximal branch). This branch should be handled with great caution because it has a very short length, and it is often surrounded by nodes. If it cannot be safely mobilized, it is advisable to loop and clamp the main PA before accidental lacerations occur. The lung is then retracted posteriorly, and the superior pulmonary vein is isolated, stapled, and divided. While doing so, it is important to make sure that the inferior vein is not included in the suture line because, on occasion, both veins will have a common origin from a single trunk. Obviously the division of both veins while doing an upper lobectomy will lead to catastrophic consequences.

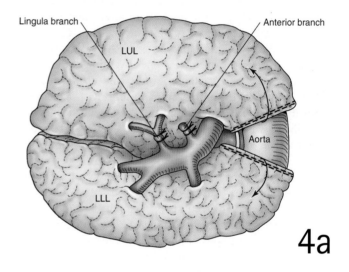

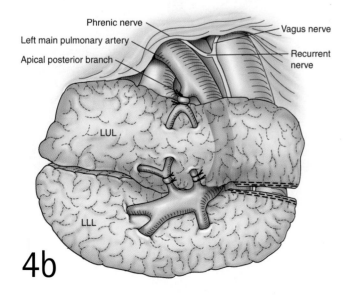

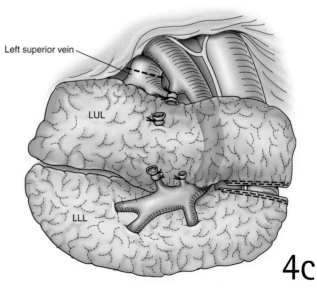

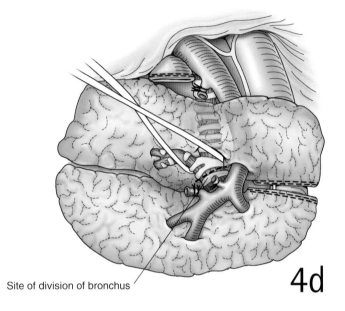

4d,e An umbilical tape is then placed around the left upper lobe bronchus to allow for traction, and a stapling device is used to secure the bronchus at its origin. The inferior pulmonary ligament is then released to allow the lower lobe (LLL) to move up and fill the space previously occupied by the upper lobe.

Site of division of bronchus

4d

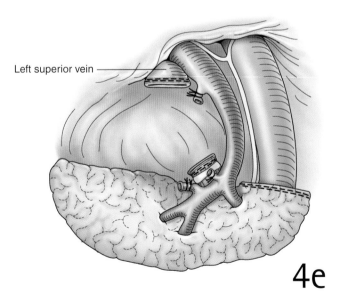

Left superior vein

4e

4f–i When performing a left upper lobe sleeve resection, the arteries and superior pulmonary vein are ligated and divided as they are in a standard left upper lobectomy. The pulmonary artery is then mobilized and retracted away from the upper lobe bronchus. A sleeve resection of the main bronchus is accomplished by dividing it on each side of the take off of the upper lobe bronchus. A circumferential anastomosis is then carried out between the proximal mainstem bronchus and lower lobe bronchus using interrupted 3-0 polyglycolic sutures. If necessary, the repair can be buttressed through the use of parietal pleura or intercostal muscle.

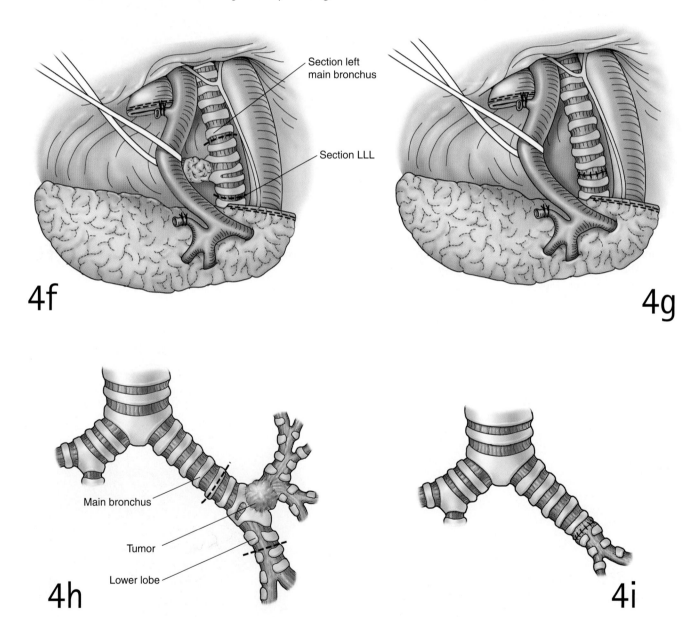

4f

Section left main bronchus

Section LLL

4g

Main bronchus

Tumor

Lower lobe

4h

4i

LOWER LOBECTOMY

5a The procedure is similar to that of left upper lobectomy. The interlobar fissure is first exposed with the assistant reclining the upper lobe superiorly and anteriorly. The visceral pleura is then opened, and both branches of the PA going to the lower lobe (basal and apical branches) are identified, dissected, and ligated. Before ligating the basal artery, it is important to clearly identify the arterial branch of the PA going to the lingula so that it can be preserved.

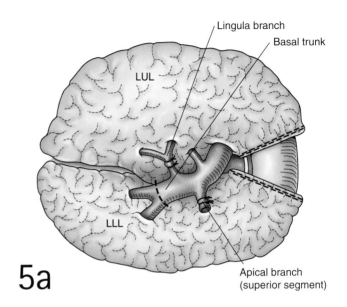

5b–e The inferior pulmonary ligament is then mobilized and the inferior pulmonary vein identified and stapled. At this stage, both anterior and posterior portions of the fissure are divided, and the lower lobe bronchus is freed right up to the origin of the upper lobe where it is stapled and divided. For proximal endobronchial lesions of the lower lobe, a sleeve resection can be done by reattaching the upper lobe to the main stem bronchus. However, this type of bronchoplasty is seldom done.

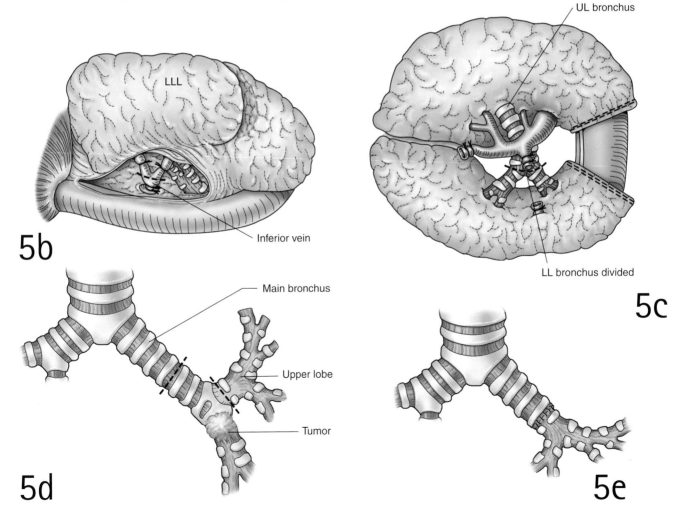

LEFT LOBECTOMY WITH CHEST WALL RESECTION

Occasionally, lung cancer locally invades the chest wall which must then be resected *en bloc* with the involved lobe. If this type of resection has been anticipated through the review of the CT scan or because the patient presents with chest pain, the pleural space is entered one or two intercostal spaces below the area where the tumor is invading the ribs. The chest wall dissection and resection is then done prior to exposure of the hilum or suturing of blood vessels. Ribs should be divided at least 5 cm away from the margins of the tumor. It is also recommended to remove one rib below and one rib above the site of involvement. This technique is facilitated by lifting the scapula away from the ribs. When the chest wall is completely freed, it falls down into the pleural space along with the rest of the lung, and the lobectomy can be carried out in the fashion previously described. The chest wall is only repaired when the scapula does not cover the defect, and in such cases, a prosthetic mesh is used.

Intraoperative maneuvers useful to decrease complications after lobectomy

One of the most common complication of lobectomies is a persistent air leak (> 7 days) with or without residual space. This problem is commonly due to incomplete lung reexpansion; and indeed, air leaks tend to be minimal when the lung is completely reexpanded because the parenchyma is in contact with the parietal pleural where it creates an inflammatory reaction which tends to seal the air leak.

When full reexpansion appears possible, prolonged air leaks can be prevented by careful suturing of parenchymal tears or by the use of staples, reinforced staples, or biological glues over suture lines and fissures. When full reexpansion does not appear possible, for example after combined left lower lobectomy and lingulectomy, one can reduce the "boundaries" of the pleural space through the use of a pleural tent (after upper lobectomy) or pneumoperitoneum after left lower lobectomy. This latter technique has never been popularized but can at times be very useful. A small catheter is inserted intraoperatively through the diaphragm into the peritoneal cavity. This catheter is brought out through a separate skin incision adjacent to the chest tube, and it is attached to a three-way stopcock. If a residual space is present despite proper pleural space drainage, air can be injected into the peritoneal cavity in order to elevate the hemidiaphragm and help collapse this space.

Although phrenic crush techniques are no longer used, the hemidiaphragm can be raised by injecting a local anesthetic agent such as marcaine in the fatty tissues located around the phrenic nerve above the diaphragm. In the majority of cases, this technique will create a temporary paralysis of the diaphragm which may be useful to collapse a potential residual space.

Pneumonectomy

STANDARD PNEUMONECTOMY

6a With the lung retracted posteriorly and inferiorly, the mediastinal pleura is opened and the left main PA identified. During this dissection, care must be taken not to injure the phrenic or the vagus nerves. If necessary, the ligamentum arteriosum can be divided in order to increase the length of the main artery available for dissection and division. In order to get around this artery one can use a Leahey clamp or finger dissection. Once freed, the artery is stapled proximally, clamped distally, and divided.

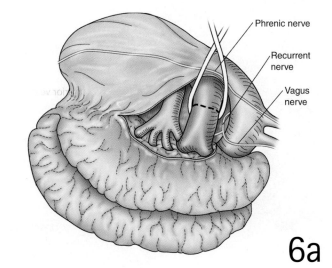

Phrenic nerve

Recurrent nerve

Vagus nerve

6a

6b–f The superior pulmonary vein is then identified in the anterior hilum when it is stapled and divided. Sometimes, it is easier to divide the superior vein first in order to gain access to the main PA. The inferior vein is then located at the base of the hilum after division of the inferior pulmonary ligament and it is mobilized, stapled, and divided. An umbilical tape is then passed around the left main bronchus which is freed posteriorly and anteriorly up to the carina where the stapler is applied and the bronchus divided. During this dissection, great care must be taken not to injure the esophagus which is located immediately behind the bronchus. Sometimes we ask the anesthetist to withdraw the double-lumen tube in the trachea in order to increase the mobility of the carina. We seldom recover the left main bronchus because its stump retracts underneath the aortic arch which acts as autologous tissue. This situation is different than on the right side where the pneumonectomy stump is free in the pleural space.

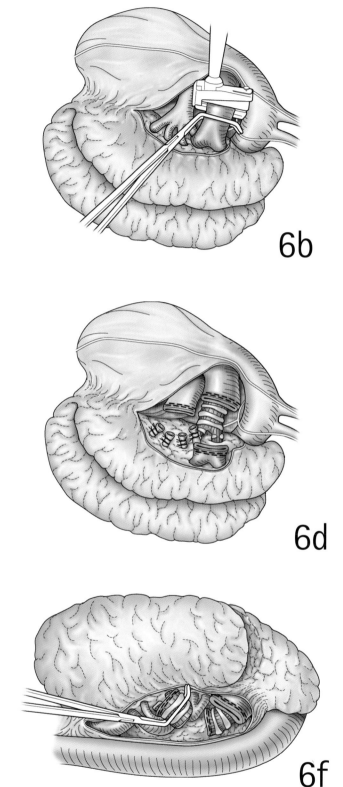

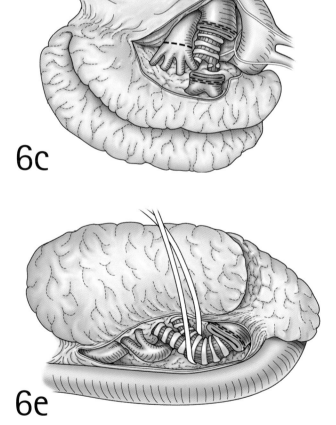

On occasion, it may be advantageous to divide the bronchus before ligating the pulmonary blood vessels (bronchus-first technique). If this technique is done, one has to be careful in freeing the bronchus which is very close to the superior vein (anteriorly), the pulmonary artery (superior border), and the lower vein (lower border). Dividing the bronchus first is particularly helpful to gain access to the superior vein and main PA in cases of completion pneumonectomies.

INTRAPERICARDIAL PNEUMONECTOMY

7 The opening of the pericardium greatly facilitates access to the main pulmonary blood vessels especially when the tumor is centrally located and/or is very large. The pericardium is usually opened anterior to the phrenic nerve, and the incision is carried upwards to the aorta. The PA is mobilized first and, to improve access, the pericardial incision is carried right up to its reflection over the PA. This maneuver will lead the operator directly to the adventitia of the artery which can be opened, and the PA is fully mobilized and stapled. Once the artery has been secured, the access to the pulmonary veins becomes much easier.

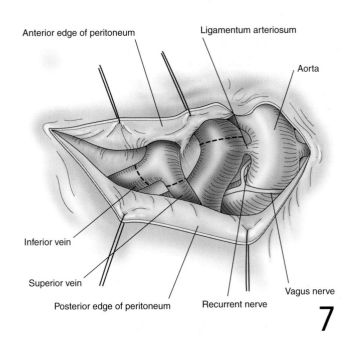

Anterior edge of peritoneum

Ligamentum arteriosum

Aorta

Inferior vein

Superior vein

Posterior edge of peritoneum

Recurrent nerve

Vagus nerve

7

In cases of intrapericardial pneumonectomy, we try to divide only one of the two pulmonary veins within the pericardium in the hope to prevent postpneumonectomy cardiac herniation (the vein which is divided extrapericardially will anchor the heart and prevent its herniation). Once the lung has been removed, it is also important to close the pericardium in order to prevent herniation of the heart which is fatal in the majority of cases. This goal is accomplished with interrupted nonabsorbable sutures.

Segmental resections of the left lung

The most commonly resected segments of the left lung are the lingula and apical segment of the lower lobe. Indications for this type of operation include lung cancer in compromised individuals and bronchiectasis or tuberculosis limited to one segment.

The principles involved in the resection of pulmonary segments are similar to those used for lobectomy, although the surgery is done in two rather than three phases. The first step is the identification of the artery and bronchus (bronchovascular pedicle), while the second step consists of retrograde dissection starting at the hilum and following the plane of the intersegmental vein which must stay with the remaining lung. Most surgeons now use staplers to divide the intersegmental plane rather than the more classic finger dissection while the anesthetist inflates the lung.

8a

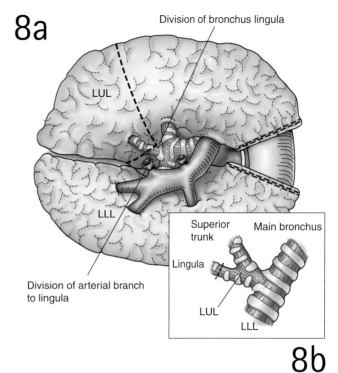

Division of bronchus lingula

LUL

LLL

Division of arterial branch
to lingula

Superior trunk

Main bronchus

Lingula

LUL

LLL

8b

8a,b The lingula is made of two segments (superior and inferior), which are usually resected together. In principle, lingulectomy is an easy operation. The interlobar fissure is opened, and the arterial branch to the lingula (the most distal branch) is first identified and ligated. The bronchus is then identified and stapled, and the segment is removed. The venous drainage is through a common trunk which is the lower part of the superior vein. This trunk is easily mobilized and divided.

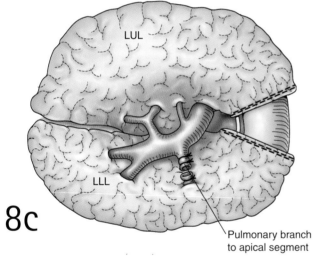

LUL

LLL

Pulmonary branch
to apical segment

8c

8c,d The surgical pedicle to the apical segment is also made up of a bronchus and an arterial branch. The artery is first mobilized from the fissure, ligated, and divided. The bronchus can also be reached through the fissure, divided, and closed (manually or with stapler). For this segment, no clear venous branch can be identified, so that on freeing the segment from the basal segments, each collateral or secondary vein is freed, clipped, and divided.

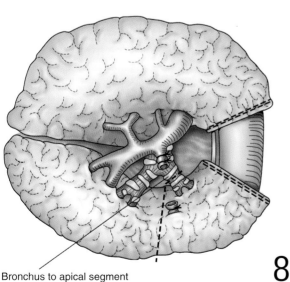

Bronchus to apical segment

8d

POSTOPERATIVE CARE

Tube drainage

After lobectomy or segmentectomy, one or two chest tubes are left in the pleural space. If two tubes are used, one is placed anteriorly and at the apex, and the second one is positioned inferiorly and posteriorly. The chest tubes are connected to an active suction system usually with −20 cm of water suction. They are removed when there is no longer an air leak and when the amount of fluid drainage is below 200 ml/24 hours.

Most surgeons do not drain pneumonectomy spaces because drainage through a water seal system can lead to an extreme mediastinal shift and overexpansion of the remaining lung. Instead of drainage, we recommend aspirating 1000–1200 ml of air from the space in order to position the mediastinum as much as possible in the midline. Other options are to leave a chest tube which is removed when the patient is turned over onto his or her back or is clamped until the following morning. Possible indications to leave a draining chest tube are a high risk of postoperative hemorrhage or bronchopleural fistula. Balanced drainage systems are currently used by only a handful of surgeons.

Analgesia

The methods used to control postoperative pain have changed considerably over the years, but their purpose has remained the same. They must provide proper analgesia so that the patient can have more efficient breathing and coughing. To do so, a proper balance must be reached between too much analgesia which will sedate the patient and not enough which will make the patient uncooperative.

The most commonly used technique is that of epidural analgesia with the drugs being administered at the lumbar or thoracic levels. For most patients, this method provides good pain control although side-effects such as nausea, itching, urinary retention, and even drowsiness are common. The epidural catheter is inserted prior to operation and left for 3–4 days postoperatively. When the catheter is removed, the patient is started on narcotics given subcutaneously or by mouth.

Drug management

All patients are given heparin subcutaneously as a prophylaxis against deep vein thrombosis. Patients are also given antibiotics for 2–3 days after operation. Oxygen is given to titrate saturation at 92% or higher. Although bronchodilation drugs can be added, the best way to improve respiratory efficacy is through active physiotherapy and use of incentive spirometry which are started the evening of the operation. If mucous and sputum retention do occur, we do not hesitate to perform bedside bronchoscopy or even insert a minitracheotomy for the sole purpose of suctioning. After left-sided resections, it is not uncommon to have vocal cord paralysis because of accidental or deliberate trauma to the recurrent nerve. Unfortunately, no early solution exists for this problem, and one must be aware that these patients are more likely to have respiratory and coughing difficulties.

Although arrhythmias are a common problem after pneumonectomy (incidence of 15–20%), it is generally not recommended to use prophylactic antiarrhythmic medication prior to surgery.

OUTCOME

Early

The accepted mortality rate for left pneumonectomy is in the range of 5–6%, and most causes of death are respiratory. These problems include infectious complications, pulmonary embolism, and postpneumonectomy edema. Fatal cardiovascular events are relatively uncommon. Risk factors for mortality after pneumonectomy include age of the patient, preoperative cardiopulmonary compromise, extent of resection, and associated comorbidities such as diabetes.

For lobectomy, whether upper, lower, or associated with sleeve resection, the operative mortality is in the neighborhood of 2.5–3%. Common complications include prolonged air leaks, arrhythmias, and respiratory events. Bronchopleural fistulae (BPF) are uncommon if bronchial closure is handled with care. The incidence is less than 3% after pneumonectomy and less than 1% after lobectomy. Once the diagnosis is made, BPF can be treated in a variety of ways. BPF are seldom a cause of death although they usually are associated with prolonged morbidity.

Late

In lung cancer, long-term results reflect the stage of disease rather than the extent of operation. Since pneumonectomies are done for higher stages of disease, 5-year survival results are worse than what is seen after lobectomy and are in the range of 20–25%. By comparison, 5-year survival after sleeve resections of the left lung is approximately 50%. The use of adjuvant treatments either as induction or postoperatively has not changed those results. In most series, patients with squamous cell carcinoma do better than those with adenocarcinomas.

In general, operation on the left lung can be done quite safely if the operating surgeon follows a methodical approach for the mobilization of bronchovascular pedicles. As a whole, they are technically easier than similar procedures on the right side, and they are better tolerated. Indeed, the incidence of major morbidity or mortality is less after left pneumonectomy than after right pneumonectomy. Special attention must be given to preserve the recurrent nerve which is much more accessible to trauma on the left side than on the right side.

FURTHER READING

Bechard D, Wetstein L. Assessment of exercise oxygen consumption as preoperative criterion for lung resection. *Annals of Thoracic Surgery* 1987; **44**: 344–9.

Dales RE, Stark RM, Sankaranakayanan R. Computed tomography to stage lung cancer. Approaching a controversy using a meta-analysis. *American Review of Respiratory Disease* 1990; **141**: 1096–101.

Klemperer J, Ginsberg RJ. Morbidity and mortality after pneumonectomy. *Chest Surgery Clinics of North America* 1999; **9**: 515–25.

Ratto GB, Piaconza G, Fiola C. Chest wall involvement by lung cancer: computed tomographic detection and results of operation. *Annals of Thoracic Surgery* 1991; **51**: 182–8.

Tronc F, Grégoire J, Rouleau J, et al. Long-term results of sleeve lobectomy for lung cancer. *European Journal of Cardiothoracic Surgery* 2000; **17**: 550–6.

Weisbrod GL. Transthoracic needle biopsy. *World Journal of Surgery* 1993; **17**: 705–11.

Tracheal resection

PETER GOLDSTRAW FRCS
Consultant Thoracic Surgeon, Royal Brompton Hospital, London; Professor of Thoracic Surgery, Imperial College, London, UK

HISTORY

Early attempts at tracheal resection were timid, limited to 2 cm or less of the trachea and frequently less than circumferential. More extensive resections were attempted, exploring the use of various prostheses and homograft techniques. The results with such techniques were poor, adversely affected by failure of healing and granulation tissue ingrowth. The modern era of tracheal surgery began when Dr H.C. Grillo and colleagues undertook a series of cadaveric studies to establish the length of trachea that could be safely resected with end-to-end anastomosis. These studies were confirmed by surgical series in which he and Dr F.G. Pearson developed and expanded surgical techniques. These pioneers established the general principles of this surgery; the length of trachea that could be safely resected, and the ancillary measures required allowing tension-free anastomosis. Although some have tried to extend these limits by developing newer prosthetic materials, these have not proven to be safe.

PRINCIPLES

Segmental resection of the trachea is appropriate for benign or malignant conditions affecting the trachea from the cricoid cartilage to the carina. Below this level carinal resection and reconstruction is possible. Such conditions include fibrous stricture following intubation or tracheostomy, benign tumors of the airways such as carcinoid tumors and malignant tumors, chiefly squamous carcinoma and adenoid cystic carcinoma. To be suitable for resection the disease process has to be limited to a length of trachea that can be safely resected, and the patient must be sufficiently fit to tolerate such surgery safely. As a general rule 50% of the trachea can be resected and repaired by end-to-end anastomosis. This

length may be slightly greater in a young child and slightly less in an older person. As one approaches these limits various release procedures are helpful to enable end-to-end anastomosis without undue tension.

A cervical approach allows resection of airway pathology affecting the distal larynx, the cervical trachea, and all but the distal 2–3 cm of the intrathoracic trachea. If this segment is involved then a thoracic approach is to be preferred, allowing carinal reconstruction, if necessary. The approach used will be influenced somewhat by the pathology. The length of airway to be resected can be more reliably determined for benign pathology. The margins of resection for malignant disease are less predictable and the surgeon will have to plan to allow for wider resection if necessary.

The choice of relieving procedure will, to some extent, also be influenced by the incision used.

In planning the surgical approach consideration must be given to the alternatives available to allow continued ventilation during resection and reconstruction. The use of cardiopulmonary bypass has been tried in the past but has been rendered obsolete by alternatives that do not require heparinization.

Prophylactic antibiotics should be given for any operation on the airway, and anaerobic cover is added if there is severe obstruction or necrotic tumor.

As the surgeon will understandably restrict the length of resection to the minimum, the use of frozen section examination is recommended when undertaking airway resection for tumors, especially adenoid cystic carcinoma with its propensity for microscopic intramural extension.

For patients who are unfit for surgery, or whose disease is too extensive to permit resection, there are many alternative techniques. The appropriate technique will vary depending upon the site, length, and pathology of the stricture, and include radiotherapy and a wide range of surgical procedures that achieve disobliteration and the maintenance of a safe airway by the use of temporary and permanent stents. These techniques are beyond the scope of this chapter. The long-term results of such therapy are less satisfactory than those achieved by an operation and the opinion of an appropriate surgical specialist should be sought before denying the patient an operation.

PREOPERATIVE ASSESSMENT

The severity of airway narrowing can be assessed clinically, by spirometry and lung function testing and by radiology. The extent of disease, particularly its intramural and extramural component, is aided by computed tomography (CT). However, bronchoscopy remains the most critical evaluation, and the use of the rigid bronchoscope under general anesthesia has the advantages of a wide field of view, temporary breath holding, and the ability to take multiple large biopsies. In the emergency situation its use can prove life saving, allowing measures to achieve rapid relief of critical stenosis. Using the rigid bronchoscope the surgeon can accurately measure the length of the trachea, the extent of the segment which would require resection, and the relationship of its proximal and distal margins from such key landmarks as the carina, larynx, and any tracheostome. This is best done by marking the bronchoscope with thin strips of adhesive applied at the level of the upper incisors. The assessment of any dynamic,

malacic component is aided by examining the airway with the patient coughing at the end of the evaluation.

Basic oncological principles apply when evaluating the feasibility of airway reconstruction for malignant disease. Distant metastases and extensive nodal disease should be excluded. Mediastinoscopy may be of value but local, mediastinal extension does not carry the same import as when evaluating lung cancer, as long as resection is deemed feasible.

Patient fitness must be assessed carefully. A greater level of fitness is necessary if a thoracic approach is needed, especially if concurrent pulmonary resection is contemplated. It is less of an issue if a cervical approach is judged suitable. Lung function testing is not representative of the patient's fitness in the presence of severe airway obstruction! Psychological and cerebral status may affect the patient's ability to cooperate with the physiotherapist in the postoperative period, and to tolerate the neck flexion necessary to safeguard the anastomosis (see later).

Tracheal resection should not be undertaken as an emergency. Surgical disobliteration will allow measured evaluation, accurate staging of malignant disease, discontinuation of steroid medication, and clearance of distal infection. The patient can then be brought to elective surgery fully appraised of the risks and benefits of surgery, and in the best physical and psychological state. The surgeon can plan the surgery carefully, ensure expert anesthetic support, and the availability of frozen section pathology services.

OPERATIONS

Segmental resection of the trachea by a cervical approach

1 Following induction of anesthesia it is helpful to repeat the bronchoscopic assessment using a rigid broncho-scope. This will allow the anesthetist to assess the size of endotracheal tube that can be negotiated through the stric-tured area. The surgeon can assess the location of the stricture relative to the skin incision by inserting a narrow-bore needle percutaneously into the lumen and viewing its relationship to the stricture through the bronchoscope. Ventilation during tracheal mobilization is safer if an endotracheal tube can be placed across the stricture. If this is not possible the airway is precarious and intermittent obstruction may be encountered. A size 5.5 or 6.0 Fr. armored endotracheal tube can usually be negotiated through the stricture into the distal, normal tra-chea. The patient is positioned supine, with the neck extended by a sandbag under the shoulders and the head secured in a ring.

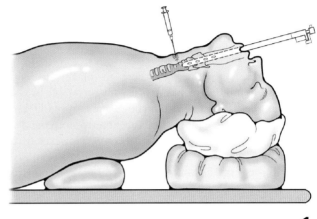

1

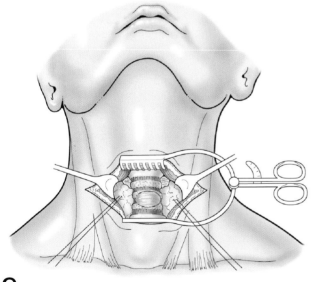

2

2 A curved, collar incision is made, centred upon the tracheostomy scar, or midway between the thyroid carti-lage and the suprasternal notch, extending between the lateral borders of the sternomastoid muscle on each side. The inci-sion is deepened through platysma muscle using the diathermy, dividing superficial veins. The sternomastoid muscles are mobilized laterally from the suprasternal notch to the level of the thyroid cartilage. The trachea is identified in the midline and mobilized along its anterior aspect for the full length of the incision. The strap muscles may be divided but are usually reflected laterally. If necessary the isthmus of the thyroid gland is divided between transfixion sutures.

3 One must now decide where to make the initial incision into the trachea. It is usually preferable to make the distal transection first as this allows one to speedily transfer ventilation to an endotracheal tube inserted into the distal trachea, if this is thought to be necessary. However, if the proximal margin of resection is easier to define one can easily start at this point. The limits of the stricture may be apparent from external examination of the trachea, but if this proves difficult identification of this important point is aided by temporarily withdrawing the endotracheal tube over a flexible bronchoscope. The light is visible through the tracheal wall, and the precise point at which to make the first incision can be identified by passing a fine gauge needle into the lumen under endoscopic control. The trachea is mobilized circumferentially at this level. Care must be taken to avoid the recurrent laryngeal nerves. Some experts would favor dissection to identify these nerves. However the surrounding inflammatory response can make this difficult and it is usually preferable to avoid damage to the nerves by keeping the dissection close to the diseased tracheal wall. The contralateral nerve is at greater risk and extreme care is needed when dissecting between the trachea and the esophagus around the far side of the trachea.

The anterior wall of the trachea is incised with a pointed blade and circumferential division undertaken using scissors. Stay sutures of 2/0 monofilament are inserted into the anterior wall of the distal trachea to prevent retraction of the distal lumen. Ventilation is not interrupted, as the cuff of the tube should lie distal to this level. A longitudinal incision is then made along the anterior wall of the trachea, until the normal lumen is identified at the other limit of resection.

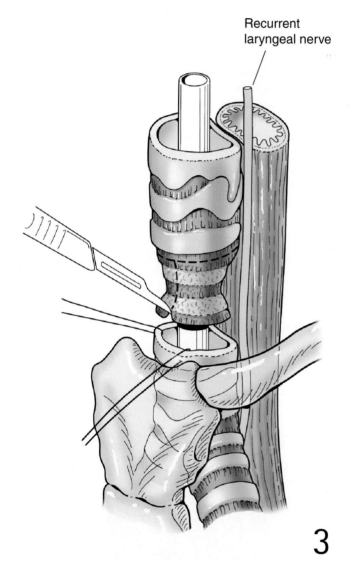

Recurrent
laryngeal nerve

3

4 The endotracheal tube can be retracted anteriorly whilst the whole circumference of the diseased segment is mobilized. If this step is difficult or prolonged, the endotracheal tube should be withdrawn into the larynx. A suture into its tip facilitates retrieval into the trachea. Ventilation is then transferred to an endotracheal tube inserted into the distal lumen across the operating field. A Bain's circuit is less intrusive for connecting this tube to the ventilator. This distal endotracheal tube is often in an unstable position and it is as well to delegate an assistant to focus entirely upon maintaining satisfactory ventilation. Liaison with the anesthetist is essential during this type of ventilation. Care is necessary to keep close to the tracheal wall whilst undertaking this circumferential mobilization, avoiding damage to the esophagus and the recurrent nerves. Once the length of the tracheal defect is known the surgeon should assess if further mobilization or release procedures are necessary to allow apposition of the tracheal ends without tension (see later). Mobilization of the distal airway should be limited to the anterior and posterior aspects of the trachea, preserving the lateral, vascular tissues.

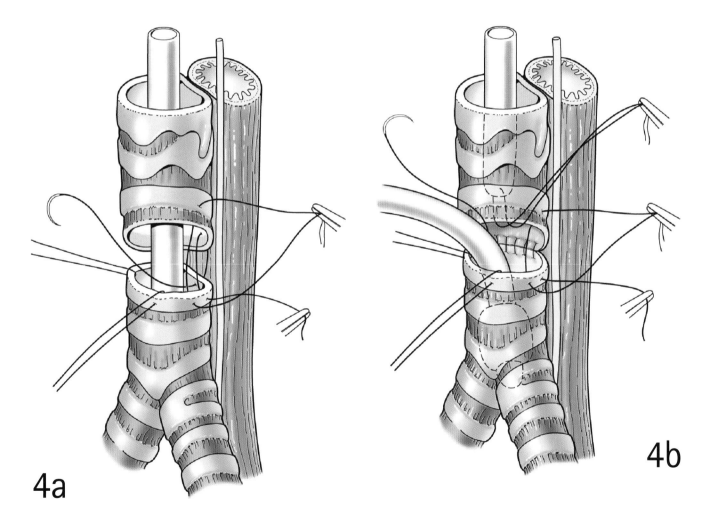

4a

4b

5 An end-to-end anastomosis is performed using continuous monofilament material, such as 3/0 Prolene on a 17 mm needle. The anastomosis is reinforced at each quadrant with interrupted sutures of 2/0 Prolene which, ideally, should pass through the cartilages of the trachea and not penetrate the lumen of the trachea. The first interrupted suture is placed at the near posterior cornu of the tracheal cartilage. The continuous suture runs, over and over, through the full thickness of the posterior tracheal wall to the opposite cornu where the second stay suture is inserted. Each of the stay sutures should be inserted just ahead of the running suture to avoid damage to the continuous suture. Once the posterior wall of the anastomosis has been completed the sandbag beneath the shoulders is removed. Traction of the two stay sutures approximates the ends of the trachea and the continuous suture is drawn tight. The continuous suture continues around the far wall of the trachea to the anterior aspect of the anastomosis. A further stay suture is inserted at this point. The standing suture at the near side of the posterior wall is then used to run in an over-and-over full thickness fashion around the nearside of the trachea to the anterior wall. The fourth stay suture is inserted at the anterior quadrant, ahead of the continuous suture. The continuous suture is tied, and the four stay sutures are tied to complete the anastomosis. If an endotracheal tube has been inserted into the distal lumen, at some point during the anastomosis it becomes intrusive. The translaryngeal tube is retrieved into the trachea to continue ventilation, and the distal tube is removed.

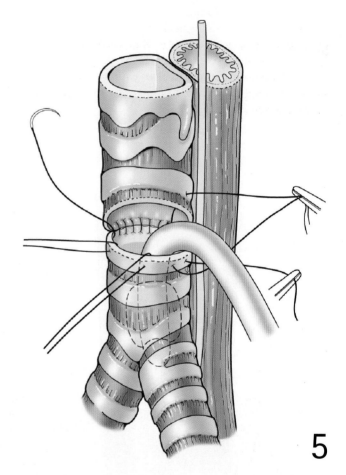

5

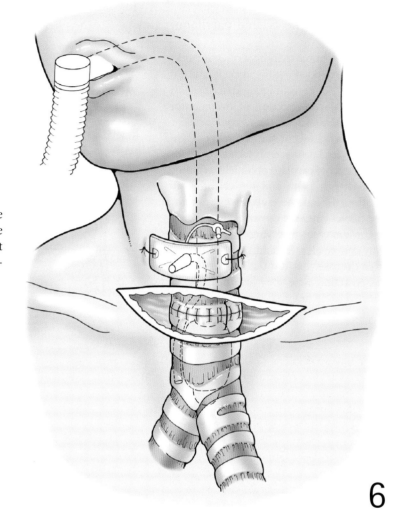

6 Postoperative problems with sputum clearance are uncommon but if this occurs there can be great difficulty inserting a minitracheostomy tube. It is best to insert such a tube, above or below the anastomosis, as a routine.

6

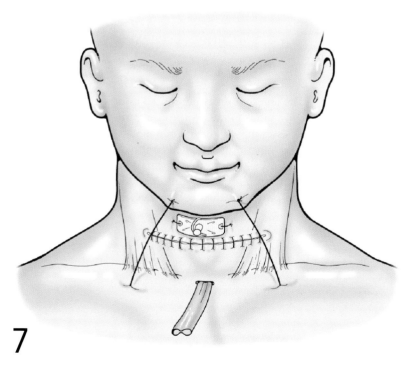

7 A corrugated drain is inserted and the strap muscles are approximated in the midline. The skin is closed with continuous subcuticular suture. The chin is fixed to the presternal skin using strong monofilament sutures with the neck in moderate flexion.

7

Resection of the cricoid cartilage

8 The proximal margin of resection may be extended into the larynx if necessary. The technique, described by Pearson, allows resection of the anterior and lateral aspects of the cricoid cartilage with preservation of the recurrent laryngeal nerves. These are protected by dividing the cricoid cartilage obliquely, avoiding the posterior plate and the cricothyroid junction, the landmark at which the recurrent nerves enter the larynx.

The mucosa overlying the posterior plate can be elevated and resected if, as is often the case, it is fibrotic. The cartilage of the posterior plate may also be partially resected using fine rongeurs to enlarge the lumen.

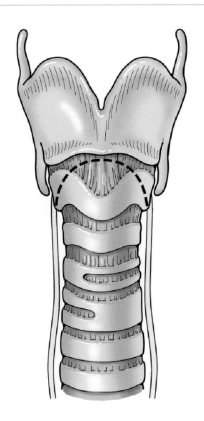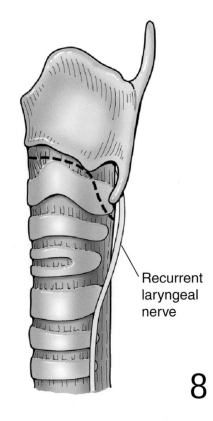

Recurrent laryngeal nerve

8

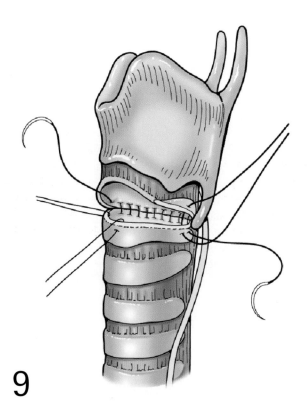

9

9 The anastomosis is performed as described above. The continuous suture along the posterior part of the anastomosis passes through the membranous wall of the distal trachea and superiorly is limited to the mucosa of the larynx, which is usually quite robust. Full thickness bites and the reinforcing sutures at each quadrant are only inserted once past the posterolateral angle on each side where the nerves enter.

10 As with all airway anastomoses it is important to avoid tension and a laryngeal release procedure may be necessary (see below). The subglottic area is narrow, and edema associated with such a high anastomosis may involve the larynx. In most such cases therefore the author prefers to protect the upper airway by inserting a T-tube at the end of the procedure, leaving the proximal limb extending above the vocal cords. It is best to bring the T-tube through the trachea above or below the anastomosis. A minitracheostomy tube is thus unnecessary. A corrugated drain is led through a stab incision and the chin is fixed in slight flexion.

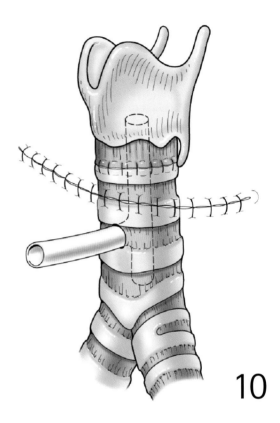

10

Release procedures

It is important to limit circumferential mobilization of the airway to the segment to be resected and a cuff at each end for anastomosis. This minimizes ischemic injury that may result in complete dehiscence or defects in the anastomosis leading to the formation of granulation tissue, a process often attributed to tissue reaction to suture material. However, tension on the anastomosis is equally undesirable. The early cadaveric studies undertaken by Dr Grillo have shown the various release procedures that can allow more extensive airway resection to be undertaken without undue tension. However, individual surgeons will have to judge from their own experience when tension on the anastomosis is excessive, requiring a release procedure, and even when it is prudent to limit any further resection and accept an incomplete resection.

11 When tension is considered excessive there are several steps that can be taken that will sequentially assist approximation of the anastomosis. First check that the maximum flexion of the neck has been achieved. Freeing the anterior wall of the proximal and distal segments will allow the airway to slide a few millimeters without adding to the ischemic injury. Mobilizing the posterior wall is more effective but also more hazardous. Grillo has emphasized the importance of preserving the lateral vascular pedicles, although this seems less imperative given the good results of slide tracheoplasty. When a thoracic approach has been used one can provide release by mobilizing the pulmonary hilum and freeing the pulmonary ligament. Additional length is achieved by incising the pericardial attachments of the pulmonary vessels. When carinal resection has been under-

taken a Barclay reconstruction (see later) may be necessary. When a cervical approach is used a laryngeal release can be added, the method now preferred being the supralaryngeal release described by Dr Montgomery. A second, circumferential skin incision is made over the hyoid bone. Its anterior surface is cleared of platysma and the attachment of stylohyoid divided. The three thin, muscular attachments to the superior surface of the hyoid, mylohyoid, geniohyoid, and genioglossus, are divided, exposing the pre-epiglottic space. The lesser cornu is divided, freeing the pharyngeal muscles attached to it and releasing the sling of digastric. Heavy scissors are used to divide the body of the hyoid bone from the greater cornu on each side, immediately anterior to the sling of the digastric muscle, allowing the central portion to slide inferiorly.

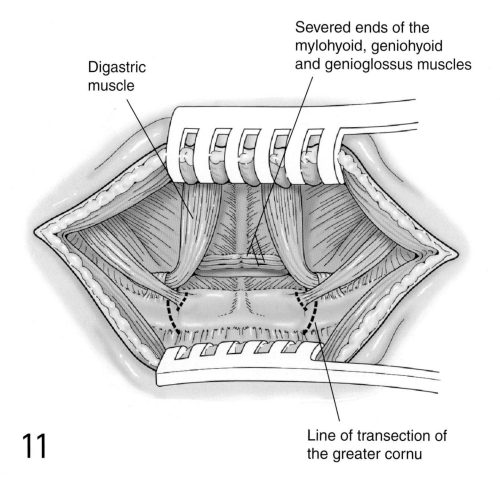

Severed ends of the mylohyoid, geniohyoid and genioglossus muscles

Digastric muscle

Line of transection of the greater cornu

11

If a laryngeal release is judged to be necessary when undertaking a thoracic approach to the trachea or carina it is logistically easier to perform this step prior to thoracotomy.

Resection of the lower trachea

A right thoracotomy through the fourth interspace or the bed of the fifth rib provides access to the intrathoracic trachea, the main carina, the whole of the right bronchial tree, and the left main bronchus to its lobar division. If the airway will accommodate a double-lumen endobronchial tube, this facilitates dissection prior to airway division.

12 The mediastinal pleura is incised over the lower trachea, the azygos vein is divided and its ends transfixed, the hilum of the right lung is circumnavigated, freeing the hilar structures and dividing the pulmonary ligament. Lymph nodes around the affected segment of the airway will be resected, and in malignant cases more extensive nodal evaluation is required. During this maneuver bronchial and mediastinal vessels will be encountered. Whilst one should divide as few as possible, it is important to accurately define the anatomy and the extent of disease.

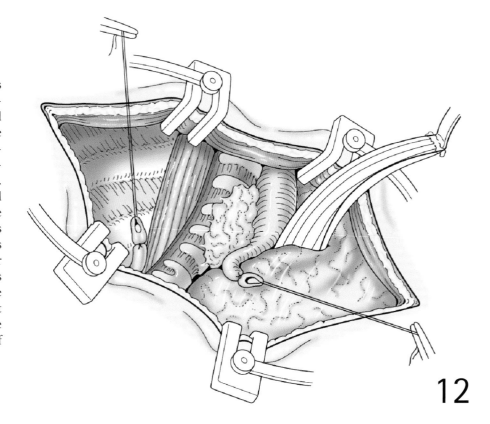

12

13 The airway is now ready to be divided. However, before doing so it should be decided how best to continue ventilation. (a) Use the existing endotracheal tube, withdrawing it temporarily whilst resecting the airway and working around it whilst undertaking the anastomosis. The bulkiness of an endobronchial double-lumen tube makes this difficult. However, if the strictured area could only accommodate a narrow endotracheal tube, this should be left full length so that it can be advanced into the distal trachea or left main bronchus to continue ventilation during the anastomosis. (b) The tube, whether endobronchial or endotracheal, is withdrawn and ventilation continued using an armored, small caliber tube across the operating field into the distal trachea or left main bronchus. This prevents blood spilling into the left lung but is obtrusive and has to be removed at some stage during the anastomosis. This method is the one of choice when undertaking a Barclay reconstruction (see later). (c) The tube, endotracheal or endobronchial, is withdrawn. A nasogastric tube is inserted through the original tube into the distal trachea or left main bronchus and used to provide ventilation using a Venturi injector. The nasogastric tube is sutured in place to prevent it flailing around. Hemostasis is important to limit the amount of blood insufflated into the left lung. This is probably the method of choice for uncomplicated segmental resection of the lower trachea or carinal reconstruction.

If the surgeon forewarns the anesthetist, pre-oxygenation will allow sufficient apnea time for the surgeon to transect the trachea, decide upon the length of resection, and restore ventilation using one of these techniques. As always the surgeon should resect to macroscopically normal airway, supplementing this assessment with frozen section histology in malignant cases.

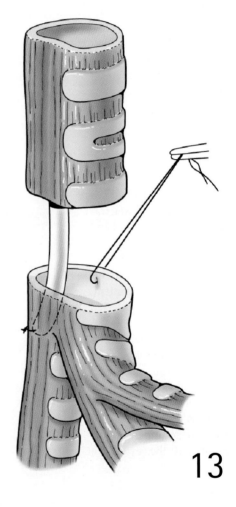

13

14 The anesthetist should flex the neck, supporting it with a pillow, before the surgeon begins the anastomosis. The anastomosis is similar to that described for segmental resection in the neck. A continuous suture commences at the far, posterior horn of the tracheal cartilage, continuing around the front wall to the posterior cornu at the near side. The standing end is then continued across the membranous wall and tied at the right posterior cornu. Reinforcing sutures are used at each quadrant, inserted ahead of the continuous suture to avoid damaging this suture.

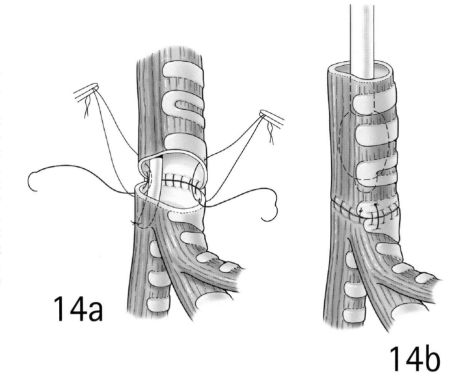

14a

14b

The mediastinal pleura is closed over the repair, a drain is inserted and the thoracotomy closed. The patient is rolled into the supine position with the neck fixed in moderate flexion. A minitracheostomy tube, a corrugated drain, and the neck restraining sutures are inserted.

Carinal resection and reconstruction

15 Resection of the carina is undertaken using a right thoracotomy approach, providing continued ventilation by the Venturi method described above. Reconstruction is achieved by first recreating a new carina using the medial third of the circumference of both main bronchi, and anastomosing this double-barreled lumen to the distal trachea as described above.

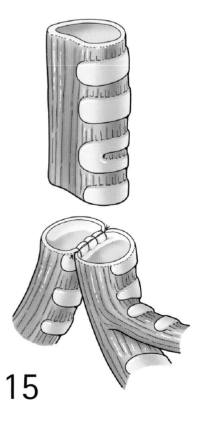

15

16 A variation of this technique allows resection of the right main bronchus and anastomosis of the intermediate bronchus and the left main bronchus to recreate the carina. If the right upper lobe bronchus can be preserved it can be subsequently anastomosed to the side of the trachea a centimeter above the main anastomosis. A small, semicircular defect is created in the cartilage of the lateral wall of the trachea, at its junction with the membranous part of the tracheal wall.

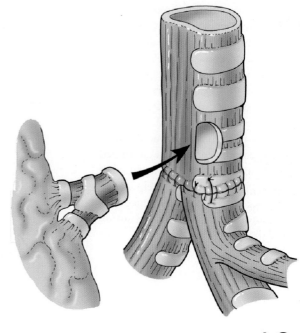

16

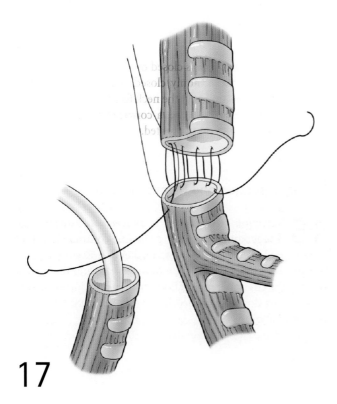

17

17 After carinal resection, elevation of the left main bronchus is limited by the aortic arch. If more extensive resection of the trachea or left main bronchus is necessary this double-barrelled reconstruction is not possible. The reconstruction described by Barclay allows an end-to-end anastomosis in such circumstances. In this, the right main bronchus, or the intermediate bronchus, is anastomosed to the distal trachea whilst the left lung is ventilated using a small armored endotracheal tube across the operative field.

18 The left main bronchus is then anastomosed to the medial aspect of the intermediate bronchus after creating a small semicircular defect in the cartilage at its junction with the membranous portion of the airway.

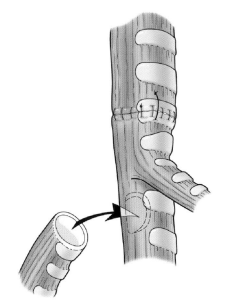

18

The mediastinal pleura is closed over the repair and the thoracotomy closed. The patient is rolled into the supine position with the neck held flexed. A minitracheostomy tube, a corrugated drain, and the neck restraining sutures are inserted.

Slide tracheoplasty

This operation was originally devised to cope with congenital funnel (stove-pipe) trachea involving greater than 50% of the total tracheal length. It was accepted at that time that this was the maximum length of trachea that could be resected with end-to-end anastomosis. Various on-lay grafts using periosteum or rib had been tried with varied success. The concept of the slide tracheoplasty is simple – one halves the length of the trachea and doubles its circumference. The initial success of this operation infers that the trachea in this condition has an unusual, circumferential blood supply. However, the operation has since been used successfully in long, benign, acquired strictures in adults.

The operation is usually undertaken through a cervical approach, allowing access to the whole of the trachea to the level of the carina. If the stenotic segment extends onto one of the main bronchi, especially when associated with an aberrant left pulmonary artery, the procedure can be undertaken through a right thoracotomy. Ventilation is difficult when operating upon such tight stenoses in a tiny patient, but the operation is possible with intermittent apnea, and cardiopulmonary bypass has been avoided.

19 Once the full extent of the stenotic area has been exposed circumferentially the trachea is divided transversely at the midpoint of the stenosis. The posterior wall of the distal segment is incised longitudinally until a normal caliber airway has been reached. The anterior wall of the upper segment is incised over a similar length. The ends of each segment may be trimmed slightly to create more of a pointed end on each flap. The proximal segment of trachea is drawn behind the distal segment, the anastomosis begins on the posterior aspect of the distal segment and spirals around each side of the reconstructed airway and is completed anteriorly.

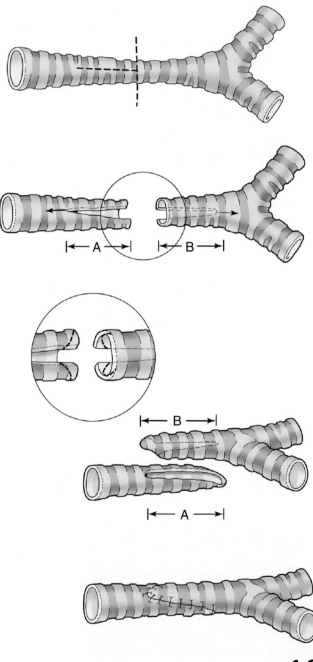

19

POSTOPERATIVE MANAGEMENT

After most airway reconstructions the patient can usually be extubated at the end of the procedure. If a supralaryngeal T-tube is inserted, the closing minutes of the operation can be conducted using Venturi ventilation through the transverse limb of the tube. If there is any need to continue assisted ventilation a laryngeal mask is preferred, thus avoiding an endotracheal tube across the anastomosis. Sputum clearance is facilitated by the minitracheostomy tube or T-tube. Prophylactic antibiotics are continued for 3–4 days.

Once speech has been assessed and adequate laryngeal function seems assured, the patient is allowed nourishing fluids, usually from the first postoperative morning. The use of a drinking straw is helpful until the patient becomes used to the neck restraining sutures. A normal oral diet is usually established within 24 hours. A supralaryngeal T-tube may require more caution but it is surprising how well patients swallow without any aspiration.

The wound drainage ceases over the first 24 hours but removal of the drain is delayed until the eighth day when the minitracheostomy tube and neck-restraining sutures are also removed. The patient should be warned to protect the anastomosis from undue neck extension for a few weeks, particularly when sleeping. A U-shaped pillow is helpful. By the time they return to the clinic at 3–4 weeks they have lost cautious approach and will be moving their necks normally.

In situations in which a T-tube is considered necessary the patient returns for endoscopic review under general anesthesia after 6 weeks. The tube is removed, and healing and laryngeal function are assessed. If there is any concern a clean T-tube is inserted for a further period, usually of 6 weeks, and the assessment repeated.

Other postoperative problems are rare, but dysrhythmias can occur.

OUTCOMES

Postoperative mortality and morbidity depend upon co-morbid conditions, patient fitness, the length of airway resected, and the complexity of the reconstruction. Emergency resection can be avoided by the measures described previously.

Most benign lesions, and almost all postintubation strictures, can be resected, unless complicated by previous failed surgery or laser treatment. The perioperative mortality for such surgery is usually less than 2%. Good to excellent functional results are obtained in 90–95% of patients.

The perioperative mortality for surgery in malignant cases, in which more extensive resections are required, is higher, in the region of 5–6%. It is difficult to give estimates of prognosis after resection of malignancy, as even in large series the numbers in subgroups become small. The natural history of adenoid cystic carcinoma is often one of slow progression. Such patients can live for several years after radiotherapy alone, and asphyxia can be prevented by disobliteration techniques, stenting, and brachytherapy. In one series mean survival after treatment of presumably more advanced disease by radiotherapy alone was 6.4 years, compared with 9.8 years after complete resection and 7.5 years after incomplete resection and radiotherapy. As in other cancer procedures the surgeon should strive for complete resection but it is clearly unjustified to imperil the patient by striving for this if wider excision complicates the reconstruction and adds appreciably to perioperative risk. Such a delicately balanced decision requires experience. There are fewer statistics on survival after resection of squamous carcinomas, but survival in the region of 35% at 5 years has been reported.

Anastomotic problems, such as dehiscence or stricture, occur in less than 5% of operations performed in experienced units.

FURTHER READING

Barclay RS, McSwann N, Welsh TM. Tracheal reconstruction with the use of grafts. *Thorax* 1957; **12:** 177–80.

Goldstraw P. Endobronchial stents. In: Hetzel M ed. *Minimally invasive techniques in thoracic medicine and surgery.* 1st edn. London: Chapman and Hall, 1994.

Grillo HC. Development of tracheal surgery: a historical review. Part 1: techniques of tracheal surgery. *Annals of Thoracic Surgery* 2003; **75:** 610–19.

Grillo HC, Wright CD, Vlahakes GJ, MacGillivray TE. Management of congenital tracheal stenosis by means of slide tracheoplasty or resection and reconstruction, with long-term follow-up of growth after slide tracheoplasty. *Journal of Thoracic and Cardiovascular Surgery* 2002; **123:** 145–52.

Kutlu CA, Goldstraw P. Tracheo-bronchial sleeve resection using a continuous anastomosis: results of 100 consecutive cases. *Journal of Thoracic and Cardiovascular Surgery* 1999; **117:** 1112–17.

Maddaus MA, Toth JLR, Gullane PJ, Pearson FG. Subglottic tracheal resection and synchronous laryngeal reconstruction. *Journal of Thoracic and Cardiovascular Surgery* 1992; **104:** 1443–50.

Shankar S, George PJ, Hetzel MR, Goldstraw P. Elective resection of tumors of the trachea and main carina after endoscopic laser therapy. *Thorax* 1990; **45:** 493–5.

Tsang V, Murday AJ, Gillbe C, Goldstraw P. Slide tracheoplasty for congenital funnel-shaped tracheal stenosis. *Annals of Thoracic Surgery* 1989; **48:** 632–5.

Lung volume reduction surgery

JOSEPH B. SHRAGER MD

Associate Professor, Department of Surgery, University of Pennsylvania School of Medicine; Chief of Thoracic Surgery Hospital of the University of Pennsylvania and Pennsylvania Hospital, Philadelphia, Pennsylvania, USA

HISTORY

Lung volume reduction surgery (LVR) is an old operation that was recently revived as a treatment for emphysema. Otto Brantigan pioneered the procedure and performed it on a group of patients in the 1950s, reporting symptomatic improvement in 75%. However, the inability to objectively document improvements in pulmonary function and the early mortality rate of 16% in Brantigan's series led to abandonment of the operation. In the early 1990s, Joel Cooper reintroduced the procedure in a series of 20 highly selected patients operated on with no mortality and with dramatic improvements in dyspnea, pulmonary function, and quality of life. Although the procedure has continued to engender significant controversy, resulting in the establishment of several multicenter randomized clinical trials in an attempt to rigorously determine its efficacy, a plethora of evidence now exists that selected patients with emphysema benefit from LVR. The National Emphysema Treatment Trial (NETT) has established that most hyper expanded patients with FEV, less than 45% predicted, who have apical predominate disease, and even some patients with homogeneous disease and very low exercise capacity as measured by bicycle ergometry are candidates for the operation.

PRINCIPLES AND JUSTIFICATION

The physiological rationale for the procedure is elegant, particularly in light of the fact that the removal of lung tissue in patients who already suffer from a lack of functioning lung appears at first glance to be counter intuitive. In emphysema, parenchymal destruction results in loss of the normal elastic recoil of the lung. This situation has the dual effect of reducing expiratory driving force and decreasing the external mechanical support provided to the airways, which results in decreased expiratory airflows. The lung progressively distends, depressing the diaphragm and forcing it and the other respiratory muscles to operate at a mechanical disadvantage, reducing inspiratory muscle force and efficiency. The overall work of breathing is markedly increased. By removing the most diseased areas of lung that provide little contribution to gas exchange, LVR improves the elastic recoil of the remaining lung and returns the inspiratory muscles and chest wall to more physiological positions. The work of breathing is diminished, and the severe dyspnea experienced by these patients is ameliorated.

LVR is offered to selected patients with severe emphysema (FEV_1 less than 45% of predicted value) and hyperinflation (residual volume greater than 180% of predicted value in my practice) that results in markedly diminished quality of life. Patient selection is as critical to a favorable outcome after LVR as the technical performance of the procedure – the latter being fairly straightforward. Criteria for patient selection continue to undergo refinement, but several principles have become clear from clinical series involving the operation.

First, NETT identified a high risk group who should not be operated upon because the mortality is 16%. This group consists of individuals with FEV less than 20% predicted and either a diffusing capacity less than 20% predicted or homogeneous distribution of disease.

Secondly, the operation is most beneficial in patients whose chronic obstructive pulmonary disease approaches the 'pure emphysematous' type. Those with predominant chronic bronchitis, with copious sputum production, inflammatory airway narrowing, and reactive airways, tend not to do well. We have found that a postbronchodilator improvement in FEV_1 of greater than 30% is a strong predictor of a suboptimal outcome. Certainly, patients whose emphysema is most severe in one portion of the lung, with other areas (usually the lower lobes) left with relatively preserved parenchyma, do better because in these patients resection can be targeted to the more diseased areas. In addition, patients with markedly elevated PCO_2, in the opinion of the author and many others, are at higher risk after the operation. Similarly, patients with markedly elevated pulmonary artery pressures and those who are severely depleted nutritionally are not good candidates. No fixed age limit exists, but the operation should be approached with caution in patients older than 70 years. Patients who have had previous thoracotomy cannot safely undergo LVR on that side, and patients who have undergone previous sternotomy are also poor candidates due to difficulty with adhesions and subsequent prolonged air leaks.

Pulmonary complications are common after LVR, and patients should be informed preoperatively of the risks of mucous plugging requiring bronchoscopy and/or minitracheostomy placement, pneumonia, and prolonged air leaks. When LVR is performed by median sternotomy, imperfect sternal healing may occur because these patients have a high work of breathing, but this problem virtually always presents as only a minor 'click' without instability. We have had one case of frank mediastinitis in over 200 LVRs performed at our institution. The most common major morbidity of the operation is respiratory failure with prolonged mechanical ventilation, and this complication often leads ultimately to the death of the patient, if not within 30 days of the procedure. Published series of LVRs report operative mortality rates of 0–10%, with a mean of 6%. These rates may be significantly higher without careful patient selection.

LVR can be performed unilaterally or bilaterally, and the surgical approach can be via median sternotomy or video-assisted thoracoscopy (VATS). A growing consensus favors the bilateral procedure in the vast majority of patients, but the question of the best incision(s) for the bilateral procedure remains unsettled. We present the bilateral operation first as it is performed by sternotomy, then as it is performed by thoracoscopy.

PREOPERATIVE ASSESSMENT AND PREPARATION

Patients must have quit smoking at least 3 months before the operation and preferably earlier. They all complete at least 6 weeks of a vigorous pulmonary rehabilitation program to maximize their physical conditioning before surgery. Nutritional deficiencies are corrected to achieve a body weight within 20% of the ideal value. Medical treatment of the emphysema is optimized; an attempt is made to wean patients off steroids, but those who are only able to get as low as 5 mg daily are accepted for surgery.

Targets to be resected are determined by careful examination of computed tomograms of the chest and quantitative perfusion scans. In addition, all patients undergo full pulmonary function testing with plethysmographic measurement of lung volumes, arterial blood gas testing, cardiac echocardiography with estimation of pulmonary artery pressures and right heart catheterization if indicated, and cardiac stress testing.

ANESTHESIA

The placement of a thoracic epidural catheter for postoperative pain management is critical to allow optimal clearance of secretions and prevent postoperative atelectasis or pneumonia. General anesthesia is provided through a double-lumen endotracheal tube with the distal balloon placed in the left main stem bronchus, which allows sequential collapse of each lung. Inspiratory pressures must be assiduously monitored and minimized (less than 25 cm H_2O) in the ventilated lung. This monitoring is particularly important during ventilation of the lung that has been operated on first and has fresh staple lines, to prevent rupture of these staple lines. Minimizing inspiratory pressures may prevent the unlikely but potentially catastrophic occurrence of an intraoperative pneumothorax prior to opening the chest. Any increase in peak airway pressures noted by the anesthesiologist after the institution of positive pressure ventilation calls for immediate assessment to rule out such an event. The inspiratory:expiratory ratio often must be decreased in these patients, as a longer expiratory phase is necessary to prevent the auto–positive end-expiratory pressure phenomenon.

OPERATION

Median sternotomy

INCISION

1 Before incision, flexible fiberoptic bronchoscopy is performed through a single-lumen endotracheal tube to rule out unexpected malignancy or active infection that would preclude proceeding with the operation. A sputum sample is sent for microbiological study for use in guiding initial antimicrobial therapy should the patient develop an infiltrate in the early postoperative period. After placement of the double-lumen tube, the patient is positioned, prepared, and draped for sternotomy. Antibiotics covering both Gram-positive and Gram-negative organisms are administered before the incision.

A median sternotomy is performed with complete division of the bone from the sternal notch to the xiphoid process. The skin incision may be kept as much as 10 cm shorter without compromising exposure. Subcutaneous flaps may be raised to expose the full extent of the bone incision. The lungs should be left unventilated for at least 10 seconds before division of the sternum to avoid injuring the lungs, which usually are so hyperexpanded that they abut in the midline. Care is taken throughout the procedure to handle the sternum gently; the divided sternum is spread slowly to avoid fracture, and devascularization is minimized by only judicious use of electrocautery, as these patients are prone to sternal healing complications because of the high stress imposed on the sternal closure by their increased work of breathing.

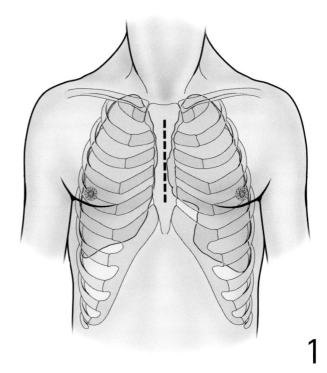

1

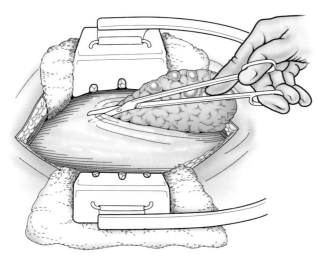

2

PLEURAL ENTRY

2 We prefer using a Buggie sternal retractor, which allows sequential elevation of each hemisternum without having to replace the retractor on the opposite side of the table after completion of one side, as is required with the type of retractors used for mammary harvest.

The side with the more severe disease is operated on first so that single-lung ventilation is maintained for the shortest possible time on this lung. Ventilation to this side is discontinued as the bone incision is being made, which provides sufficient time for the slowly deflating, emphysematous lung to collapse. Usually by the time the pleural space is entered, the areas with the most perfusion are well deflated by absorption atelectasis, whereas the most severely diseased areas, usually at the apex, remain partially inflated.

The pleura on the side of interest is opened close to the anterior chest wall to be as far from the phrenic nerve as possible. The pleural opening is begun inferiorly and extended superiorly. At the craniad end of the incision, where the phrenic nerve is most anterior and, thus, most at risk, the pleura is bluntly reflected off the anterior chest wall for several centimeters before it is incised. This maneuver facilitates identification of the nerve and careful avoidance of injury to it. Electrocautery should not be used during the incision of the craniad portion of pleura.

EXPLORATION AND LYSIS OF ADHESIONS

3 Sternal retraction is gradually increased until sufficient room has been created to insert a hand or sponge stick into the thorax. Most patients have scattered areas of filmy adhesions, which may be vascular, resulting from past inflammatory processes. Taking care not to tear these, the surgeon carefully retracts the lung, and the adhesions are divided with electrocautery as they are encountered. Overly aggressive retraction may cause the lung, rather than the adhesion, to tear and this occurrence may result in a prolonged postoperative air leak. On rare occasions, we have encountered severe, dense adhesions that had not been anticipated preoperatively and that caused us to abort the procedure on that side. We do not, as a routine, incise the inferior pulmonary ligament.

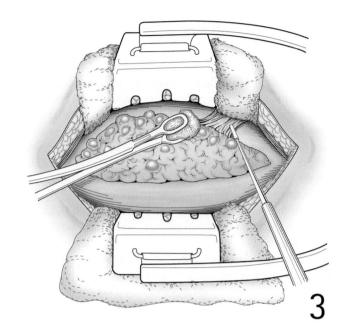

3

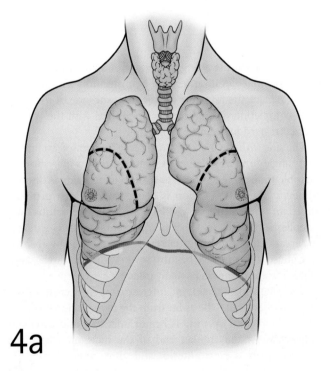

4a

PARENCHYMAL RESECTION 1

4a Once the lung is fully mobilized, the areas for resection are chosen. Ideally, a single, large oblique, somewhat u-shaped strip of tissue from the upper lobe (in the ideal patient who has upper-lobe-predominant disease) can be resected with several firings of the stapler, with a single continuous staple line created from the most caudad portion of the upper lobe to the extreme apex. This strip generally constitutes approximately 40–50% of the upper lobe. In patients who have disease that by ventilation-perfusion scan and computed tomography is not localized to the apices, we target the areas of resection to the regions of worst disease and often resect portions of the middle or lower lobes.

As mentioned, the target areas usually remain inflated and sometimes must be deflated to obtain enough space to insert a stapler. In these cases, once the portion of lung is deflated by incising into the lung, resection proceeds more expeditiously. In patients who have minimal function in the right upper lobe, we have rarely performed a formal right upper lobectomy on that side.

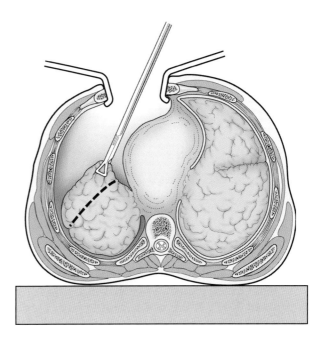

4b Because the chest is typically extremely deep in these patients, filling the hemithorax with saline and rotating the table slightly to the side of interest is often useful to float the lung up into the operative field, which facilitates the resection.

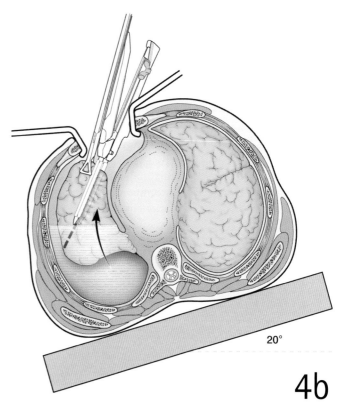

20°

4b

PARENCHYMAL RESECTION 2

5 The lung in the target area is grasped with either a Duval clamp or a ring clamp – lung not to be resected is left undisturbed – and the staple line is begun beneath the clamps. For the median sternotomy technique, we use an 80-mm Endo GIA stapling device with 4.8-mm staples and 0.35-mm polytetrafluoroethylene(PTFE) inserts to buttress the staple lines to minimize postoperative air leaks (see inset). As the staple line is progressively created, each reloaded stapler is placed exactly at the 'crotch' created by the previous staple line. We believe that some postoperative air leaks occur at points where staple lines cross.

How much parenchyma to remove cannot be easily quantitated, but approximately 20% of the volume on each side is targeted. More is removed, certainly, in hemithoraces containing more areas of severely diseased lung; less is removed in hemithoraces containing less severely diseased lung. If too much is resected, postoperative oxygenation may be compromised; if too little is resected, one fails to accomplish the intent of the operative procedure. One index that can be used is that the resection should result in a small to moderate residual apical space when the lung is reinflated. If no such space is visible after initial reinflation, one should consider removing more tissue. Not uncommonly, we resect additional tissue from the superior segment of the lower lobe in those with primarily apical disease. Early in the surgeon's experience, the most likely outcome is the resection of too little parenchyma.

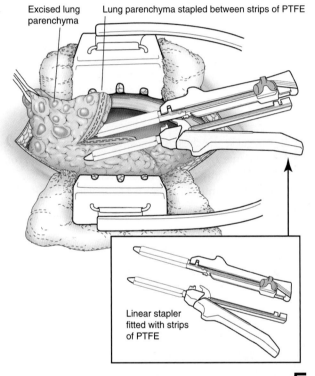

Excised lung parenchyma

Lung parenchyma stapled between strips of PTFE

Linear stapler fitted with strips of PTFE

5

EVALUATION FOR AIR LEAKS

6 Once the resection on the first side is completed, the lung is gently re-expanded while the staple line is submerged in saline to evaluate for air leaks. We are extremely careful to keep peak inspiratory pressures at less than 25 cm H_2O at the time of lung re-expansion and from this point forward during the procedure. Ideally, no air leaks are identified at this time. Occasionally, leaks occur adjacent to the buttressed staple line. Small leaks are tolerated if found, as attempts to repair them often lead to worsening of the air leaks. The rare large air leak may be repaired by restapling the area or occasionally by careful placement of 000 absorbable suture incorporating strips of buttress material. Needless to say, the emphysematous parenchyma is not a particularly hospitable environment for suture placement. For this reason, once more effective sealant materials are developed than those currently available, they may find application in LVR. Although others routinely create a pleural tent, we have not noted a high enough rate of prolonged air leaks to justify the time required for and potential morbidity of this additional procedure.

Once the procedure on the first side is completed, we check arterial blood gas as the patient is ventilated with both lungs. If severe hypercarbia is identified (P_{CO_2} higher than 70 mmHg in patients with no preoperative CO_2 retention), we ventilate both lungs for several minutes to reduce the CO_2 toward normal before reinstituting single-lung ventilation. The opposite lung is then collapsed, and the procedure described earlier is repeated on the second side. Peak pressures on the previously operated lung, which is now being ventilated, are kept at a minimum.

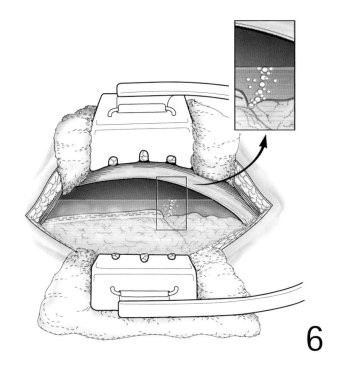

6

CLOSURE

7 Generally, one 28-Fr thoracostomy tube is placed on each side via separate lateral inframammary incisions and positioned at the apex posteriorly. A mediastinal tube is placed only if an unusual amount of bleeding occurs. The tubes are left to water seal with no suction applied.

The sternum is closed with three wires in the manubrium and no less than four others in the body of the sternum. These wires are secured tightly but without tearing through the sternum. A Robicsek-type weave with the sternal wires may be necessary in some patients with fragile sterna, such as older, osteoporotic women. This maneuver involves weaving a single wire longitudinally around all of the costal cartilages proceeding from superior to inferior and back on each side; transverse wires are then placed around the longitudinal wire struts. The upper abdominal fascia is closed with a few interrupted 0 nylon sutures. The presternal fascia is closed with running 0 absorbable suture, the subcutaneous tissue with running 00 absorbable suture, and the skin with running subcuticular 000 absorbable suture.

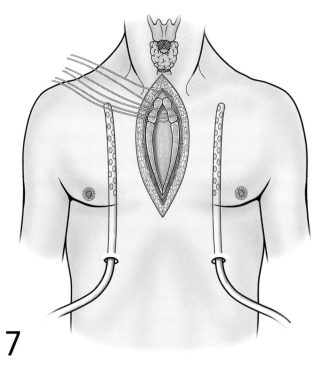

7

Video-assisted thoracoscopy

The goal of the operation remains the same whether the procedure is performed via median sternotomy or VATS. We tend to favor VATS over sternotomy in those older than 65 years and in others who appear to be more severely compromised by a variety of clinical criteria but who nevertheless remain reasonable candidates for the procedure. Epidural analgesia is as important with VATS as with the median sternotomy incision.

We perform the VATS procedure with the patient in the lateral decubitus position, even though this approach requires that the patient be repositioned before working on the second side. The operation *can* be performed with the patient supine and the arms positioned over the head without the need for repositioning, but we see no advantage to this approach because all patients benefit from a period of two-lung ventilation to reduce P_{CO_2} before beginning on the second side.

INCISIONS

8 The incisions pictured are optimal for the usual patient with upper-lobe-predominant disease. The locations of the ports must be altered if the target areas are not apical. The initial incision is placed just posterior to the level of the anterior superior iliac spine in approximately the sixth intercostal space. An introducer for the 30-degree, 10-mm videothoracoscope is placed here. Two additional incisions are made as pictured for placement of a ring clamp used for grasping the lung and the linear stapler. No introducers are used for these instruments – they are placed directly through the incision into the chest. The port for grasping is made one or two ribs superior and slightly posterior to the first incision; the port for the stapling is made at the same level but approximately 8 cm anterior to the first incision.

We have found that this arrangement of ports facilitates visibility and gives a reliable angle allowing removal of large wedges of parenchyma from the upper lung.

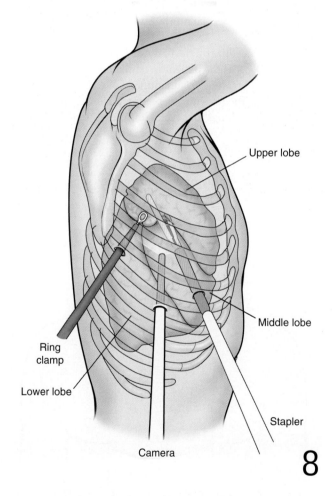

Upper lobe

Middle lobe

Ring clamp

Lower lobe

Camera

Stapler

8

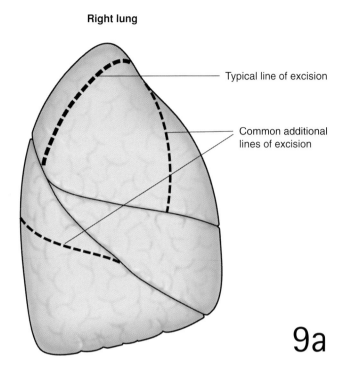

Right lung

Typical line of excision

Common additional
lines of excision

9a

PARENCHYMAL EXCISION

9a,b Just as with the median sternotomy approach, we excise a large oblique strip of lung parenchyma, proceeding from the inferior aspect of the upper lobe to its apex. Because the VATS approach is lateral rather than anterior, however, we have found it most effective during VATS to remove the initial strip from the *posterior* aspect of the upper lobe, beginning near the confluence of the fissures and proceeding around the apex.

The tendency to remove too little tissue is compounded during the VATS approach by the magnification provided by the video camera and the limited jaw opening of endoscopic staplers. Thus, removing additional wedges of tissue is more common with VATS. Common sites for these additional excisions in the patient with apical-predominant disease are as shown from the anterior aspect of the upper lobe and the superior segment of the lower lobe. Furthermore, either increasing or compressing the poorly collapsing lung tissue with a long Kelly clamp to facilitate placement of the stapling device is often useful.

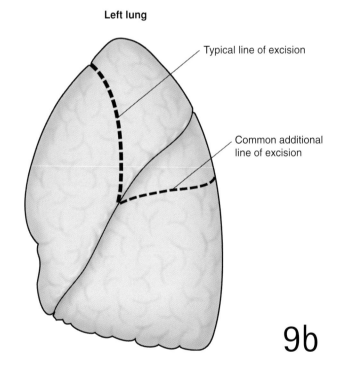

Left lung

Typical line of excision

Common additional
line of excision

9b

We have chosen to buttress the staple lines when using the VATS approach with Seemguard (Goretex, Inc). The literature indicates that buttresses do reduce the mean duration of air leaks but at a cost approximately equal to the cost of the extra days spent in the hospital.

Most adhesions that are encountered can be taken down during VATS as during sternotomy. If very dense adhesions are encountered, conversion to an open procedure may be necessary, and we prefer to use a vertical axillary muscle-sparing thoracotomy incision to accomplish this conversion. As previously discussed, great care must be taken to avoid tearing the fragile lung parenchyma while lysing adhesions in patients with emphysema, and this goal can be more difficult to achieve when working via a VATS approach.

CLOSURE

10 A single 28-Fr chest tube is tunneled submuscularly then into the chest at the intercostal incision made for the camera (because placing the tube directly through the port incision without a tunnel can lead to air entry when the tube is removed in these frequently very thin patients). The tube is positioned at the apex of the chest posteriorly and left to water seal. The lung is carefully re-expanded under direct vision. The incisions are closed with interrupted 00 absorbable suture on the muscle, running 000 absorbable suture on the subcutaneous tissue, and a running 0000 absorbable subcuticular stitch.

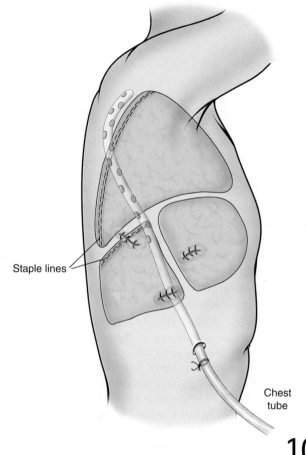

Staple lines

Chest tube

10

After the first side is completed, the patient is repositioned while both sides are ventilated, with inspiratory pressures minimized. The procedure is completed on the second side in similar fashion, and the patient is then awakened and extubated.

POSTOPERATIVE CARE

The patient can virtually always be extubated in the operating room, and this maneuver is of great importance to minimize prolonged positive pressure on the staple lines in the fragile emphysematous lung tissue. Occasionally, one must wait up to 30 minutes in the operating room after the placement of the dressings for a significant respiratory acidosis with CO_2 narcosis to improve before extubation. It is fairly routine, however, for these patients to be extubated with PCO_2 levels in the 80s. These values typically return to the patients' preoperative values within several hours of operation.

Chest tubes are placed to water seal and not to suction. The highly compliant emphysematous lung does not require negative suction in the pleural space for it to expand, and air leaks tend to be more severe and persistent when the tubes are placed to suction. We tolerate an initial postoperative pneumothorax (typically an apical space) of up to 20% without placing the tubes to suction in an effort to resolve the space. Generally, such small pneumothoraces resolve over the first 2–4 postoperative days if no large air leak is present. If a pneumothorax of greater than 20% is present, we place the chest tube on that side to –10 cm H_2O temporarily. Once air leaks have resolved, we remove chest tubes despite the presence of a small residual space. If any question exists of a small, persistent air leak, we clamp the tube for several hours and check for stability on chest radiogram before tube removal.

Unilateral persistent air leaks beyond 1 week after operation occur in about 10% of patients. In these remaining patients, if they are otherwise clinically well, we cut the chest tube close to the chest and place a Heimlich valve. The patients can be discharged to home with the valve in place, on oral antibiotics, with follow-up in the office twice weekly until the air leak resolves and the tube can be removed.

All patients are instructed and aided in vigorous pulmonary toilet from the time they arrive in the recovery room. They are encouraged to cough and use the incentive spirometer, and chest physiotherapy is used when indicated for difficulty in clearing secretions. Although it is unusual, we occasionally perform bronchoscopy on a patient who is unable to clear secretions; and if this procedure is required more than twice, we place a minitracheostomy tube through the cricothyroid membrane to allow suctioning on a regular basis.

Thoracic epidural catheters are kept in place for 5 days before converting to oral narcotic analgesia. Nebulized bronchodilators are used routinely for 5 days before converting to whatever inhaled bronchodilators the patient was taking preoperatively. Although we do not routinely administer antibiotics beyond the perioperative period, we have a low threshold for restarting them in those patients with any indication of tracheobronchitis or pneumonia. The cultures that are routinely sent from the preoperative bronchoscopy are useful to direct this therapy.

Patients are made to ambulate at least three times per day beginning on postoperative day 1, and our physical therapists work closely with them to maximize physical activity as early as possible.

OUTCOME

We have collated data from all pre-NETT published series of LVR that use the now-standard stapled, bilateral approach (including both median sternotomy and thoracoscopic incisions). The mean increase in FEV_1 from these reports is 52%. The mean decrease in residual volume in those studies that measured this parameter is 28%, and scores on the 6-minute walk test increased an average of 25%. These benefits were achieved with a mean operative mortality of 6.0% and a mean length of stay of 15 days. Furthermore, all studies that have looked at quality of life or dyspnea scores have shown marked improvement in these measures. The author's personal experience corroborates these results.

The impressive results of the NETT trial are readily available to readers and will not be reviewed in detail here. Suffice it to say that this study proved that appropriately selected patients with heterogeneous disease and low exercise capacity not only benefit from dramatic improvements in quality of life but also from greater survival. Even patients with homogeneous disease, if their exercise capacity is low, may benefit from a dyspnea and quality of life standpoint.

FURTHER READING

Brantigan OC, Kress MB, Mueller EA. The surgical approach to pulmonary emphysema. *Diseases of the Chest* 1961; **39**: 485–501.

Cooper JD, Trulock EP, Triantafillou AN, *et al*. Bilateral pneumectomy (volume reduction) for chronic obstructive pulmonary disease. *Journal of Thoracic and Cardiovascular Surgery* 1995; **109**: 106–19.

Fishman A, Martinex F, Naunheim K, Piantadosi S, Wise R, Ries A, Weinmann G, Wood DE. National Emphysema Treatment Trial Research Group. A randomized trial comparing lung-volume-reduction surgery with medical therapy for severe emphysema. *New England Journal of Medicine* 2003; **348**: 2059–73.

Hazelrigg SR, Boley TM, Naunheim KS, *et al*. Effect of bovine pericardial strips on air leak after stapled pulmonary resection. *Annals of Thoracic Surgery* 1997; **63**: 1573–5.

National Emphysema Treatment Trial Research Group. A randomized trial comparing lung-volume-reduction surgery with medical therapy for severe emphysema. *New England Journal of Medicine* 2003; **348**: 2059–73.

Shrager JB, Kaiser LR. Lung volume reduction surgery. *Current Problems in Surgery* 2000; **37**: 253–317.

18

Videothoracoscopic bullectomy for spontaneous pneumothorax

TOMÁS ANGELILLO MACKINLAY
British Hospital of Buenos Aires, Capital Federal, Buenos Aires, Argentina

HISTORY

No specific milestones exist in the evolution of bullectomy except for the advent of video assisted thoracic surgery (VATS). In the past posterolateral thoracotomy was usually indicated for persistent leaks after tube thoracostomy. Subsequently, during the 1970s and 1980s a tendency towards limited thoracotomies emerged, and bullae were preferably resected through small axillary thoracotomies. In the 1990s the advent of VATS introduced a radical change in the surgical approach for this disease. Different methods of producing bullae disappearance and air leakage control were implemented, such as endostapling, YAG laser, argon beam, and endo-looping. Of all of these techniques, endostapler bullae resection prevailed as the most effective and rational surgical technique.

PRINCIPLES AND JUSTIFICATION

Bullectomy is the surgical removal of a bulla or bleb usually performed during a spontaneous pneumothorax episode with the expectation that the bulla represents the leaking source. A bulla has been defined as an emphysematous space more than 1 cm in diameter during the distended state. Unruptured bullae do not have surgical indication unless they progress in size to the degree that they compress the adjacent normal lung parenchyma. When this phenomenon occurs, the giant bulla occupies more than one-third of the entire hemithorax. Blebs are small intrapleural collections of air representing forms of interstitial emphysema and have no epithelial lining. Rupture of bullae or blebs produces spontaneous pneumothorax.

The aim of the operation is threefold:

1 To eliminate the leakage point
2 To re-establish negative pressure within the chest restoring normal ventilation
3 To avoid septic contamination of the pleural cavity.

Spontaneous pneumothorax may be primary (PSP) or secondary (SSP). Primary spontaneous pneumothorax occurs in young patients, 85% of whom are less than 40 years of age. Apart from the pain and mild dyspnea, the patients tolerate the episode fairly well without jeopardizing their respiratory capacity. Ruptured blebs are usually responsible for this situation, which rarely leads to tension pneumothorax or to hemorrhage from a torn adhesion.

Secondary pneumothorax usually is the consequence of a ruptured bulla and occurs in older people (50–65 years of age). They have a worse functional tolerance because of co-morbid pathology and poorer cardiorespiratory reserve, since most of them suffer from chronic obstructive pulmonary disease (COPD). This group comprises a population at high risk and should be treated accordingly by prompt drainage of the pneumothorax by means of a thoracostomy tube in the emergency room. The incidence of tension pneumothorax and hemopneumothorax is also higher in these patients. Mortality rates as high as 16% have been reported in this population. The size of the pneumothorax is not as important as the cardiorespiratory response to it. Definitive treatment should wait until medical and cardiorespiratory stability have been reached.

The options for treatment of spontaneous pneumothorax are:

1 Clinical observation with optional oxygen therapy
2 Tube thoracostomy (which can be associated with talc slurry pleurodesis in selected cases)
3 Bullectomy, either by thoracotomy or videoassisted thoracic surgery (VATS) with or without pleurodesis.

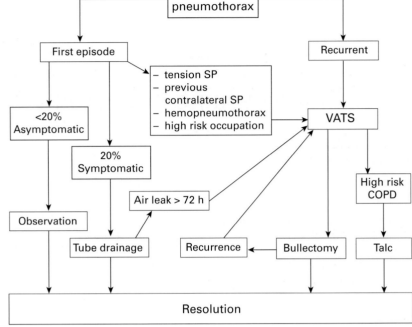

1 The timely selection of each particular treatment varies according to different clinical conditions, which are roughly expressed in the algorithm.

PREOPERATIVE ASSESSMENT AND PREPARATION

Preoperative assessment and preparation for bullectomy in primary spontaneous pneumothorax patients usually does not represent a problem since they are, by and large, healthy young individuals with a good cardiorespiratory reserve. In a second episode of pneumothorax, basic routine presurgical tests will suffice in such patients.

Secondary pneumothorax in elderly patients represents a great challenge. They should be drained as soon as they arrive in the emergency room because they are at great risk of tension pneumothorax and sudden death. In fact, 5% of them die before a chest tube is inserted. The internal diameter of the tube should not be less than 6.88 (28 French), which is capable of draining flows as high as 15–16 L/min when connected to a –10 cm H_2O suction source. Once the patient is stable, accurate cardiorespiratory risk can be assessed, and a final therapeutic decision can be made. After proper preparation, the great majority of these patients tolerate a VATS procedure on one-lung ventilation. Some extremely high risk COPD patients are not candidates for surgery. In this situation 5 g of asbestos free talc slurry introduced through the tube thoracostomy might be an option. This therapeutic modality should be reserved only for those patients who cannot be candidates for lung volume reduction surgery.

ANESTHESIA

These patients should be operated on under general anesthesia with a double-lumen endotracheal tube, which is a standard procedure in VATS surgery. Better control of the respiratory function is obtained in patients under general anesthesia than when local anesthesia is used.

A note of caution: when using double-lumen endotracheal tubes, never ventilate the lung which is going to be operated on, unless the hemithorax has been previously drained, and the drainage tube system is still open. Otherwise, the risk of tension pneumothorax is very high, and intraoperative death may result.

Postoperative pain control is obtained by infiltrating the corresponding intercostal nerves with bupivacaine 0.5% before the surgical field is set and the trocars are introduced. Intravenous and oral analgesics during the postoperative period will suffice. Opioids are seldom needed.

OPERATION

This operation has three phases:

1 The liberation of the pleural space (if necessary) and thorough lung exploration with identification of the leaking source

2 Resection of the bulla or bleb
3 Consolidation and drainage of the pleural space. By "consolidation" we mean pleural abrasion, occasionally talc pourage, and rarely parietal pleurectomy.

For the first phase two ports are enough; in the second phase a "holder" port (usually a 5 mm trocar) should be added either in the axillary rim or in the auscultatory triangle, while the other two are reserved for the camera and stapler.

2 For port placement, a triangular-shaped scheme is used: incisions should be separated from each other for a distance of at least 10 cm in order to avoid "swording." The first incision is placed in the sixth or seventh intercostal space (i.s.)

at the level of the posterior axillary line (caudal port). After digital exploration, a 5 or 11 mm diameter trocar is introduced, in order to speed up the spontaneous lung collapse. We do not use CO_2 insufflation. For the initial visual exploration a 30 degree telescope is preferred – either 5 or 10 mm in diameter – so as to rule out pleural adhesions or other abnormal findings. The second incision, 2 cm long, is made in the periareolar line in the male while in the female patient a similar location is placed (fourth intercostal space) in the submammary line by retracting the breast medially (ventral port). This incision, like any other one, should be watched videoscopically. Its wider extension (2 cm) allows digital palpation and easy specimen retrieval. These two incisions are the key ones through which the endostapler and the telescope will be introduced alternately in each phase of the operation.

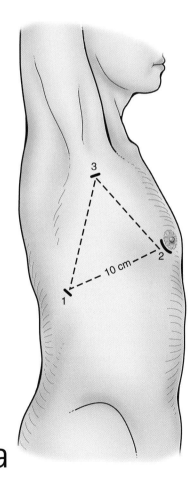

2a

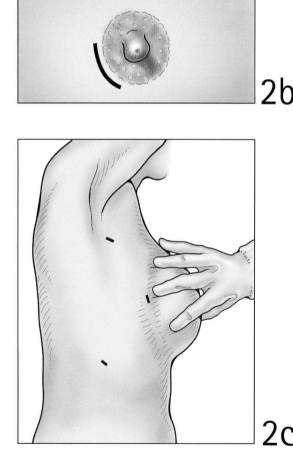

2b

2c

3 Once both entries are usable, instrument-driven exploration begins, looking for pleural adhesions which, if found, are cut and coagulated with endo-scissors. The best instrument to manipulate the lung is an endo-Pföerster; or when the distance between the port and the target is adequate, a regular curved Pföerster forceps will do. By exchanging the location of the camera and the endo-Pföerster, the whole pulmonary surface can be explored. Even when obvious bullae or blebs are readily seen, careful search for additional pathology should always be accomplished initially. Special attention should be paid to the dorsal aspect of the upper and lower lobes which can be exposed by grasping the lung in its lateral aspect and dragging it ventrally from the periareolar entry keeping the camera in the caudal port. Interplaying with the telescope and the grasper between these two entries generally renders excellent results.

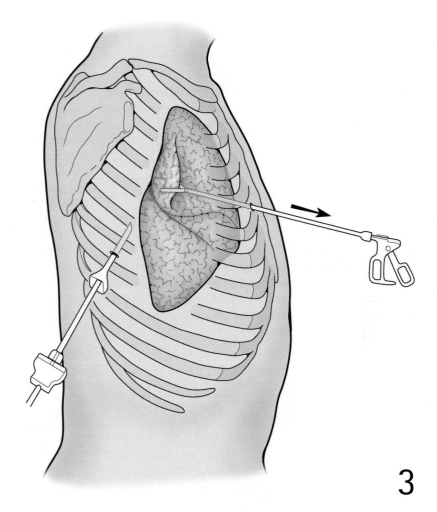

3

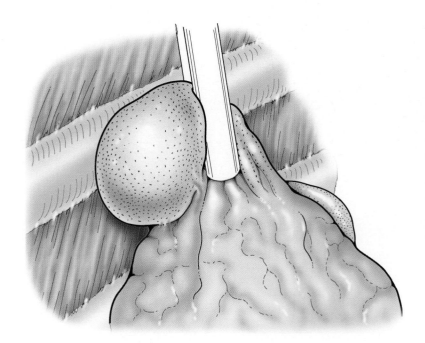

4

4 A bulla on the collapsed lung can either be seen deflated as a "whitish" plane area applied over the pulmonary surface or as an inflated balloon. In any case, it is wise to ventilate the lung with small tidal volumes in order to determine the exact site of leakage and/or to make evident any other accompanying lesion.

5 The endograsp is removed, and an endoretractor is inserted to restrain its full expansion while a sufficient amount of saline is poured into the cavity so as to make the leaking point evident. This maneuver should be repeated after the bulla resection is completed in order to rule out any leakage from the suture line and to be sure that no leaking points are left behind.

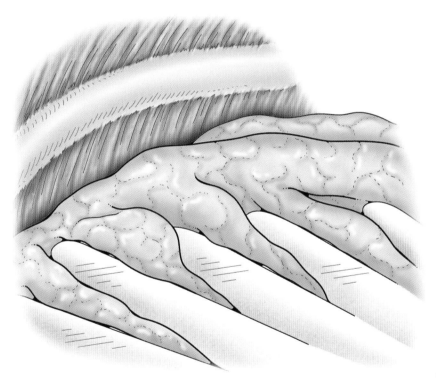

5

6 When the leaking source has been identified, the third incision is done according to its placement in the lung's surface. For apical lesions, a small 5 mm trocar is inserted in the axillary rim; for more dorsal lesions, an auscultatory triangle 5 mm port will do. Sometimes this incision has to be extended to 11 mm whenever a good alignment angle for the endostapler cannot be acheived. Whether three or four incisions are needed is not important. The goal is to obtain a good complementary angle with the first endostapler "firing."

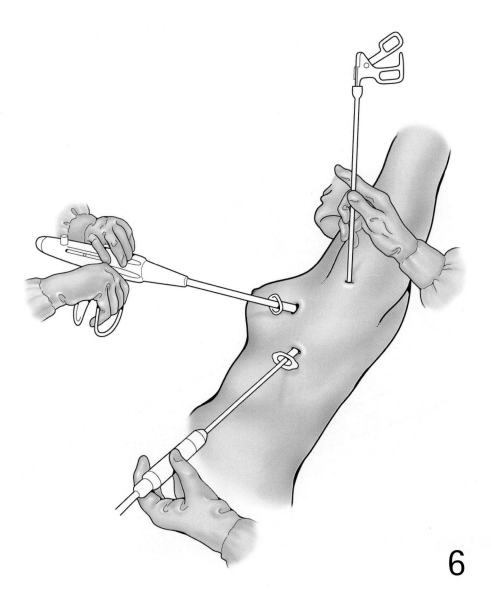

6

7 In any case, 5 mm diameter holding instruments like an endograsp or endoclinch are used. Sometimes during the exploration phase an obvious leaking bulla is found at the apex of the lung, hanging from a parietal pleural adhesion. At this instance the surgeon can be tempted to apply the endostapler directly onto the neck of the bulla without cut- ting the adhesion in an attempt to avoid another incision. Such a maneuver is to be condemned since frequently leads to troublesome consequences, either bleeding from an unseen vascularized pedicle or the presence of some concealed pathology on the dorsal area of the parenchyma.

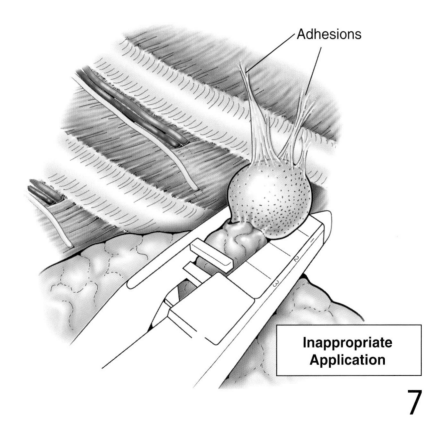

Adhesions

Inappropriate Application

7

8 Once the lung is totally freed from the adhesions and the leaking source has been truly identified, the operation enters its second phase: resection of the compromised tissue. The bulla is grasped by a 5 mm diameter endoclinch inserted through the axillary port or the auscultatory triangle. The endostapler is introduced through the periareolar entry; the trocar is pulled back, and the stapler is progressed beyond the target tissue to get full opening of both jaws.

The stapler is retracted a bit so as to encompass the base of the bulla between the wide-opened jaws. Note that the bulla has to be resected with a thin rim of normal parenchyma. Therefore, the angle of incidence should be almost parallel to the pulmonary surface. **Avoid acute angles and thick bits of lung tissue. Resect only the bulla and its base.** It is very important to line the stapler to the desired angulation by exchanging ports, if necessary, in order to avoid "the banana peel" phenomenon. The endostapler should be positioned over the long surface close to the bulla's base, making sure that a rim of normal parenchyma is removed together with the specimen. Do not place the stapler on the bulla itself.

Occasionally, in small bullae the leaking point can be sutured only with the unbladed Endogia 30 or Endo TA 30, leaving six rows or staples *in situ* without sectioning. Stapling is a much safer method than endolooping ligation and equally expensive. **We do not recommend endoloop ligation.**

When the leaking source cannot be found, it is advised to blindly resect the apex of the lung or the most suspicious area according to the CT scans. This situation usually occurs in young people with primary spontaneous pneumothorax. In elderly patients this situation should be treated by inducing pleurodesis with talc poudrage or pleural abrasion without resection.

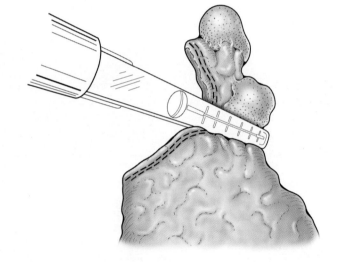

8

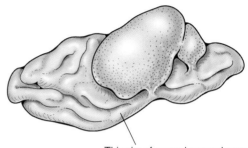

Thin rim of normal parenchyma 9

9,10 Once the bullae has been completely resected and it is hanging freely from the endoclinch within the pleural cavity, the specimen is removed through the ventral port with a Kaiser–Pilling forceps protected by a conventional polyethylene camera sleeve or any commercially available device and sent to pathology and bacteriology.

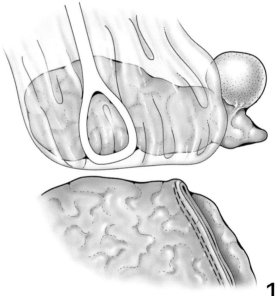

10

11 The pleural cavity is then filled with saline to check aerostasis. The third phase or consolidation is generally carried out by abrading the apical parietal pleura with a gauze sponge held by a Kaiser–Pilling curved ring forceps until the pleura becomes petechyal. The visceral pleura should also be sponged, although less vigorously. In chronic obstructive pulmonary disease (COPD) patients with multiple blebs, 4 g of asbestos free talc are insufflated and spread over the lung surface as a fine cloudy suspension, leaving a thin talc film over the whole pleural surface. **Avoid bulky (gross) deposits of talc.** The drainage tube is introduced through the caudal port and inserted, piercing the immediate cephalad "virgin" intercostal space placed under videoscopic guidance. The port wound is closed in planes around the tube, which is secured by a strong stitch to the surrounding skin and connected to a water-sealed continuous suction device.

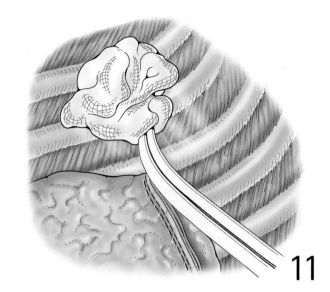

11

POSTOPERATIVE CARE

On returning to the recovery room, an immediate postoperative chest radiograph is obtained to determine the completeness of lung expansion. Suction ($-10/-15\,\text{cmH}_2\text{O}$) should be applied if there is any incomplete re-expansion or air leakage. Prophylactic antibiotics are normally stopped after 24 hours. Physiotherapy is started in the immediate postoperative period, and prompt patient deambulation is strongly encouraged. Pain control is achieved by indicating oral analgesics which interact with the preoperative bupivacaine intercostal nerve blockage. Epidural analgesia is not recommended for this type of procedure. Drainage tube removal is indicated after any 24 hour period once air leakage ceases and full lung expansion has been attained. A chest X-ray is obtained 12 hours after tube removal, and the patient is discharged 12 hours later.

OUTCOME

The treatment of choice for a ruptured bulla and its ensuing pneumothorax, persistent air leak and septic complication of the pleural cavity is surgical resection. This goal can be accomplished by two modalities: open thoracotomy or videothoracoscopy. Full posterolateral thoracotomy constitutes a procedure too formidable for the management of a small offending lesion. A semiblind approach such as a 6 cm limited thoracotomy is acceptable in terms of anatomical disarrangement but markedly reduces the field of vision, which may result in missing other leak sources and failure of the procedure.

In the early 1990s, several initial experiences with VAT bullectomies compared its results to the historical series of thoracotomy bullectomies. The recurrence rate for VAT procedures was 6–8% while for thoracotomy it was much lower, between 0 and 1%. Most of these failures were due to inexperience, or a "learning curve." VAT bullectomy's failures, occurring during the first three days may be solved by re-exploring the pleural cavity using the same incisional ports; later than that we create new entries, in order to avoid pleural infection. Some surgeons prefer to use an open thoracotomy to treat VATS failures, in the understanding that the patient will be more willing to accept a procedure different from the one which failed originally. We do not share this policy and re-explore prolonged bullectomy leaks by VATS. Nowadays acceptable recurrence rates should be 1–2%.

Complications are infrequent, ranging between 5% and 15%. The most frequent complication is prolonged air leakage. Localized empyema is exceptional and is usually associated with talc instillation. Chest wall bleeding and hemorrhage after parietal pleurectomy is possible but very rare. All these complications can be treated by VATS. Postoperative pain is seldom a problem if intercostal nerves have not been compressed by improper trocar insertion. Most of these complications result from a faulty surgical technique. Mortality depends on the patient's condition but by proper management should be nil. Strict adhesion to the strategic algorithm is recommended.

Our own experience comprises 472 episodes of spontaneous pneumothorax treated between February 1985 and January 2000. Ninety-five of these cases were dealt with before February 1992 when we incorporated VATS equipment and techniques into our practice ("pre VATS era"), and 377 were treated after that date ("VATS era"). In the "pre VATS era" 76 cases were resolved by simple tube drainage, and another 19 required thoracotomy and bullectomy. None of these thoracotomy-treated cases recurred. Morbidity was 9.1% and mortality 0% in the first subset.

During the "VATS era" 234 cases were treated by tube

drainage; 126 by VATS; 10 giant bullae were resected through axillary thoracotomy; and 15 small pneumothoraces were managed by simple observation. In the VATS group three recurrences (2.3%) occurred during the first part of the experience and were probably due to faulty technique ("learning curve"). The morbidity was 10.9% and the mortality 0%. None of the patients required conversion into an open thoracotomy.

In summary, VAT bullectomy emerges as the gold standard procedure for the treatment of recurrent pneumothorax during its second or subsequent episodes. It renders:

1 Excellent visualization of the entire lung and pleural cavity
2 A high rate of success
3 Little anatomical disarrangement
4 Low postoperative pain
5 Good cosmesis
6 Reduced hospital stay
7 Earlier return to work.

FURTHER READING

Baumann MH, Strange C, Heffner JE. AACP Pneumothorax Consensus Group. Management of spontaneous pneumothorax: an American College of Chest Physicians Delfi consensus statement. *Chest* 2001; **119**: 590–602.

Boutin C, Viallat JR, Aelony Y. Practical Thoracoscopy. Springer-Verlag, Berlin, 1991.

Deslauriers J, Beaulieu M, Després JP, Lemieux M, Leblanc J, Desmeules M. Transaxillary Pleurectomy for Treatment of Spontaneous Pneumothorax. *Annals of Thoracic Surgery* 1980; **30**: 569–74.

Henry M, Arnold T, Harvey J. Pleural Diseases Group, Standards of Care Committee, British Thoracic Society. BTS guidelines for the management of spontaneous pneumothorax. *Thorax* 2003; **58** Suppl 2: 39–52.

Killen DA, Gobbel WG. Spontaneous Pneumothorax. Little Brown, Boston, 1968.

Light RW. Pleural Diseases. 2nd Ed. Lea & Febiger. Philadelphia, 1990.

19

Pulmonary hydatid cysts

ANDRES VARELA MD, PhD
Professor, Department of Surgery, Autonomous University of Madrid; Section Chief of Thoracic Surgery and Lung Transplantation,
Department of Cardiovascular and Thoracic Surgery, Hospital Puerta de Hierro, Madrid, Spain

RAUL BURGOS MD, PhD
Associate Professor, Autonomous University of Madrid, Department of Cardiovascular and Thoracic Surgery, Hospital Puerta de Hierro,
Madrid, Spain

EVARISTO CASTEDO MD, PhD
Professor of Surgery, Autonomous University of Madrid, Department of Cardiovascular and Thoracic Surgery, Hospital Puerta de Hierro,
Madrid, Spain

HISTORY

Hydatid disease, which was known in medicine in the times of Hippocrates, was described by Goze in 1782. This disease is thought to have been brought to Europe by dogs accompanying whaling boats in the eighteenth century. Echinococcosis is endemic to the Mediterranean region, South America, Australia, New Zealand, the Middle East, Alaska, and Canada, where it is widespread among Indian tribes. In the adult stage, the parasite lives in the intestinal tracts of carnivores.

Humans contract the disease from contaminated water or food or by direct contact with dogs. Once the eggs reach the stomach, the hexacanth embryos are released. They pass through the intestinal wall and reach the tributary veins of the liver, where they undergo a vesicular transformation and develop into the hydatid. Hexacanth embryos can reach the thorax, mainly after passing through the portal system. The lymphatic system or bronchi can also serve as the pathway for infestation, although this route is less common. Within the thorax, the lung is the organ most frequently colonized. If parasites advance beyond the lung, they may reach any organ, carried by the bloodstream.

PRINCIPLES AND JUSTIFICATION

1 Surgery, when feasible, is the principal definitive method of treatment of hydatid disease. The objective of surgical treatment is to eradicate the parasite, to prevent the intraoperative rupture of the cyst with subsequent dissemination of its contents, and to remove the residual cavity.

Planning of the surgical technique is based on a good knowledge of the anatomical relations of the cyst with vascular and bronchial elements. Three topographical regions must be differentiated:

- External layer (fibrous whitish aspect) (Part A)
- Medium layer (lung parenchyma with small vessels close to the pericystic membrane) (Part B)
- Internal layer (bronchial openings and vessels close to the pericystic membrane) (Part C)

The treatment of choice is to completely eradicate the parasite while preserving the lung parenchyma.

Small and medium-sized cysts (up to 4–5 cm) are best treated by enucleation and partial resection of the pericystic layer. Giant cysts and those at risk of rupture may be treated with needle aspiration or a trocar-suction device.

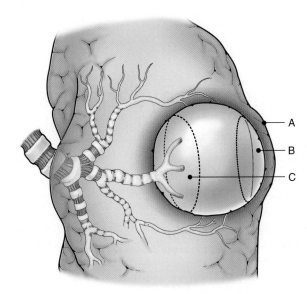

1

PREOPERATIVE ASSESSMENT AND PREPARATION

Imaging studies

Because a period of 5–20 years often elapses before cysts enlarge sufficiently to become symptomatic, they are frequently detected incidentally on a routine radiograph or ultrasonographic scan.

The finding of a cystic tumor in the chest radiograph of a patient in good clinical condition who comes from an area where the disease is endemic, has been in contact with dogs, or has eosinophilia strongly suggests the diagnosis of pulmonary hydatidosis. In fact, the combination of a positive finding on chest radiograph and a suggestive clinical history has a sensitivity of 95% in our series.

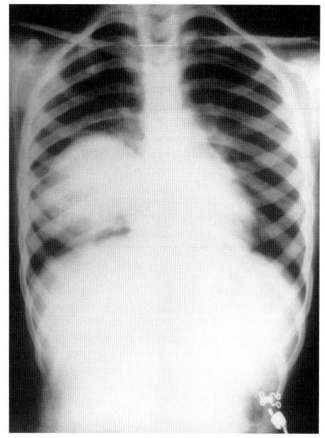

2a On a plain chest radiograph, intact pulmonary cysts are usually defined as round or oval-shaped irregular masses, of uniform density, and with a perfectly defined margin. Ruptured or complicated cysts, however, may have the membrane floating in fluid resembling the water-lily sign, an incarcerated membrane folded back in the form of a barricade. Evidence of cyst wall calcification, pneumothorax, empyema, pleural effusion, pneumonitis, or atelectasis also may be found.

2a

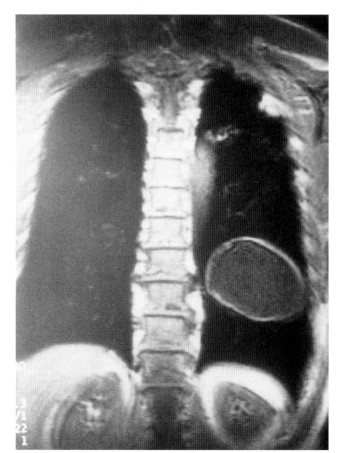

2b Ultrasonography, computed tomography (CT), and magnetic resonance imaging usually reveal well-defined cysts with thick or thin walls, which may contain fragments of the hydatid membrane. Repeated evaluation of cysts by CT and magnetic resonance imaging is also especially useful in evaluation of the response to treatment. Differential diagnosis should be made with pulmonary carcinoma, sarcomas, or tuberculosis.

CT-guided aspiration of hydatid cysts for diagnosis is not recommended, because of the risk of cyst rupture and fluid leakage, which results in either dissemination of infection or anaphylactic reaction.

2b

Serological tests

A specific diagnosis can be made by serological assays, although a negative test result does not exclude the diagnosis of hydatidosis. Cysts in the liver elicit positive antibody responses in 85% of infected individuals, but up to 50% of patients with lung cysts may have negative serological results, especially if the cysts are not ruptured. The Casoni test has a high sensitivity but a poor specificity. Immunoblotting has the highest specificity, although false-positive findings may be obtained in cases of cysticercosis. Indirect hemagglutination, indirect immunofluorescence, and enzyme immunoassay also may be used. Results of serodiagnostic assays usually become negative in a mean interval of 2 years after surgical cyst removal.

Definitive diagnosis

Definitive diagnosis can be established either after surgery, when scolices or daughter cysts are detected in the subsequent histopathological study, or preoperatively, with the examination of sputum, feces, or urine if a rupture of the cyst has occurred. Scolices can be demonstrated with a Ziehl-Neelsen stain.

ANESTHESIA

General anesthesia is always required. Valsalva maneuvers or cough must be avoided during induction to reduce the risk of cyst rupture. Use of a double-lumen endotracheal tube is mandatory to prevent dissemination. Caution should be taken to prevent anaphylactic reaction or shock.

OPERATION

Unilateral cysts

For simple or multiple unilateral cysts, a sparing muscle thoracotomy incision is used. In appropriate patients with uncomplicated pulmonary hydatid cysts, a surgical approach via minithoracotomy with the help of video-assisted thoracoscopy may be a possibility. Selective unilateral lung ventilation is begun. Protection of the operative field and surrounding tissues is accomplished with surgical sponges soaked in 3% hypertonic saline solution.

ENUCLEATION

Small or medium-sized cysts up to 4–5 cm in diameter and those close to the surface of the lung can be treated by enucleation.

3a, b
Almost always the cyst is visible on the lung surface as a white protruding area. The incision in the lung parenchyma encircles the area with care so that the pericystic membranes are spared. The dissection between the lung parenchyma and the pericystic membrane involves small vessels and bronchi that must be carefully ligated (Figure 3b).

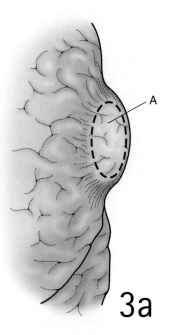

3a

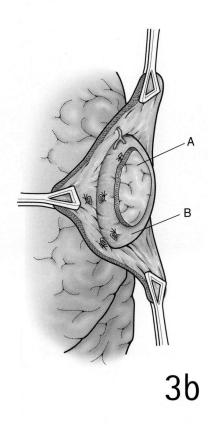

3b

3c, d, e, f

The pericystic membrane may sometimes be opened spontaneously rather than incised with scissors. Blunt forceps are used to hold open the pericystic membrane, but herniation of the cyst is avoided. Dissection of the cyst is completed digitally. Tension on the pericystic membrane is reduced by making star-like incisions.

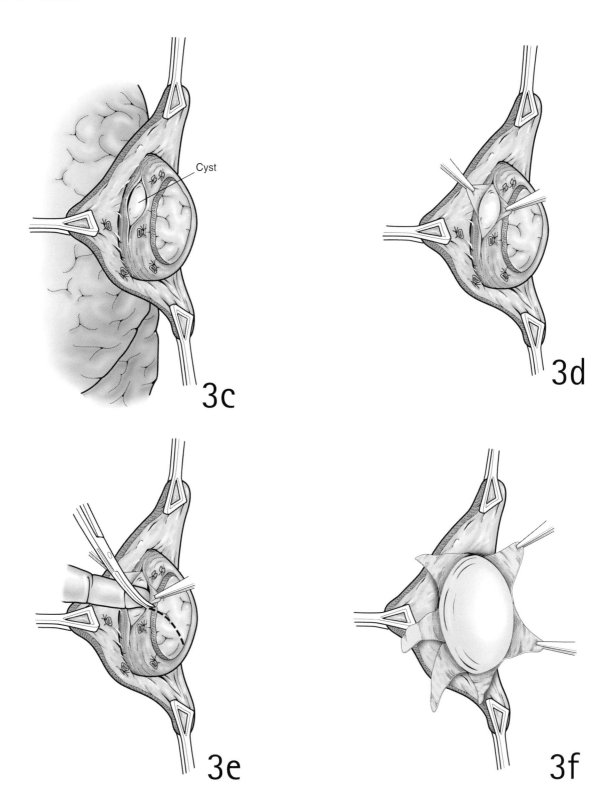

Cyst

3c

3d

3e

3f

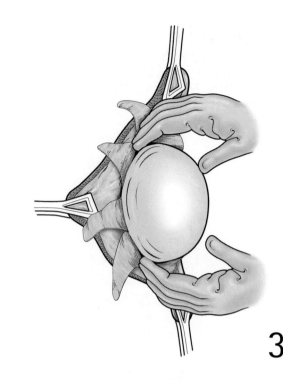

3g

3g, h
Thereafter, the cyst is evacuated by cupping of the hands or by direct enucleation if the topography of the lesion permits.

3h

3i
With small cysts, total resection with the pericystic membrane is a better alternative.

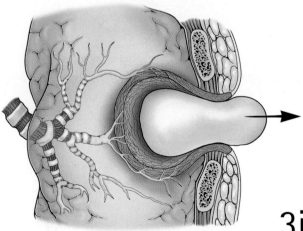

3i

ASPIRATION OF THE CYST

4a In our experience, giant cysts (larger than 5 cm) or cysts in a location at risk of rupture are best treated by needle aspiration or by use of a trocar-suction device. The use of the latter instrument prevents the rupture of the cyst, eradicates the parasite, and makes it possible to excise the residual cavity.

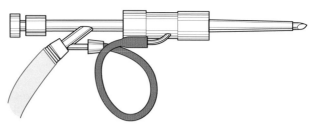

4a

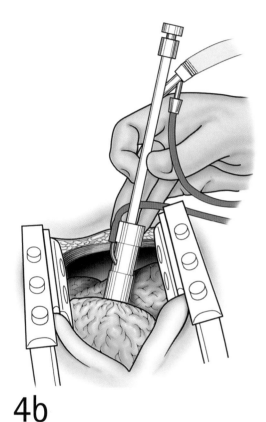

4b

4b This device is composed of a trocar containing a needle connected to a system of negative pressure aspiration and surrounded by a suction cup that fits over the convex part of the cyst wall. When the device is applied to the cyst, the negative pressure makes the suction cup adhere hermetically to the cyst wall, which impedes the extravasation of the content as it is suctioned out and eliminates the possibility of intraoperative contamination. The cystic contents are partially aspirated and replaced with the same amount of 3% saline solution. This maneuver is repeated several times with a wait of 3–5 minutes between applications.

4c Cystectomy is then performed and the membrane removed.

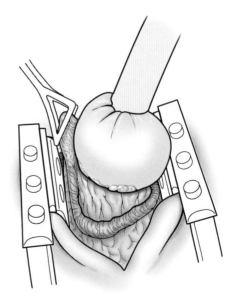

4c

MANAGEMENT OF THE RESIDUAL CAVITY

Management of the residual cavity involves the partial resection of the pericystic layer and capitonnage.

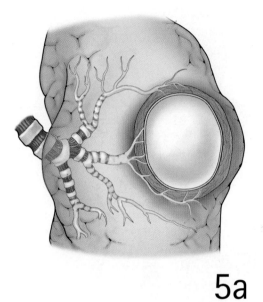

5a

5a, b The partial pericystectomy leaves intact the internal layer. The bronchial openings should be closed with individual sutures, and the free portion of the pericystic membrane should be resected.

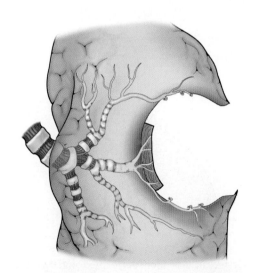

5b

5c, d
The capitonnage is the obliteration of the residual space by placement of concentric rows of sutures.

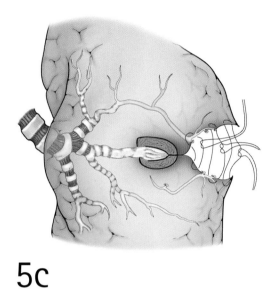

5c

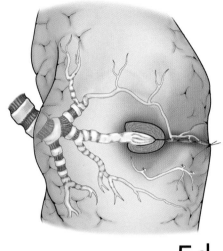

5d

5e, f
The visceral pleura is sewn over the incision.

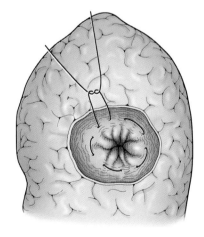

5e

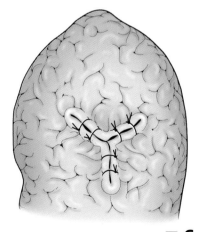

5f

Bilateral cysts

6 A bilateral 'clamshell' thoracosternotomy is used when dealing with cysts in both lungs. This is the approach of choice for cysts that involve both the heart and lungs.

A median sternotomy is usually sufficient when the cysts are not located in the left lower lobe.

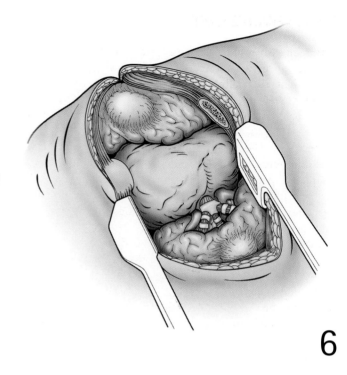

6

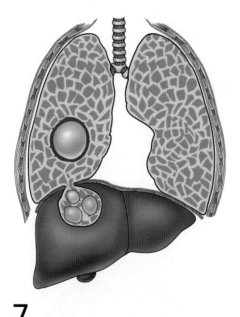

7

Hepatic and lung cysts

7 The decision as to which cysts should be removed first is based on the size, location, and risk of rupture. With apical liver cysts and cysts of the right lower lobe, the best approach is a lateral seventh to eighth intercostal thoracotomy that goes through the diaphragm with simultaneous resection of all cysts.

Occasionally, involvement of the bile duct may mandate extension of the thoracotomy to a laparotomy for placement of a T tube.

Complicated cysts

Rupture of the cyst prior to the operation can be a serious complication. Precautions to be taken include maintenance of the airway free of secretions and cystic contents by appropriate bronchoscopy suction. Anaphylaxis may occur during induction of the anesthesia or during the operation, due to communication of the cyst into the bronchi or the pleural space. If this situation occurs, the cyst is opened, the contents are evacuated, and the cavity is thoroughly irrigated with 3% saline solution. The bronchial openings are closed, and the residual cavity is closed by partial resection of the pericystic layer and capitonnage. Pulmonary lobectomy is a safer treatment when the cyst is associated with severe pulmonary changes such as abscess, atelectasia, or fibrosis.

POSTOPERATIVE CARE

Although early results with surgical treatment were quite satisfactory, surgery is not free of complications. In our series of 240 patients surgically treated for pulmonary hydatid disease between 1966 and 1988, three patients (1.25%) died in the immediate postoperative period due to tension pneumothorax, hemoptysis, and thromboembolic pulmonary disease, respectively. The mean hospital stay was 14.6 ± 4.8 days. Pneumothorax, pleural effusion, wound infection, bronchopleural-cutaneous fistula, and empyema were the most frequent postoperative complications. Data concerning these and other complications that arose during the early postoperative period are shown in **Table 19.1**.

Medical treatment of pulmonary hydatid cysts has been used as adjuvant therapy to surgical removal. New drugs such as the imidazoles (flubendazole and albendazole) are the agents for this treatment. When the cyst is intact and there appears to be no risk that it will rupture during the surgical procedure, the treatment is administered for 1 month. When the cyst is ruptured or possible intraoperative dissemination is suspected, treatment is continued for 3–6 months. When dissemination is confirmed and total or partial resection of the lesions is not feasible, one must excise as many of the cysts as possible while attempting to conserve a maximum of lung parenchyma, and administer imidazoles until no radiological evidence of the lesions is seen.

Table 19.1 *Postoperative complications associated with pulmonary hydatidosis*

Complication	No. of patients	%
Pneumothorax	24	8.8
Pleural effusion	20	7.4
Wound infection	18	6.6
Bronchopleural (cutaneous) fistula	12	4.4
Empyema	10	3.7
Atelectasis	6	2.2
Phrenic nerve palsy	2	0.7
Hemorrhage	2	0.7
Transcervical palsy	1	0.4
Deep venous thrombosis	1	0.4

OUTCOME

8 When surgery is approached correctly, long-term results after operation are excellent. In our series, overall survival after a mean follow-up of 17.8 years (range, 8–22 years) was 94.6%. Of the surviving patients, 95.1% were free of hydatid disease, and 98.3% were free of pulmonary hydatid disease.

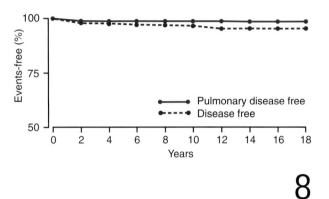

8

FURTHER READING

Burgos R, Varela A, Castedo E, *et al.* Pulmonary hydatidosis: surgical treatment and follow-up of 240 cases. *European Journal of Cardio-Thoracic Surgery* 1999; **16**: 628–35.

Heleg H, Best LA, Gaitini D. Simultaneous operation for hydatid cysts of the right lung and liver. *Journal of Thoracic and Cardiovascular Surgery* 1985; **90**: 783–7.

Jerray M, Benzarti M, Garrouche A, Klabi N, Hayouni A. Hydatid disease of the lungs. Study of 386 cases. *American Review of Respiratory Disease* 1992; **146**: 185–9.

Kir A, Baran E. Simultaneous operation for hydatid cyst of right lung and liver. *Thoracic and Cardiovascular Surgeon* 1995; **43**: 62–4.

Oto O, Silistreli E, Erturk M, Maltepe F. Thoracoscopic guided minimally invasive surgery for giant hydatic cyst. *European Journal of Cardio-Thoracic Surgery* 1999; **16**: 494–5.

Salik OK, Topenoglu MS, Celik SK, Ulus T, Tokcan A. Surgical treatment of hydatid cysts of the lung: analysis of 405 patients with pulmonary hydatidosis. *Journal of Thoracic and Cardiovascular Surgery* 1995; **19**: 714–19.

20

Bronchopleural fistula after pneumonectomy and lobectomy

DAVID P. JENKINS BSc, MS, FRCS (CTH)
Formerly Specialist Registrar, Department of Thoracic Surgery, Harefield Hospital, Middlesex, UK: Consultant Cardiothoracic Surgeon, Papworth Hospital, Cambridge, UK

EDWARD R. TOWNSEND FRCS
Consultant Thoracic Surgeon, Thoracic Surgery Unit, Royal Brompton & Harefield Hospital NHS Trust, Harefield, Middlesex, UK

HISTORY

Bronchopleural fistula is defined as a communication between the bronchial lumen and pleural space after an operation for lung resection. However, the term is often used loosely, and incorrectly, to refer to persistent alveolar air leaks in patients with a pneumothorax. This chapter deals with the former, and the correct terminology should always be encouraged as it implies a specific etiology and a major difference in the degree of morbidity and prognosis for the patient. Formation of a bronchopleural fistula after lobectomy is extremely rare; and therefore, the majority of this chapter refers to pneumonectomy. Despite the advances in surgical technique, anesthesia, instrumentation, and postoperative care, bronchopleural fistula remains a significant complication after lung resection.

PRINCIPLES AND JUSTIFICATION

The pathophysiology is relatively simple: the bronchial closure breaks down to form a communication with the pneumonectomy space. This complication allows contamination of the space, with resultant empyema, and passage of fluid from the space into the trachea and opposite bronchus to impair gas exchange in the remaining lung. In the most extreme case in which a large fistula develops early when the space contains several liters of fluid, the condition can be rapidly fatal due to drowning and respiratory arrest.

The incidence in recently published series is between 1% and 3% after pneumonectomy, and no difference is found for sutured closures and parallel staple gun closures. Even with meticulous surgical technique and the most advanced stapling devices, this complication is impossible to prevent entirely. The reported mortality after fistula development ranges from 6% to 67%, but most units expect a mortality of at least 20%. Right-sided fistulae are more common than left-sided. Predisposing factors include the use of postoperative positive pressure ventilation, the presence of disease (tumor or mycobacterial infection) in the main bronchus, and treatment with neoadjuvant chemotherapy or radiation. Bronchial mucosal blood flow and stump healing have been demonstrated to be significantly reduced after chemoradiation in particular.

Traditionally, the timing of fistula formation has been described as early or late, and the dividing time in most series is approximately 7–10 postoperative days. Although this distinction is necessarily artificial, the principle does contribute to the management of the condition; repair of an early fistula is commonly attempted via the original thoracotomy, whereas most sources recommend an alternative approach for repair of late fistulae. Most fistulae become evident in the first 30 days after operation, and for a fistula to present after 90 days is very rare. The other classification of importance is between small and large fistulae. The division point is around 2 mm, with smaller fistulae having a greater chance of closing spontaneously or responding to endobronchial treatment.

The development of a large fistula during the in-hospital postoperative phase results in such a dramatic insult to the patient that the diagnosis is not difficult to make as long as a high level of suspicion and vigilance is maintained. Smaller fistulae arising later, however, especially after the patient has left the hospital, may be more difficult to diagnose. Symptoms vary according to the size of the fistula and the rate of fluid movement into the trachea. Classical symptoms include cough, which may be postural, and bloody sputum, followed by varying quantities of space fluid, which is often pink. Respiratory distress may be extreme, with tachypnea and cyanosis. Cardiovascular compromise may be present, with tachycardia, atrial fibrillation, peripheral vasoconstriction, and sweating. The differential diagnosis includes myocardial infarction, pulmonary embolus, pulmonary edema, and severe pneumonia. Diagnosis is usually confirmed by the appearance of the chest radiograph. Comparison with previous films shows a change in the shape of the apical airspace and a reduction in the fluid level. In patients with very small 'pinhole' fistulae, symptoms may be remarkably minor, and the only abnormality may be absent space fluid on a follow-up chest radiograph. Bronchoscopy is necessary as a therapeutic intervention for larger fistulae but may be confusing in the diagnosis of smaller fistulae as tiny holes are often not visible unless bubbles of air are seen. Other reported methods to confirm the diagnosis include isotope ventilation scanning and, more recently, injection into the pleural space of diethylenetriamine penta-acetic acid labeled with technetium 99m.

PREOPERATIVE ASSESSMENT AND PREPARATION

Emergency intervention

The immediate treatment of a large fistula arising early during postoperative recovery is concerned with prevention of damage to the remaining lung. The patient should be turned to lie with the pneumonectomy side dependent and given oxygen to maintain arterial saturation while preparations are made for insertion of an intercostal drain. A basal intercostal drain is then inserted to drain the pneumonectomy space to dryness. Care must be taken, especially on the left side, as mediastinal shift and elevation of the hemidiaphragm after the pneumonectomy can make drain placement hazardous, even in positions usually considered safe.

Bronchial toilet should follow drainage and can often be performed under local anesthetic, even with a rigid bronchoscope. If the latter is used, adequate anesthesia is necessary and is best accomplished by injection of 1% lignocaine through the cricothyroid membrane. The rigid endoscope allows a large-bore suction device to be used. The stump should be inspected to assess the extent of disruption, fol-lowed by suction of the contralateral bronchial tree. Aspirates should be sent for culture and broad-spectrum intravenous antibiotics commenced until results of sensitivity tests are available.

ANESTHESIA

The pathophysiology of bronchopleural fistula makes the use of general anesthesia especially hazardous. Although drainage of the pneumonectomy space should reduce the risk of space fluid aspiration to the remaining lung, every precaution must be taken. Patients are thus induced to sit upright, and a double-lumen endotracheal tube is carefully positioned to isolate the bronchus before the patient is positioned supine and positive-pressure ventilation is commenced. For a right-sided fistula, a long single-lumen endotracheal tube positioned in the left main bronchus is an alternative. An additional theoretical problem with large fistulae and a poorly isolated bronchus is loss of tidal volume into the pneumonectomy space.

OPERATIONS

The objectives of all the operative interventions are to locate the fistula, reclose the bronchus, buttress the new closure, isolate it from the infected pneumonectomy space, and finally to deal with the empyema.

Management of early fistulae via the left or right thoracotomy approach

INCISION

The patient is placed in a lateral position after bronchial isolation with a double-lumen endotracheal tube. The original thoracotomy skin incision is reopened. The best approach, however, is often to use a different intercostal space to enter the thoracic cavity. Usually the fifth interspace will have been used in the first operation; and therefore, we would recommend the fourth interspace. This maneuver not only allows easier access away from scar tissue but also permits the preparation of an undamaged intercostal muscle and bundle for use in buttressing the new bronchial closure and better positioning for access to the superior hilum where the bronchus will be lying.

1 The periosteum covering the fourth and fifth ribs is incised longitudinally along the center line of the outer surfaces with diathermy. The periosteum is then stripped with the elevator above and below to isolate the muscle and bundle of the fourth interspace. The muscle and bundle are transfixed and divided anteriorly just before the costal cartilage, but at the posterior limit near the neck of the fourth rib the bundle must be preserved. The muscle is wrapped in a warm saline swab. The fourth rib can now be removed, if necessary, to improve exposure.

Any residual fluid or material is removed from the thoracic cavity to leave as clean a space as possible. Identification of the bronchus and fistula may be easy, but considerable difficulty may be encountered if retraction has occurred. Sometimes one must cover the area with a small volume of saline and allow the anesthetist to partially deflate the bronchial cuff of the contralateral bronchus to see bubbles betraying the fistula location.

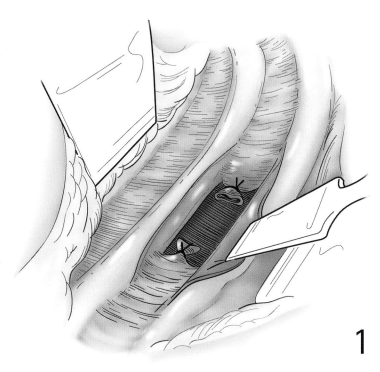

1

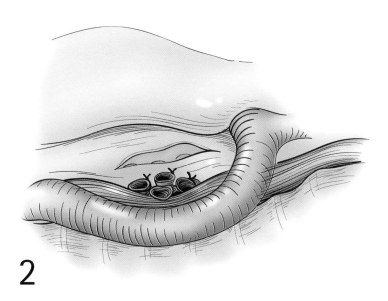

2

LEFT HILUM DISSECTION

2 On the left side considerable dissection may be necessary to achieve access to the bronchial stump. If the bronchus is visible or palpable, it should be separated from the pulmonary artery by sharp dissection. To prevent catastrophic hemorrhage from inadvertent damage to the pulmonary artery stump, the best method is to open the pericardium just posterior to the phrenic nerve to secure a clean plane around the artery. When the bronchus has retracted deeply into the mediastinum, direct dissection is difficult and dangerous, as the remainder of the left pulmonary artery is in close apposition. One alternative is to approach a left-sided bronchopleural fistula from a right-sided thoracotomy. Although this approach requires another incision and intermittent or jet ventilation of the right lung, in the authors' experience good access to the left bronchus can be obtained by dividing the azygous vein and retracting the esophagus posteriorly and to the right.

3 For a retracted left bronchus stump to be reached from the left thorax, the aorta must first be mobilized and retracted anteriorly. The pleura overlying the posterior border of the descending thoracic aorta is divided, and the incision is extended superiorly to free the proximal few centimeters of the left subclavian artery. The thoracic duct lies just deep to the subclavian artery at this point. The vagus and recurrent laryngeal nerves pass over the aortic arch anterior to the origin of the subclavian artery and should be reflected forward undisturbed with the pleura. The posterior intercostal arteries arise from the posterior surface of the aorta and should be preserved when possible. It is sometimes necessary to divide the first and/or second intercostal artery if their origin is proximal, but the fourth must be retained to vascularize the intercostal muscle pedicle for the bronchus repair. The aorta is reflected anteriorly by a combination of sharp and blunt digital dissection. This maneuver is aided by the assistant's maintaining gentle upward traction on a sloop or tape running around the aorta and the surgeon's holding the esophagus and distal trachea down. The trachea can now be followed distally to the left main bronchus and fistula. One must remember that the membranous trachea is thin, and care must be exercised to avoid puncture, especially if the tissues are inflamed and edematous.

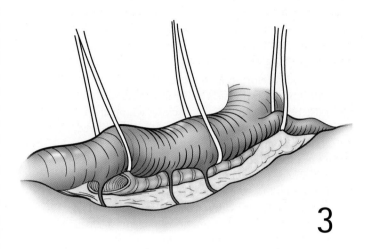

3

4

RIGHT HILUM DISSECTION

4 The bronchus is more accessible on the right than on the left, but care is still needed to avoid damage to the remainder of the right pulmonary artery, which lies just anterior to the bronchus. If any difficulty in their separation is encountered or anticipated, the best alternative is to open the pericardium anterior to the superior vena cava to ensure proximal control of the artery. The trachea is usually easily palpable in the posterior mediastinum. Dissection begins by dividing the overlying pleura of the distal trachea proximal to the carina. Dissection close to the tracheal wall is then extended distally to the carina and bronchus. Adhesions from a previous mediastinoscopy or from clearance of the right paratracheal nodes at the time of pneumonectomy may increase the difficulty.

CLOSURE OF THE FISTULA

5 Stay sutures are inserted into the mobilized left or right bronchus to allow traction up into the operative field. Even if the fistula appears small, attempting direct closure with an extra suture is not advisable. If the bronchial stump is of sufficient length, the surgeon may be able to apply a parallel-closure staple gun and achieve a more proximal staple closure. After staple closure, we recommend the addition of interrupted sutures to appose the mucosa distal to the staple line. The more likely case, however, is that the stump is not long enough to allow introduction of the staple gun. The previous closure line must be excised by a scalpel blade back to a clean part of bronchus. The bronchus is then sutured with interrupted monofilament sutures (3/0 or 4/0 polypropylene) to assure as much approximation of bronchial mucosa as possible. If the bronchial tissues are very friable, pledgets of pericardium or pleura may be used to buttress each suture. The easiest method is to place all sutures before tying down to get an even, tension-free closure. The closure should be tested with saline to an endobronchial ventilation pressure of 40 cm H_2O in the usual fashion.

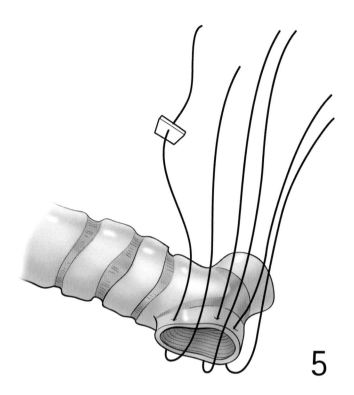

5

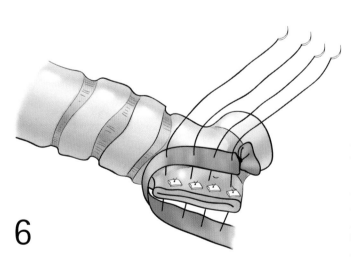

6

BUTTRESSING OF THE CLOSURE LINE

6 The repaired bronchial closure should be covered to isolate it from the contaminated pneumonectomy space. Many methods have been reported to give good results, including the use of omentum, extrathoracic muscle flaps (latissimus dorsi, serratus anterior, pectoralis major, or trapezius), and intrathoracic muscle flaps (intercostal muscle, pedicled internal thoracic artery, or diaphragm). If a good intercostal muscle flap can be procured at rethoracotomy, we would recommend its use. Extrathoracic muscles may have been damaged at the original thoracotomy and require careful dissection by surgeons familiar with the pedicle origin of their neurovascular bundles, which would require collaboration with a reconstructive surgical team. The previously prepared intercostal muscle should be long enough to reach the bronchus and is sutured anterior and posterior to the bronchial closure to completely cover the new stump.

TREATMENT OF THE SPACE AND CHEST CLOSURE

The space must be assumed to be contaminated. If the bronchus has been successfully closed at an early stage, however, sterilization of the space may be possible. All fluid and fibrinous debris should be removed and the cavity generously irrigated with sterile saline and/or an antibiotic solution, depending on the culture sensitivity. The space is then filled with the same solution and the chest closed with multiple layers of continuous 1 Dexon to maintain a seal. Some authorities recommend leaving a small intercostal drain or nasogastric tube to allow later aspiration of fluid for culture or instillation of appropriate antibiotics.

If the pneumonectomy space fails to sterilize despite successful treatment of the bronchopleural fistula, the resulting empyema should be managed as described in Chapter 21 on postpneumonectomy empyema.

EXPOSURE OF THE LEFT MAIN BRONCHUS

7 Mediastinal shift toward the side of the pneumonectomy may be marked, and rotation of the table to the right can help exposure. The pericardial incision is extended superiorly to the point at which it becomes reflected on the ascending aorta. The pulmonary trunk is retracted gently to the right by traction on a tape passed through the transverse sinus using a blunt-ended Semb-type forceps. This maneuver allows blunt dissection behind the bifurcation of the pulmonary trunk and division of the pericardium to isolate the origin of the left pulmonary artery.

Management of late fistulae via the transsternal approach

The advantage of the transsternal approach (as popularized by Perleman) is that the bronchus can be closed in a sterile field without traversing the infected space. The empyema cavity should be drained by an intercostal tube or open thoracostomy as described in Chapter 21 on postpneumonectomy empyema.

An endotracheal tube is placed as previously described, and the patient is positioned supine. A median sternotomy is performed, and the pericardium opened by an inverted T incision and sutured to the sternal edges to provide upward traction of the mediastinum. The key to the safe completion of left or right bronchial closure is careful dissection of the pulmonary artery stump.

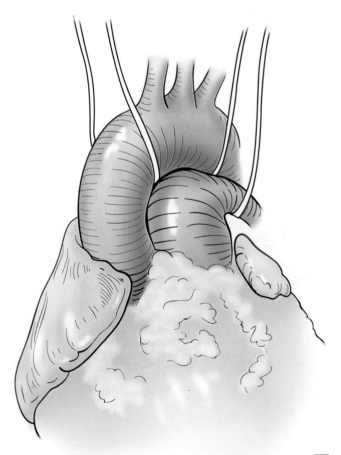

7

8 The pulmonary artery stump closed at the time of the pneumonectomy is adherent to the other side of the pericardium in the infected left chest; and therefore, the artery stump must be redivided to gain access to the bronchus. Various methods of ligation or suture have been described, but the space is small, and the proximal closure is often flush to the trunk. Therefore, the modern vascular staple guns (white 2.5 gauge) designed for endoscopic use are very convenient as they produce a triple staple line on each side and also divide the artery. The heart can then be retracted toward the right by placing swabs between the pericardium and the left ventricle to expose the left superior pulmonary vein which is divided with the vascular staple gun as described for the artery.

The trachea should now be palpable beneath the posterior pericardium and pleura. The origin of the left main bronchus is identified and the overlying pleura incised. The bronchus can now be stapled proximally flush with the carina, with care taken to avoid narrowing the right main bronchus. The distal bronchus leading to the infected space is also stapled, and then the bronchus is divided in between, at which point the distal bronchus retracts away toward the pneumonectomy space. The new staple lines are buttressed with pleura or pericardium and as much healthy tissue as possible is packed around the bronchus closure.

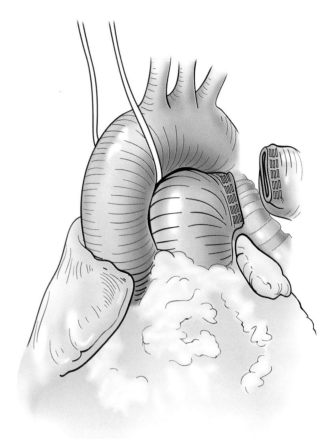

8

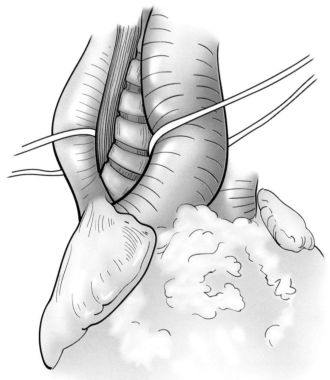

9

EXPOSURE OF THE RIGHT MAIN BRONCHUS

9 The ascending aorta is retracted toward the left after passing a tape around it with a Semb forceps. The pericardium around the superior vena cava is then incised to allow passage of another tape around it and retraction to the right, which thus opens up the space between the aorta and vena cava. Care must be taken to avoid damage to the azygous vein entering the posterior lateral border of the vena cava. The posterior pericardium overlying the right pulmonary artery is now exposed. The right pulmonary artery is much longer than the left, and it is usually easier to dissect out a suitable length for staple closure and division as described earlier for the left artery.

The trachea is then palpable under the pleura deep to the divided pulmonary artery. The pericardium and pleural layers are opened, and the bronchus is dissected. The bronchus can be reclosed as described earlier.

CHEST CLOSURE

Drains are inserted; and after careful hemostasis, the sternum is closed in routine fashion with interrupted stainless steel wires.

Endoscopic treatment of small fistulae

In some cases of very small fistulae, the patient remains well, and management can be expectant with close follow-up. A more satisfactory method of dealing with this problem is bronchoscopic closure. This method is worth attempting in cases of small fistulae, fistulae in very ill patients who would not tolerate reoperation, and fistulae developing later in the postoperative recovery period when the formation of a more fibrous thorax makes significant aspiration less likely. Many methods have been reported with varying success, including insertion of decalcified autologous bone, application of local irritants (caustic soda), or adhesion with fibrin glue. The basis of most methods is induction of inflammation and formation of scar tissue to close the hole. Multiple applications may be necessary, and reported success ranges from closure rates of 35% to over 60%.

Bronchopleural fistula after lobectomy

As stated earlier, fistula formation after lobectomy is rare in our experience. In the reported series of lung resections for carcinoma or infection, the two situations in which post-lobectomy bronchopleural fistulae are encountered are after sleeve lobectomy and bilobectomy (middle and lower) in high-risk patients, with an incidence of 6% and 11%, respectively.

Often the patient is asymptomatic, but a chest radiograph reveals a pneumothorax and fluid level. The consequences of fistula formation after lobectomy are less significant than those after pneumonectomy as long as the residual lobe is viable. If the remaining lobe is not expandable, then a complete pneumonectomy is the only option, and the mortality approaches that with fistula formation after pneumonectomy.

The initial management is insertion of an intercostal drain with an underwater seal. This maneuver may be all that is necessary if the remaining lobe is able to expand and obliterate the space. When simple drainage for a week is unsuccessful, the thoracotomy should be re-explored. The empyema cavity is débrided, and a decortication of the remaining lung is performed. The bronchial stump is amputated and reclosed with interrupted 4/0 polypropylene sutures. The expanded lobe should seal the closure and obliterate any residual space so that muscle buttressing of the closure is unnecessary. Apical and basal intercostal drains are placed, and the chest is closed in routine fashion with layers of polyglycolic acid sutures.

OUTCOME

The overall mortality in patients with bronchopleural fistula after pneumonectomy is high. In most cases the cause of death is aspiration pneumonia. The mortality tends to be highest in those developing fistulae early in the postoperative phase. This fact is probably due to the fluidity of the space contents and the higher risk of significant aspiration. Reported mortality after operative intervention to reclose a fistula is between 20% and 30%. In those patients surviving, however, recurrent fistulae are rare, and the late prognosis is determined by the stage of the malignancy. Recurrent fistula formation seems to be a uniformly fatal event. Finally, one should remember that, in cases of malignancy in which postoperative histological analysis has identified stage III disease, the medium-term prognosis is poor, even in patients who do not experience the complication of bronchopleural fistula. Therefore, before performing major reintervention in patients who present later with more chronic symptoms, one should consider a more conservative approach, with an attempt at bronchoscopic closure of the fistula and permanent intercostal drainage for the empyema space.

FURTHER READING

Deschamps C, Bernard A, Nichols FC 3rd, Allen MS, Miller DL, Trastek VF, Jenkins GD, Pairolero PC. Empyema and bronchopleural fistula after pneumonectomy: factors affecting incidence. *Annals of Thoracic Surgery* 2001; **72**: 243–7.

Deschamps C, Pairolero PC, Allen MS, Trastek VF. Management of postpneumonectomy empyema and bronchopleural fistula. *Chest Surgery Clinics of North America* 1996; **6**: 519–27.

Lois M, Noppen M. Bronchopleural fistulas: an overview of the problem with special focus on endoscopic management. *Chest* 2005; **128**: 3955–65.

Perelman MI, Rymko LP. Management of empyemas: the problem of associated bronchopleural fistula. In: Thoracic Surgery: Surgical Management of Pleural Disease, eds. Deslauriers J, Lacquet L. In: International Trends in General Thoracic Surgery, Vol 6, CV Mosby, St Louis 1991: 301.

Puskas JD, Mathisen DJ, Grillo HC *et al.* Treatment strategies for bronchopleural fistula. *Journal of Thoracic and Cardiovascular Surgery* 1995; **109**: 989.

Sirbu H, Busch T, Aleksic I, Schreiner W, Oster O, Dalichau H. Bronchopleural fistula in the surgery of non-small cell lung cancer: incidence, risk factors, and management. *Annals of Thoracic and Cardiovascular Surgery* 2001; **7**: 330–6.

Sonobe M, Nakagawa M, Ichinose M, Ikegami N, Nagasawa M, Shindo T. Analysis of risk factors in bronchopleural fistula after pulmonary resection for primary lung cancer. *European Journal of Cardiothoracic Surgery* 2000; **18**: 519–23.

21

Postpneumonectomy empyema

PETER H. HOLLAUS
Consultant, General and Thoracic Surgeon, Department of Thoracic Surgery, Pulmologisched Zentrum Wien, Vienna, Austria

PRINCIPLES AND JUSTIFICATION

Postpneumonectomy emphema (PPE) associated with bronchopleural fistula (BPF) is the most dreaded complication in thoracic surgery. The reported incidence ranges from 2–13%, reaching its peak in the second and third postoperative weeks and declining rapidly thereafter. However, PPE has been reported even 35 years after operation.

PPE is associated with a bronchopleural fistula in approximately 40% of all cases and occurs in our experience in the membranous part of the main bronchus in the majority of cases. Its size ranges from 1 mm to total stump dehiscence.

Mortality ranges from 20–70%, the most common cause of death being aspiration pneumonia with subsequent adult respiratory distress syndrome (ARDS).

The predominant causative organism is *Staphylococcus aureus.* Whether infection starts intrathoracically and leads to perforation of the bronchial stump, or primary breakdown of the bronchial stump allows secondary invasion of the thorax from the bronchial system, is not clearly established. Both pathophysiological mechanisms seem to play a role. Especially in late PPE, hematogenous spread to the postpneumonectomy space is assumed to cause infection.

The reasons why and when PPE occurs remain unclear. Risk factors for BPF have been investigated intensively. Smith et al showed that the pneumonectomy stump heals by second intention in 50% of cases. Thus, poor local blood supply together with overzealous dissection may be responsible.

Advanced age (>70 years), preoperative irradiation, diabetes, malnutrition, malignant invasion of the bronchial stump, male sex, right-sided resections, and completion pneumonectomy are proven risk factors for PPE associated with BPF. The presence of tumor cells in the stump normally is a result of nonradical resection in early BPF. In late fistulas local recurrence leads to bronchial stump breakdown either by itself or via irradiation damage.

While malignant cells, irradiation damage, diabetes, and malnutrition definitely lead to impaired wound healing, these problems are only relevant in a minority of patients. The remaining "risk factors" offer no pathophysiological explanation for the formation of BPF. Technical flaws may be responsible for very early fistulas. Some authors postulate that a long bronchial stump forms a blindsac in which secretions are pooled and become infected if the patient is not capable of removing retentions by coughing. However, this theory has never been challenged by any study and is not proven. Additionally, it does not offer an explanation for the predominance of the right side and of male sex, two proven risk factors for BPF. Some authors even prefer a long stump because it offers more therapeutic options if BPF occurs. Lymphadenectomy is thought to enhance the risk of BPF but does not explain sex and side differences either. Again, statistical confirmation is missing.

BPF mostly occurs after pneumonectomy. Although a high TNM stage has been reported to promote fistula occurrence, it is more probable that the real problem is pneumonectomy itself, which is carried out more often in advanced tumors and, therefore, leads to accumulation of high TNM stages in a selected group compared to patients with lesser resections. Postoperative ventilation also has been accused of promoting fistula formation. However, aspiration pneumonia may be the initial symptom of bronchopleural fistula, which is already present when the patient is referred to the intensive care unit (ICU). Diagnosis of BPF follows later on and may be misinterpreted as a consequence of ventilation.

The sequelae of BPF are aspiration pneumonia, empyema and, in the rare case of total bronchial stump insufficiency, massive air loss with respiratory insufficiency. Aspiration remains the main cause of death if a fistula occurs in the early postoperative period and does not depend on fistula size. Patients still suffer from ventilation/perfusion mismatch and mucous congestion in the remaining lung caused by the procedure and anesthesia. Due to pain, their ability to cough is reduced. If pneumonia occurs in this time, ARDS is nearly inevitable and even results of mechanical ventilation are disastrous. Therefore, the interval between operation and onset of BPF is the most important factor that influences clinical course and outcome. The incidence of aspiration pneumonia reaches its peak during the first two postoperative weeks, until the patient is free of pain and has regained his or her capability to cough, and drops dramatically after the ninetieth postoperative day, when the formation of fibrothorax is completed. Fibrothorax with its multiple small fluid compartments seems to offer an effective protection against fistula formation and aspiration in the late postoperative period. Mortality sharply declines as soon as the risk of aspiration diminishes.

In late fistulas empyema becomes the main problem to deal with. If adequate treatment is delayed, the patient develops sepsis.

With special regard to prognosis and postoperative time BPF can be classified as:

1 Early fistulas, occurring during the first two postoperative weeks with a maximum risk of aspiration pneumonia and, thus, highest mortality.
2 Fistulas occurring between 2 weeks and 3 months after operation. Mortality resulting from aspiration pneumonia is declining due to the patient's postoperative recovery. In this period the patient is already discharged from hospital and may fail to seek adequate treatment. Mortality is still high, though decreasing.
3 Late fistulas occurring later than 3 months after operation. The formation of fibrothorax is completed, and the main problem of BPF becomes empyema of the postpneumonectomy space with sepsis. The mortality is low. The most dangerous postoperative complications comprise fistula or empyema recurrence and persisting infection.

PREOPERATIVE ASSESSMENT AND PREPARATION

The following symptoms occur in cases of bronchopleural fistula: subcutaneous emphysema, dyspnea, fever, fetid breath, serosanguineous expectoration, and productive cough. Lying on the healthy side may lead to cough and expectoration, because in this position the bronchial stump becomes situated under the fluid level in the postpneumonectomy space. Very rarely, patients feel non-neuritic pain in the empty thoracic cavity. In some cases sudden onset of pneumonia is the only sign of bronchopleural fistula and heralds an ominous prognosis.

Clinical symptoms (drop of oxygenation, dyspnea) may be misdiagnosed as pulmonary edema, and diuretics are applied, while the patient is literally drowning in fluid aspirated from the postpneumonectomy space. In cases of late empyema patients complain about fatigue, weight loss, fever, and productive cough. Late PPEs are frequently overlooked until empyema necessitatis occurs.

C-reactive protein (CRP) and white blood count (WBC) rise dramatically and may be the first sign of beginning postpneumonectomy empyema, before clinical symptoms appear. In this early phase aspiration of the pneumonectomy space may yield positive bacterial cultures or a positive gram stain and establishes the diagnosis, but as many as 20% of cases will prove sterile, even when frank pus is drained, probably as a result of previous antibiotic treatment.

In case of an early bronchopleural fistula chest X-ray shows a drop in the fluid level in the postpneumonectomy space. In late empyema multiple fluid levels are visible radiologically after the thoracic cavity had been obliterated in previous films. A computerized tomography (CT) scan provides important diagnostic information on intrathoracic topography in late fistulas or isolated postpneumonectomy empyema. The persistence of air bubbles within the thoracic cavity suggests empyema if clinical symptoms are present. Although big fistulas may be visible, CT is not useful for fistula diagnosis itself.

Often symptoms are rather nonspecific, and a high grade of suspicion is necessary to make the correct diagnosis. If there is any doubt, diagnostic chest tube drainage is justified. If air escapes through the drain, BPF is evident. When pus is evacuated and no air bubbling is visible, a concomitant BPF must be ruled out endoscopically, because the fistula may be covered with fibrin or debris which prevent air leakage temporarily.

Bronchoscopy is performed under general anesthesia with jet ventilation and a rigid bronchoscope. Endoscopic visualization allows assessment of fistula size, identification of local tumor recurrence, and collection of intrabronchial cultures. If a very small fistula is suspected but not visible, indirect diagnosis is achieved by contrast media instilled via the bronchial stump during endoscopy and radiological examination (fistulography). If malignancy is suspected, biopsies should be taken to confirm the diagnosis.

Broad spectrum antibiotics are given parenterally. Debilitated patients require adequate nutrition in terms of calories, protein, and micronutrients.

ANESTHESIA

All operations are performed under general anesthesia with single-lung ventilation via a double-lumen endotracheal tube to avoid air loss through the leakage and further aspiration from the postpneumonectomy space.

OPERATION

Primary treatment

Immediate thoracic drainage must be performed if PPE is suspected. The goal of primary treatment is to prevent aspiration and sepsis originating from empyema. Both goals can be achieved by chest tube drainage.

Until a chest tube is inserted, the patient is turned on the operated side to prevent aspiration. The drain must be placed cranial to the thoracotomy scar to avoid intraabdominal damage. For early PPE, the procedure is carried out under local anesthesia.

In late PPE a thick fibrous layer covers the inner surface of the postpneumonectomy space. Due to scarring, the topography of the inner organs may have changed dramatically making chest tube drainage a dangerous intervention. CT scan provides excellent information on the intrathoracic topography. Rib resection and drain insertion under general anesthesia should be considered in selected cases. Further management depends on whether a fistula is present and the patient's general condition.

Sterilization of the pleural space can only be achieved if a concomitant fistula of the bronchial stump is closed. Fistula treatment options are bronchoscopic sealing with fibin glue and surgical procedures. While surgery remains the primary option, patients in a bad general condition or suffering from metastatic disease may undergo bronchoscopic treatment if their fistula is smaller than 3 mm. If the pleural space is loculated, sepsis may progress despite chest tube drainage. Immediate open window drainage (i.e. fenestration) allows evacuation of empyema, debridement of the postpneumonectomy space, and control of sepsis.

Definitive treatment

The basic goals of operative treatment are debridement of the postpneumonectomy space, closure of the fistula, and sufficient drainage of the thoracic cavity. In our experience obliteration of the postpneumonectomy space is not mandatory and should be reserved for recalcitrant cases. Late PPE is more difficult to treat, because the empyema cavity is thick-walled and the bronchial stump is covered by extensive fibrosis, making dissection of the fistula impossible. Although numerous methods are available to close a BPF, the initial operative steps remain the same, no matter how a fistula is closed.

Surgical principles of fistula repair

In our experience waiting until the mediastinum is fixed is not necessary. We prefer immediate operation and immediate start of antibiotic instillation after surgery. After pneumonectomy, the diaphragm moves upwards. To avoid opening of the abdominal cavity by mistake, secondary thoracotomy should be performed through the original incision or cranially to it. At the beginning of the procedure the thoracic cavity is thoroughly debrided, and bacteriological cultures are taken. After rinsing of the postpneumonectomy space with saline, the bronchial stump is dissected. On the right side the azygous vein is ligated to gain better access to the stump. On the left side the bronchial stump retracts deeply into the mediastinum and is much more difficult to approach.

If the fistula is not visible, the thoracic cavity is filled with water and the patient ventilated under 40 cmH$_2$O positive end-expiratory pressure (PEEP), to locate the fistula. If possible, the stump is refreshed and closed with interrupted sutures (PDS, 3.0 or 4.0). A covering flap (muscle or omentum) is sutured circumferentially around the stump with interrupted sutures (Vicryl 3.0, 4.0), regardless of whether the fistula had been previously closed. At the end of the operation the thoracic cavity is again filled with saline and the endobronchial pressure increased to 40 cm PEEP to assure air tightness.

After irrigation of the entire hemithorax with saline, one or two chest drains are inserted at the most caudal point of the thoracic cavity. Due to the natural organizing process of obliteration after successful empyema eradication, surgical reduction of the postpneumonectomy space should only be considered in cases of fistula or empyema recurrence or in empyemas recalcitrant to conservative measures.

Postpneumonectomy empyema with bronchopleural fistula

If a fistula smaller than 3 mm is present, bronchoscopic closure by submucosal injection of fibrin glue should be considered, especially in patients whose condition is too bad to tolerate surgical intervention. Several tries may be necessary until fistula closure is achieved. Bigger fistulas require surgery.

If the patient is fit enough for surgery, immediate operation should be performed, before aspiration occurs. Several different techniques of closure of the bronchial stump have been described; and to date, no option has proven to be superior to the others. Thus, the use of a particular operation depends on the surgeon's preference.

SIMPLE RE-RESECTION OF THE BRONCHIAL STUMP AND CLOSURE WITH INTERRUPTED SUTURES

This method may be used if the intervention takes place very early, before empyema has occurred. If intrathoracic infection is manifest, the closed stump should be covered.

1a The bronchial stump is approached via the original thoracotomy. On the right side the azygos vein is divided to gain better access to the bronchial stump. On the left side mobilization of the bronchial stump may be difficult due to the fact that it is retracted deeply into the mediastinum. The stump is then isolated from adjacent tissues and reamputated.

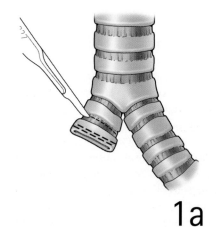

1a

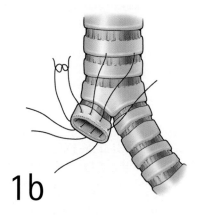

1b

1b,c Only very rarely is the stump long enough to allow the use of a stapling device. After amputation, the stump is closed with interrupted sutures (Vicryl, PDS). If the stump is too short to allow re-amputation, fistula closure is technically impossible, or empyema has already occurred, coverage with viable tissue is indicated.

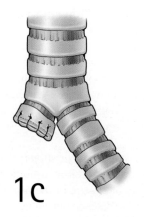

1c

Muscle flap closure of the bronchopleural fistula

Virtually every muscle flap long enough to allow intrathoracic transposition can be used. The most popular techniques comprise the m. pectoralis major, the m. latissmus dorsi, the m. serratus anterior, the diaphragm, and the intercostal muscle.

Muscle flaps also can be used from the m. rectus abdominis and the m. erector spinae.

PRINCIPLES OF MUSCLE FLAP CLOSURE

The survival of a muscle flap depends on the preservation of the vascular pedicle contained in its base. Therefore, precise anatomical knowledge of the supplying arteries is crucial. The vascular pedicle must be identified during operation so that damage of the vessels is avoided.

To avoid tension, extrathoracic muscle flaps require a route of entry into the thoracic cavity which is facilitated by an additional minithoracotomy combined with rib resection over a length of 5–10 cm. The choice of the rib to be resected depends on which flap is chosen and on the location of the vascular pedicle after completed mobilization of the muscle. The opening for the flap must be big enough to prevent kinking or compression. The flaps are fixed circumferentially around the bronchial stump with interrupted sutures.

INTRATHORACIC MUSCLE FLAPS

The advantage of intrathoracic flaps lies in the fact that no functional impairment of the upper extremity occurs.

DIAPHRAGMATIC MUSCLE FLAP

Except for the rare case of diaphragmatic resection, the diaphragm is always available and is never damaged by thoracotomy. Technically, it is the easiest way to close a BPF with a muscle flap. To approach the diaphragm, an additional thoracotomy two intercostal spaces below the original incision is useful.

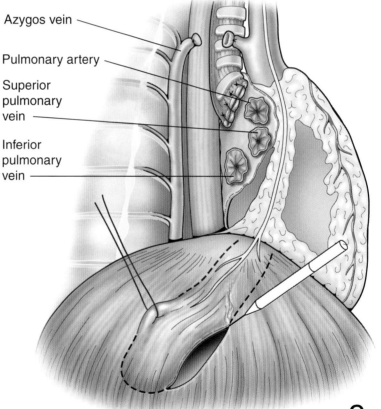

Azygos vein

Pulmonary artery

Superior pulmonary vein

Inferior pulmonary vein

2a The basis of the flap lies at the base of the mediastinum thus preserving branches of the phrenic artery. The diaphragm is elevated with tension sutures and excised with electrocautery. On the right side care has to be taken not to damage the underlying surface of the liver.

2a

2b The diaphragmatic incision is closed during flap excision with interrupted sutures, before tension sutures are removed.

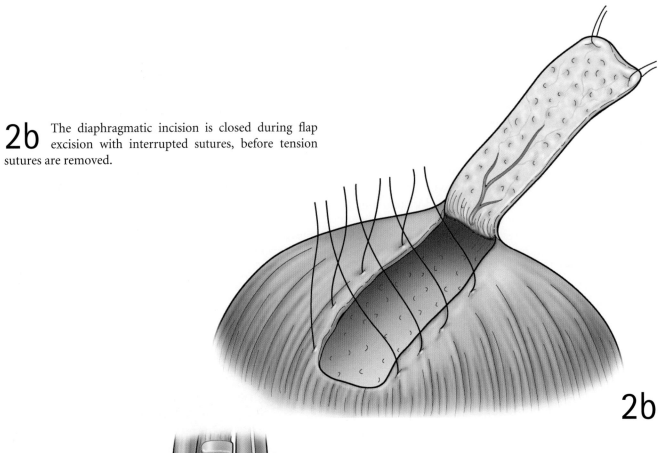

2b

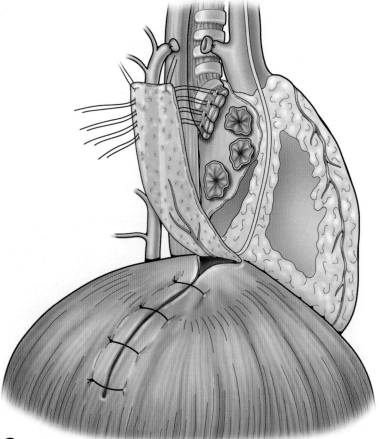

2c The flap is bent upwards and fixed around the bronchial stump with interrupted sutures.

2c

2d The lateral margins of the flap are sutured to the mediastinum.

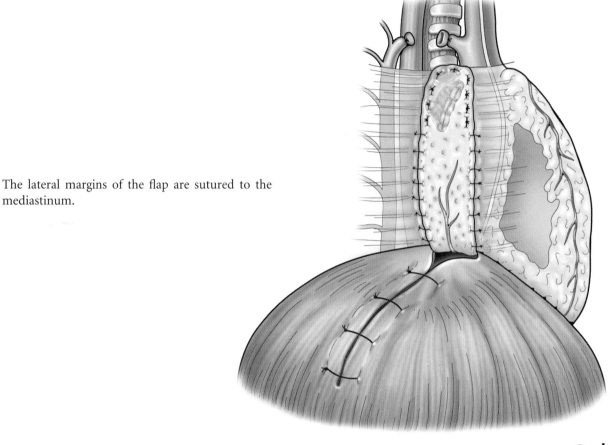

2d

THE INTERCOSTAL MUSCLE FLAP

The advantage of the intercostal muscle lies in the fact that it can reach every position within the thorax, and it has a multiplicity of uses (except in cases of thoracic wall resection). Although ossification originating from the periosteum, which is attached to the flap, was reported, this development does not hamper flap function. The pleura covering the intercostal muscle provides an epithelial surface at the site of the tracheal or bronchial repair and should therefore be left in place. When the intercostal muscle is used, the preparation of the flap is the initial procedure because the

rib spreader might damage the neurovascular bundle of the muscle.

Which intercostal space for the flap is chosen depends on the local situation resulting from rib resection, shrinkage of the chest cavity, and reduction of the intercostal spaces due to scarring.

After rib resection, the neurovascular bundle may be damaged, endangering the function of the muscle. If the muscle adjacent to the primary thoracotomy scar is used, it must be considered that scarring of adjacent structures reduces the mobility of the flap.

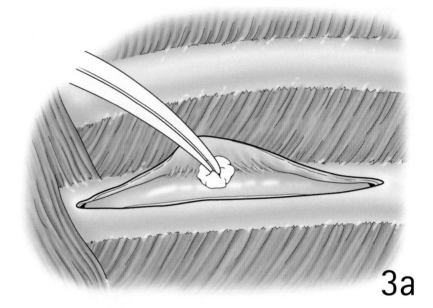

3a

3a,b After incision of the periosteum, the rib is bluntly dissected. Due to the proximity of the neurovascular bundle, the use of electrocautery should be avoided.

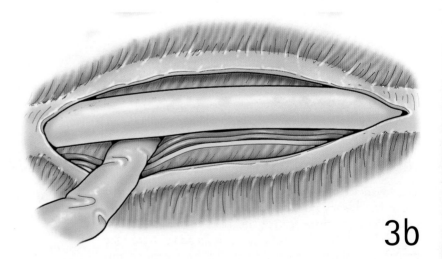

3b

3c After isolation of the rib, it is resected.

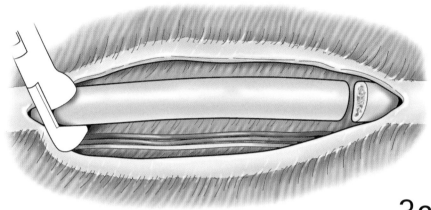

3c

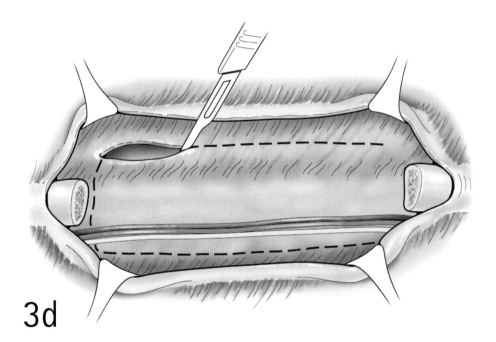

3d

3d The flap is excised from the upper margin of the inferior rib and the lower margin of the superior rib.

3e After ligation, the ventral end of the flap is divided.

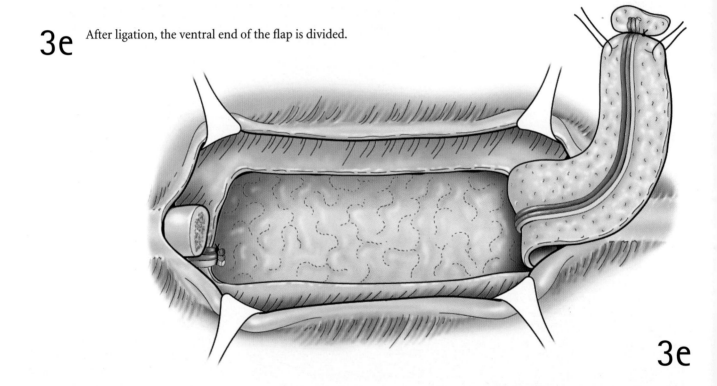

3e

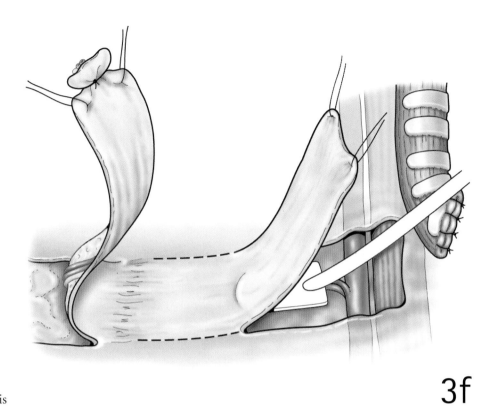

3f

3f,g The parietal pleura is removed along the intended course of the flap.

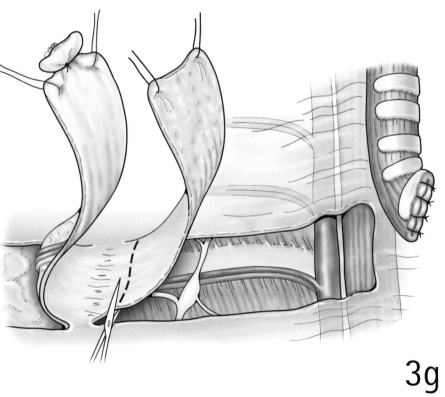

3g

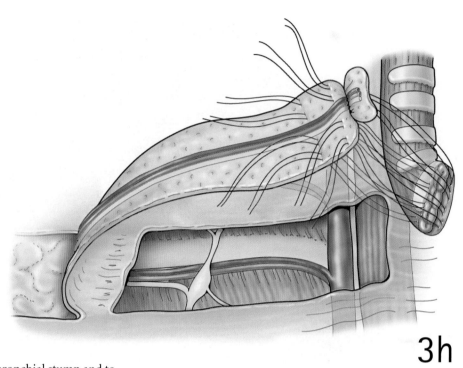

3h

3h,i,j
The flap is fixed to the bronchial stump and to the thoracic wall with interrupted sutures.

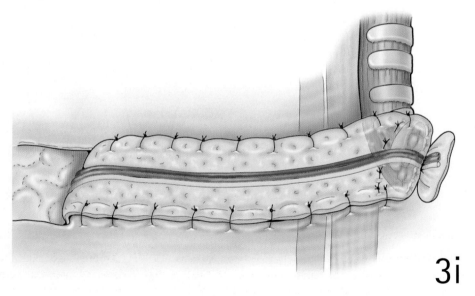

3i

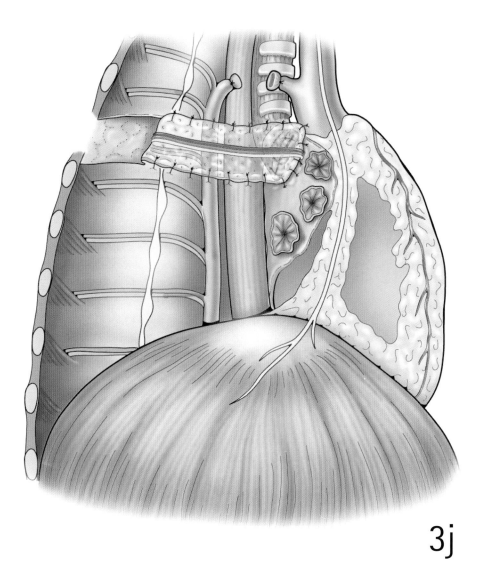

3j

EXTRATHORACIC MUSCLE FLAPS

All extrathoracic flaps can also be used to obliterate the pleural space in case of recalcitrant empyema or fistula recurrence. Closed suction drains are left in the body wall donor sites.

THE PECTORALIS MAJOR MUSCLE FLAP

Like the diaphragm, the m. pectoralis major usually is not damaged by thoracotomy. If this muscle is used, the loss of the anterior axillary fold has to be accepted as a cosmetic handicap.

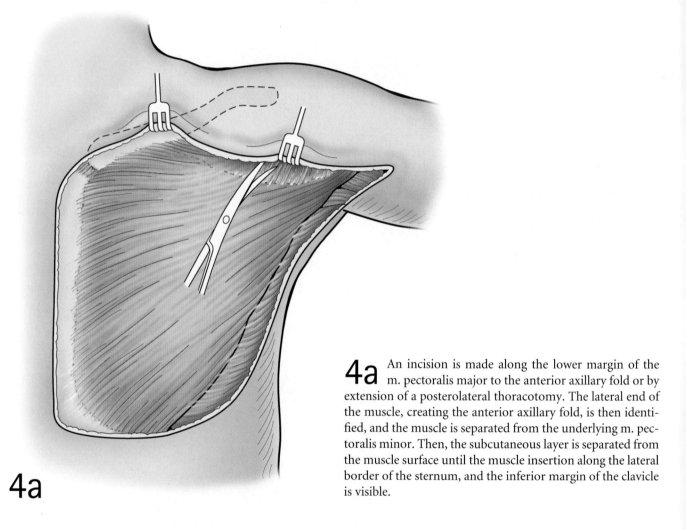

4a An incision is made along the lower margin of the m. pectoralis major to the anterior axillary fold or by extension of a posterolateral thoracotomy. The lateral end of the muscle, creating the anterior axillary fold, is then identified, and the muscle is separated from the underlying m. pectoralis minor. Then, the subcutaneous layer is separated from the muscle surface until the muscle insertion along the lateral border of the sternum, and the inferior margin of the clavicle is visible.

4a

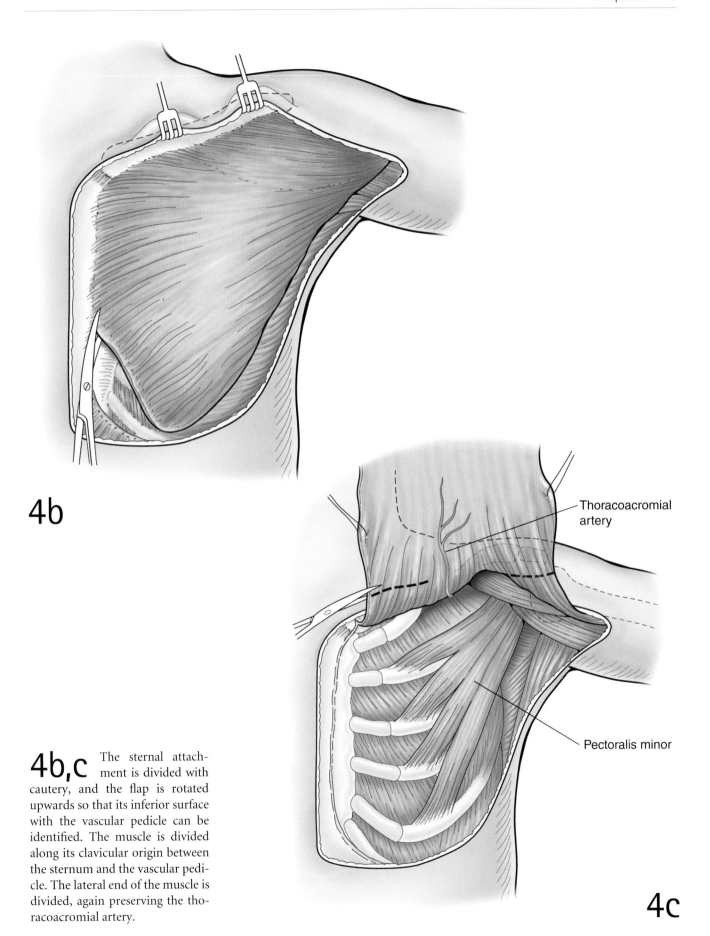

4b

4b,c The sternal attachment is divided with cautery, and the flap is rotated upwards so that its inferior surface with the vascular pedicle can be identified. The muscle is divided along its clavicular origin between the sternum and the vascular pedicle. The lateral end of the muscle is divided, again preserving the thoracoacromial artery.

Thoracoacromial artery

Pectoralis minor

4c

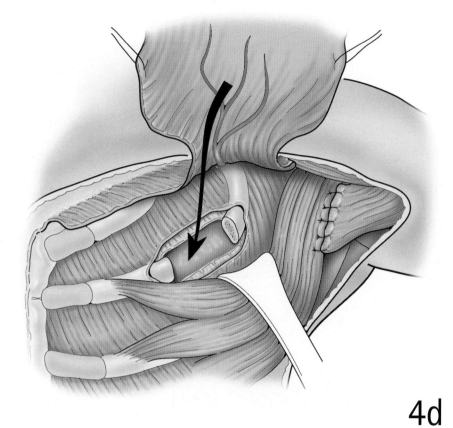

4d

4d–e The lateral muscle stump is oversewn to prevent hematoma. Then, 5–10 cm of the second or third rib are removed in the midclavicular line to allow tension-free intrathoracic transposition of the flap.

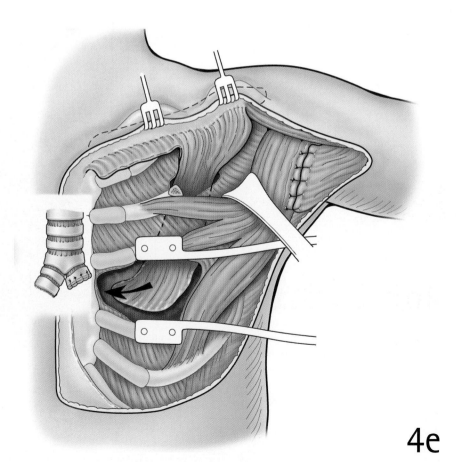

4e

THE LATISSIMUS DORSI FLAP

5a Normally, this muscle is divided during dorsolateral thoracotomy. However, sometimes the portion proximal to the division can still be used as a flap. The latissimus dorsi muscle is approached via a dorsolateral thoracotomy, and the skin is separated from the muscle surface.

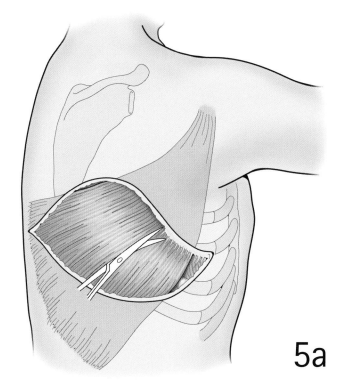

5a

5b The anterior border of the muscle is identified and the plane between the latissimus and the serratus bluntly dissected.

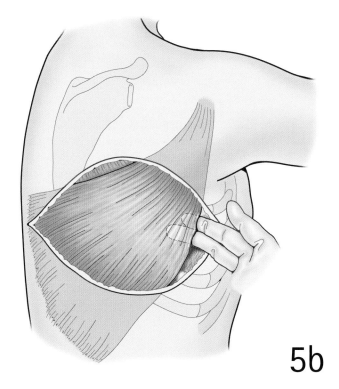

5b

5c The muscle is divided at its posterior and the inferior attachment.

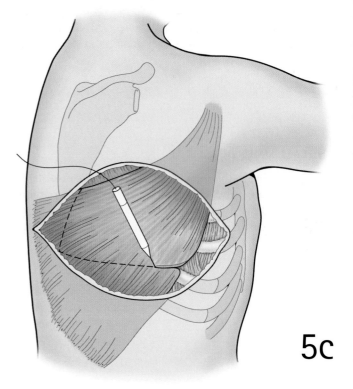

5c

5d The flap is elevated towards the axilla, where the thoracodorsal artery is visualized on its costal surface. The branches of the thoracodorsal artery to the serratus anterior muscle can be divided. Between 5 and 10 cm of the second or third rib are resected in the posterior axillary line as a portal of entry into the thorax.

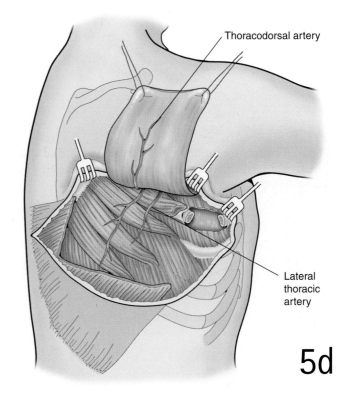

Thoracodorsal artery

Lateral thoracic artery

5d

THE SERRATUS ANTERIOR FLAP

During primary thoracotomy, the serratus anterior muscle may have been divided in its lower fifth. Usually, enough muscle is left to allow intrathoracic transposition. If necessary, the branch of the thoracodorsal artery to the serratus can be divided. Although winging of the medial border of the scapula may occur after flap dissection, very few patients complain about that problem. If possible, the most cranial two to three attachments of the serratus anterior should be preserved to avoid scapular winging.

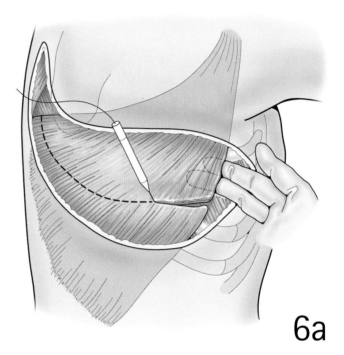

6a

6a After posterolateral thoractomy, the anterior margin of the latissimus dorsi is elevated and bluntly separated from the underlying serratus anterior muscle. Then, the latissimus dorsi muscle is transected.

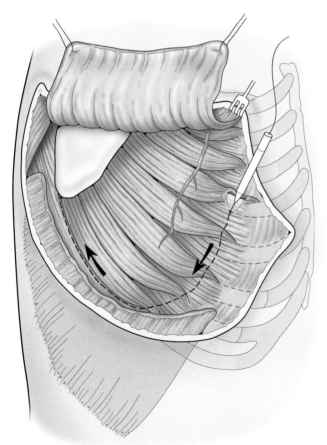

6b After the latissimus has been turned upwards, the lateral thoracic artery is identified on the surface of the serratus anterior. Then, the chest wall attachments are divided with cautery, preserving the lateral thoracic artery and the most cranial insertion at the first and second ribs.

6c The serratus anterior muscle is transected at the lower margin and mobilized from anterior to posterior and from inferior to superior to the scapular tip.

6b,c

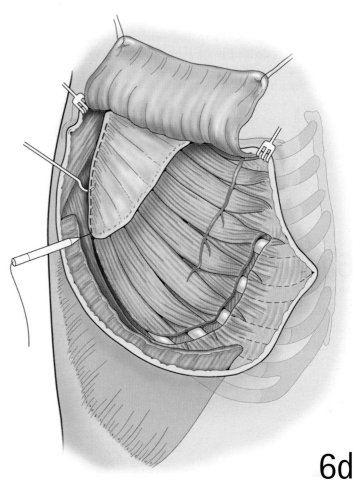

6d

6d After incision of the muscular attachment at the scapular tip, the scapula is elevated.

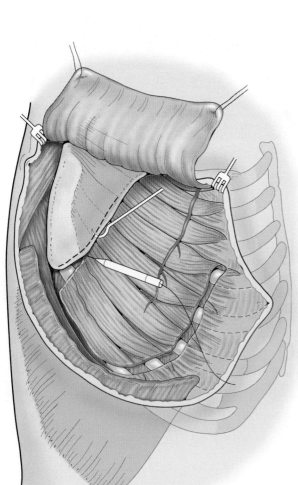

6e

6e Now, the muscular attachments on the costal surface of the scapula are divided with cautery from distal to proximal. Again, the most proximal attachment should be preserved. At the end of this step only the vascular pedicle is left. The most cranial insertions on the first two ribs and the upper part of the costal surface of the scapula should be preserved to avoid winging of the scapula.

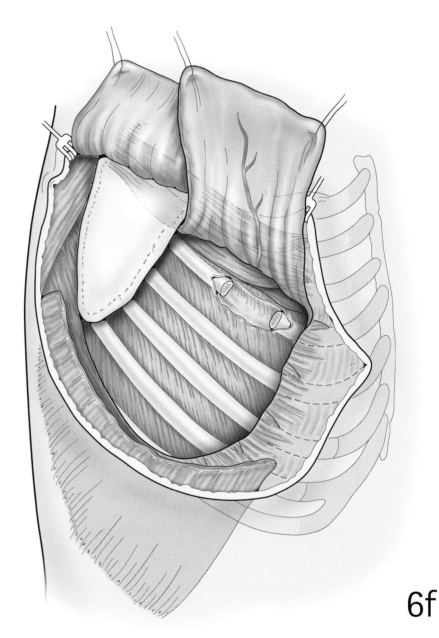

6f Between 5 and 10 cm of the second or third rib are resected in the midaxillary line as a portal of entry into the thorax.

6f

THE OMENTUM FLAP

The disadvantage of omentopexy is the lack of bulk and the necessary laparotomy. The greater omentum may not be available if prior abdominal surgery has been performed, particularly gastric or colonic procedures.

The right gastroepiploic artery is larger than the left one and, therefore, should be preserved. However, in left-sided fistulas it is sometimes beneficial to preserve the left gastroepiploic artery. The omentum is brought up into the thoracic cavity through an opening made around the costal origin of the diaphragm. Rib resection may be necessary to prevent compression.

7a After a superior subcostal incision, the omentum is reflected over the stomach. The posterior fold of the omentum is released from the colon.

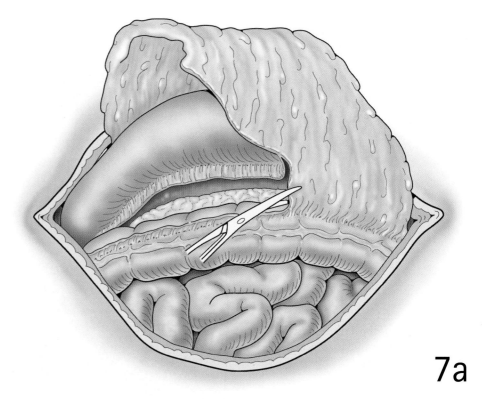

7a

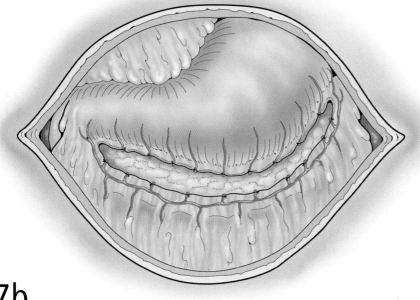

7b

7b The omentum is returned to the inferior abdominal cavity, and the anterior fold is released from the greater curvature of the stomach, preserving the gastroepiploic arch. Depending on the side of the fistula, the contralateral gastroepiploic artery is divided and the flap mobilized. On the right side the omentum is mobilized to within 5 cm of the gastric pylorus to preserve the blood supply of the antrum. On the left side immobilization is performed to within 3 cm of the avascular zone.

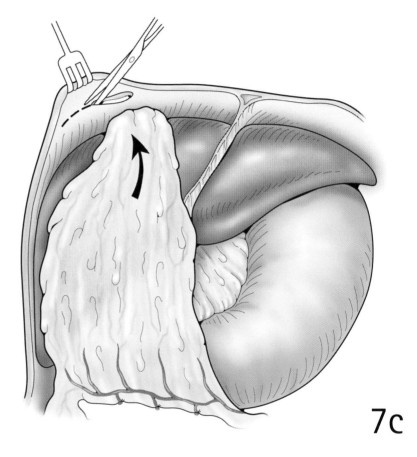

7c An opening at the diaphragmatic insertion is created.

7c

7d The omentum is pushed into the thorax and fixed to the bronchial stump, the mediastinum, and the diaphragmatic gap with interrupted sutures.

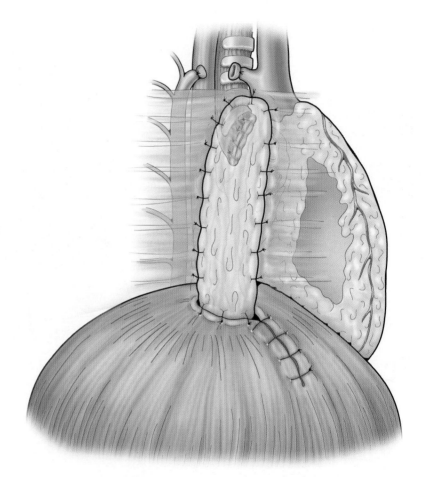

7d

Open window thoracostomy

This method is the procedure of choice to control sepsis originating from empyema. Even debilitated patients may undergo this minor operation. Window thoracostomy may also be combined with muscle flap closure of a bronchopleural fistula. In the latter case the initial rethoracotomy is left open (modified Clagett procedure).

8a Two ribs are resected over a length of 10–12 cm, and the thoracic cavity is opened and debrided. The opening should be big enough to allow insertion of wet dressings up to the apex thoracis once or twice a day, until the pleural space granulates.

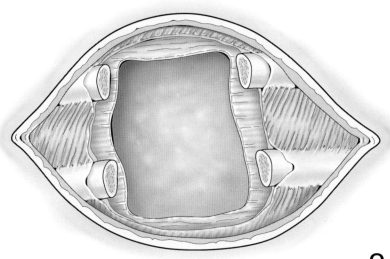

8a

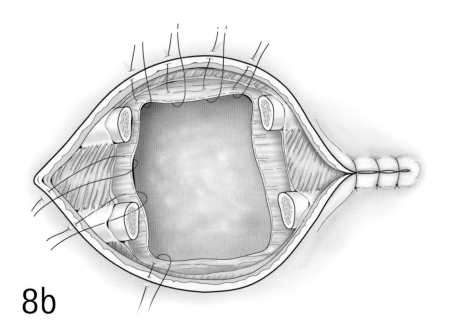

8b

8b The skin is then sutured to the thick fibrous layer that covers the inner surface of the postpneumonectomy space. The rib stumps should be short enough so that they can also be covered with skin fixed to the inner surface of the thorax.

At the end of the operation the thoracic cavity is packed with gauze dipped in an antiseptic solution. The dressing is changed once or twice a day depending on the severity of infection, and this procedure can be performed in bed with anesthesia. When infection has subsided, the thoracostomy can be closed.

THE CLAGETT PROCEDURE

The Clagett procedure requires open window thoracostomy with daily change of dressings until infection subsides and the thoracic cavity starts to granulate. After filling the hemithorax with an antibiotic solution, the thoracostomy is closed. Although very popular in the United States, the Clagett procedure has the disadvantage of a long duration of treatment, the need for a second surgical intervention and a high recurrence rate of 40%. When multiple bacterial organisms cause the infection, the success rate is about 20%. Up to a third of all patients will not be amenable to chest wall closure because of tumor recurrence or respiratory failure.

POSTPNEUMONECTOMY EMYPEMA WITHOUT BRONCHOPLEURAL FISTULA

If BPF is ruled out, a less aggressive approach is justified.

Simple drainage with antibiotic irrigation

After chest tube drainage, the tube is irrigated with antibiotics according to culture sensitivity between two and three times a day. After instillation, the drain is clamped for several hours. One major drawback of simple irrigation is the fact that debridement of the empty hemithorax is not achieved. Even if infection has subsided, the remaining intrathoracic debris still harbors organisms as a potential source for late recurrence. Additionally, antibiotic irrigation of the postpneumonectomy space can be a lengthy procedure until sterility of the thoracic cavity is achieved.

Videothoracoscopy

Videothoracoscopic debridement of the postpneumonectomy space is a simple procedure which is well tolerated by any patient. Videothoracoscopy alone does not allow the exclusion of a fistula diagnosis, as the bronchial stump is often covered with a thick layer of granulation tissue, making visual localization impossible, especially if the fistula is small. Therefore, bronchoscopy is mandatory before videothoracoscopy. If a fistula is diagnosed, open operation should be performed.

Videothoracoscopy is performed in the supine position. A camera port and a working port are inserted cranially to the thoracotomy scar. Intrathoracic debris is mobilized and removed with a long plastic suction unit, endoscopic forceps, a swab on a stick, or with a sharp spoon. The pleural space is rinsed at the end of the procedure, and a chest tube is inserted at the most caudal point of the thorax. If videothoracoscopy or irrigation fail, infection is controlled by open wide debridement, total thoracoplasty, or muscle plombage of the postpneumonectomy space.

POSTOPERATIVE CARE

Postoperative pulse oximetry is mandatory. A decrease in oxygen saturation may result from fistula recurrence with consecutive aspiration and requires bronchoscopy and reoperation. The most probable reason for this complication is flap necrosis due to kinking or tension, both technical flaws, or progressive stump necrosis.

If the bronchial stump is tight, empyema may still recur or persist. This situation is heralded by fever and a rise of WBC and CRP and also requires reoperation.

In the ward the empty hemithorax is irrigated with antibiotic solution via the chest tube according to culture results twice a day, starting on the first day after operation. After instillation, the drain is clamped for 3 hours; and the patient, if capable, is encouraged to leave bed. Repeated radiological examination of the chest reveals pneumonia due to silent aspiration and the development of multiple fluid levels in the empty hemithorax, which may be an early sign of empyema recurrence. The drainage volume is recorded every 24 hours. A decrease of drainage volume indicates successful empyema control.

Cultures should be obtained twice a week. After three consecutive negative cultures, the infection may be considered eradicated, and the drain is removed. Thereafter, the patient is kept in hospital for another week, CRP and WBC being measured regularly. If no clinical signs of infection or fistula recurrence exist and the blood results are within normal levels, the patient is discharged.

OUTCOME

If the patient escapes aspiration pneumonia, early BPF can be successfully closed by muscle or omentum in 80–90% of cases. In late fistulas the success rate by various treatments lies within 60%.

The results of treatment of isolated PPE are difficult to interpret, since very few cases are published. Wong et al achieved permanent healing in eight of 13 patients after a mean irrigation time of 12 weeks. Videothoracoscopic treatment of simple PPE was successful in five consecutive patients without recurrence.

FURTHER READING

Hollaus PH, Lax F, El-Nashef B, Hauck HH, Lucciarini P, Pridun NS. Natural history of bronchopleural fistula after pneumonectomy: a review of 96 cases. *Annals of Thoracic Surgery* 1997; **63**: 1391–7.

Hollaus PH, Lax F, Wurnig PN, Pridun NS. Videothoracoscopic treatment of postpneumonectomy empyema. *Journal of Thoracic and Cardiovascular Surgery* 1999; **117:** 397–8.

Pairolero PC, Phillip GA, Trastek VF, Meland NB, Kay PP, Arnold PG. Postpneumonectomy empyema: the role of intrathoracic muscle transposition. *Journal of Thoracic and Cardiovascular Surgery* 1990; **99:** 1958–68.

Smith DE, Karish AF, Chapman JP, Takaro T. Healing of the bronchial stump after pulmonary resection. *Journal of Thoracic and Cardiovascular Surgery* 1963; **46:** 548

Wong PS, Goldstraw P. Post-pneumonectomy empyema. *European Journal of J Cardiothoracic Surgery* 1994; **8:** 345–50

Empyema, spaces and fistula. *Chest Surgery Clinics of North America* 1996; **6:** 503–71.

22

Decortication of the lung

C. PETER CLARKE MB, BS, FRACS, FACS
Professorial Fellow, Department of Surgery, University of Melbourne; Senior Thoracic Surgeon, Austin Health, Heidelberg, Victoria, Australia

HISTORY

Jason of Greek mythology developed a fever and wasting and, fearful of dying in bed, led his force into battle. An assailant speared him in the chest, releasing a gush of pus, and with renewed energy he ungratefully slew his nameless surgeon and went on to make a complete recovery. Hippocrates (460–377 BC) gave a remarkably accurate account of empyema. He noted that if patients survived two weeks, they should have dependent drainage and packing of the wounds. Serefeddin Sabuncouglu (1385–1470) was a military surgeon in the Persian Empire who had a good understanding of empyema occurring after penetrating chest wounds and at the age of 80 wrote a masterly text on surgery entitled 'Imperial Surgery'.

After this promising start, surprisingly little progress was made in the understanding and management of empyema until the nineteenth century. In 1843, Trousseau introduced the concept of thoracentesis by needle aspiration, and Hewitt proposed closed pleural drainage in 1876.

In chronic situations when the lung was trapped and would not re-expand, the initial approach was to manage the cavity by open drainage or thoracoplasty. In 1893, Fowler reported the first successful decortication for empyema. The term *decortication* was popularized in 1896 by Delorme, who gave a clear description of the procedure designed to remove the thick parietal and visceral pleura, and allow the lung to re-expand to fill the thoracic space and the chest wall to regain its mobility.

PRINCIPLES AND JUSTIFICATION

Decortication is most commonly performed for established empyema or fibrothorax, and less commonly for trapped lung in patients with an effusion and malignancy. The usual cause of an empyema is parapneumonic infection, and an empyema occurs in approximately 5% of cases of pneumonia with an associated effusion. Other causes are trauma, complications of surgery, and specific infective situations, for example, tuberculous or a lung abscess. A hemothorax after trauma, if undrained, eventually results in a trapped lung due to a thick fibrous layer, the so called 'fibrothorax'.

1a, b, c

An empyema classically progresses through three phases:

1 Exudative
2 Fibropurulent with loculations
3 Organizing with a thick fibrin wall

An exudative empyema is watery with a leucocyte count of less than 6 400 per mL. At this stage it can be conveniently drained by a wide-bore needle, an image-guided catheter placed under radiographic or ultrasonographic control, or an intercostal catheter.

If the effusion is not completely drained, it then evolves into a multi-loculated fibropurulent lesion, which requires a more formal approach for management. Often the empyema is sterile after treatment by appropriate antibiotics, and the patient is no longer toxic; but if the lesion is left, the underlying lung becomes entrapped, which leads to the ongoing danger of recrudescence of local infection.

At this stage, the insertion of an intercostal catheter, even with the adjunctive use of streptokinase, is ineffective, and the treatment choice is between a muscle-sparing minithoracotomy or a video-assisted thoracoscopic clean-out of the space and removal of peel from the underlying lung.

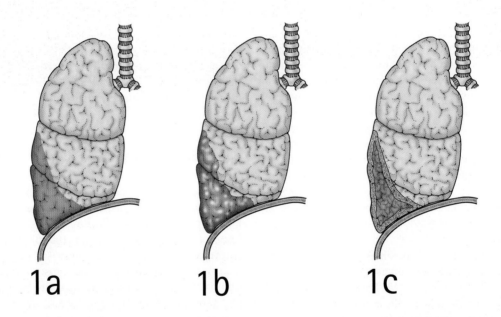

1a   1b   1c

PREOPERATIVE ASSESSMENT AND PREPARATION

A video-assisted thoracic surgery (VATS) approach results in a shorter hospital stay and less postoperative morbidity and is the procedure of choice. The exact stage at which an empyema becomes mature and the peel can no longer be handled by a VATS approach is often blurred, and the surgeon should not hesitate to open the chest and proceed with a formal decortication if necessary. In my hands the conversion rate has been 30%, but the rate inevitably varies depending on the enthusiasm with which the VATS approach is used.

OPERATION

Video-assisted thoracoscopic approach

2a, b The best studies for detecting and localizing a fibropurulent empyema are the computed tomographic scan and percutaneous ultrasonography. Figure 2a is a computed tomographic scan that shows a loculated empyema treated by decortication using VATS. Figure 2b is an ultrasonogram of a basal right loculated collection.

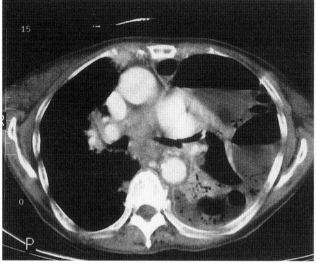

2a

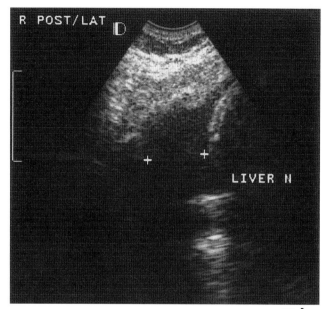

2b

3 The operation is carried out under an anesthetic using a double-lumen tube, which allows protection of the dependent lung. The patient is placed in the full lateral position with the scapula pulled well forward. A three-point triangular approach is used, and modified sponge holders and large-bore suction devices are used to evacuate the pleural space of debris. Usually only one port for the telescope is required as the other instruments are easily introduced through short incisions. The port for the telescope is moved along with the instrument for better lateral views.

If the peel over the parietal pleura is soft, it can be safely worked off the underlying structures with the modified sponge holders. The space is then irrigated with an antibiotic saline solution, and two or more drainage tubes are left *in situ* via the port sites. Care should be taken to check that the underlying lung re-expands to fill this space. Gentle suction is applied postoperatively.

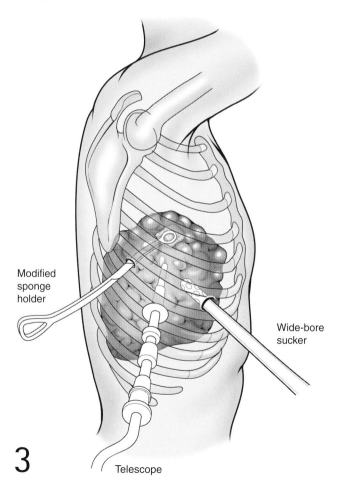

Modified sponge holder

Wide-bore sucker

3

Telescope

Decortication

Mature empyemas with a thick rind require a formal decortication via a thoracotomy unless the patient is too frail or has significant comorbidity that rules out a major procedure in which case a rib resection and drainage is preferable. It used to be advised that it was necessary to wait six weeks for the peel to mature and strip more easily, but modern imperatives mandate proceeding with treatment expeditiously.

4 The peel over the parietal pleura splints the chest wall and causes the ribs to become contracted as it matures. The peel over the lung entraps it and prevents it from re-expanding. If the ribs are contracted, then a full rib resection during the approach is helpful and aids in starting to strip the parietal pleura from the chest wall before inserting a rib spreader.

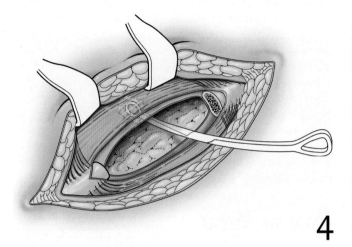

4

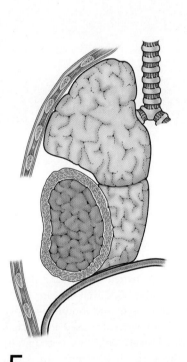

5

5 The aim of the procedure is to perform a total empyectomy. This goal is often not feasible because of difficulties at the apex and over the diaphragm, and frequently the cavity must be opened and the visceral pleura approached directly.

6 The peel should be stripped from the lung with care using a peanut on a long artery forceps for blunt dissection to avoid air leaks as far as possible.

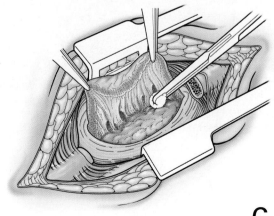

6

7 The fissures should be cleared and, in extreme cases in which the peel is adherent to the lung without an apparent plane, it can be cut in a crosshatched manner and the anesthetist asked to vigorously reinflate the lung.

Obtaining full reinflation of the lung is important, as any residual space will lead to a further empyema, and this goal can usually be accomplished with persistence. On rare occasions a small space will remain despite the surgeon's best efforts, in which case it can be filled with a muscle flap. Small superficial air leaks can be ignored as they will stop when the lung abuts the chest wall, but any tears in the lung should be sutured with an absorbable suture or treated with tissue glue. Oozing from the raw chest surface can be a problem and must receive attention. Two or more intercostal catheters are left *in situ* and placed on gentle suction, and physiotherapy is started as soon as the patient is awake. Antibiotics should be continued to cover at least the early postoperative period.

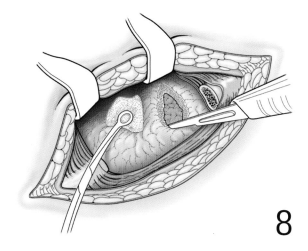

7

POSTOPERATIVE CARE

Postpneumonic empyemas are generally easier to treat than specific empyemas such as those due to tuberculosis, but the principles are the same. Similarly, although children have remarkable powers of healing compared with adults, they should not be left with thickened pleura and splinted chest walls, and an aggressive approach using a VATS technique in early cases and open decortication in later cases is justifiable.

8 A small number of patients exist with trapped lung and malignant effusions when the peel is infiltrated with tumor which prevents easy dissection yet where decortication is useful. These include patients with stable carcinoma of the breast who have neglected malignant effusions and patients with localized malignant mesothelioma who are having debulking of the tumor before adjunct phototherapy. In these cases the tumor cells grow directly into the lung, which prevents simple removal of the rind and requires careful excision with a scalpel.

This procedure results in superficial air leaks; but if the lung can fully re-expand, these leaks generally cease within a few days. The lung should be tested by re-expansion under saline, and any large leaks should be managed by direct suture, superficial diathermy, or tissue glue. Two or more drain tubes are then introduced and gentle suction is applied.

8

OUTCOMES

The earlier an empyema is treated, the better the outcome, as there is less likelihood of ending up with residual pleural thickening leading to splinting of the chest with impaired pulmonary function.

The best results can be expected in younger patients and those without significant co-morbidities. In older patients, and particularly when there are associated problems, a balance has to be struck between the desire to end up with a good functional result and the dangers of major operative procedures.

FURTHER READING

Angelillo-Mackinlay T. Empyema and haemothorax. In: Yim APC, Izzat MB, Landreneau RJ, Mack MJ, Naunheim KS eds. *Minimal access cardiothoracic surgery.* Philadelphia: WBSaunders, 2000: 48–57.

Maskell NA, Davies CW, Nunn AJ, *et al.* First Multicentre Intrapleural Sepsis Trial (MIST) Group. UK Controlled Trial of intrapleural streptokinase for pleural infection. *New England Journal of Medicine* 2005; **352:** 865–74.

Shields TW. Decortication of the lung. In: Shields TW ed. *General thoracic surgery.* Baltimore: Williams & Wilkins, 1994: 710–13.

Striffeler H, Gugger M, Im Hof V, Cerny A, Furrer M, Ris HB. Video-assisted thoracoscopic surgery for fibrinopurulent pleural empyema in 67 patients. *Annals of Thoracic Surgery* 1998; **65:** 319–23.

Thurer RJ. Decortication in thoracic empyema. *Chest Surgery Clinics of North America* 1996; **6**(3): 461–90.

23

Thoracic incisions

M. BLAIR MARSHALL MD
Chief, Division of Thoracic Surgery, Georgetown University Medical Center, Washington DC, USA

PRINCIPLES AND JUSTIFICATION

In approaching the chest, numerous options are available to choose from as a means of entry into the thorax. These approaches can be modified to fit special circumstances. The art of thoracic surgery starts with the decision-making for each approach with or without modifications to suit each particular situation.

OPERATION

Posterolateral thoracotomy

The posterolateral thoracotomy has been the incision of choice for many thoracic procedures and continues to be the most frequently used incision. The incision gives full exposure of the entire thoracic cavity and has stood the test of time. When made through the fifth intercostal space, the hilum can be readily accessed for exposure and control of the pulmonary artery, veins, the distal trachea, and bronchi.

A sandbag is placed on the operating table prior to putting the patient on the table. The patient is induced with general anesthesia after placement of a thoracic epidural catheter. A Foley catheter and pneumatic compression stockings are placed. The endotracheal tube is positioned, and bronchoscopy is performed evaluating the trachea, right and left bronchi down to the subsegmental level. We then change the endotracheal tube to a double-lumen tube, and the patient is placed in the full lateral decubitus position. The patient's superior posterior iliac spine is positioned at the level of the break in the table. The free arm is brought up, flexed at the elbow, and supported with a padded armrest. The bottom leg is flexed at the knee, and pillows are placed between the legs. Frequently, the bottom foot will need additional padding. The bed is maximally flexed to stretch the intercostal space. The axilla is usually adequately protected by the beanbag, although in some cases additional protection is required. The chest is prepped and draped.

1a The standard skin incision follows an arc between two anatomical points, the first being 2 cm below the inferior border of the scapula and the second being the mid-point between the thoracic spine and the medial margin of the scapula. From this arc, the lateral extension of the incision continues across horizontally as needed. The posterior extent of this incision may be continued up to the base of the neck paralleling the spine for a posterior approach to superior sulcus tumors and other chest wall resections. The length of the incision is determined by the extent of the procedure being performed.

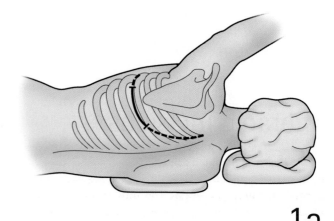

1a

Once the skin and subcutaneous tissues have been divided, the latissimus dorsi is divided. Small vessels are cauterized. In the case of a limited incision, we try to spare the serratus anterior. The areolar tissue along the posterior edge of the serratus is divided obliquely extending inferiorly toward the anterior margin of the latissimus. The incision is continued between the latissimus and serratus allowing for further mobilization. When a more extensive posterior incision is required, as for first rib resections, it may be necessary to divide the inferior border of the trapezius and the rhomboids to lift the scapula away from the chest wall.

Next, the thoracotomy is made by dividing the intercostal muscles along the top border of the sixth rib through the fifth intercostal space (ICS). The fifth ICS is identified by counting the ribs beneath the scapulae. We use the insertion of the posterior scalene onto the second rib as the starting point for counting. Relying on palpation of the first rib may be misleading. We do not routinely resect a posterior margin of rib although this maneuver may be helpful in reoperative surgery. One must keep the mammary vessels in mind to avoid their inadvertent injury during the anterior division of the intercostal muscles. Posteriorly, the intercostals can be divided to the angle of the rib. We try to elevate the thoracicus iliacus and sacrospinalis off the posterior ribs and spine rather than dividing them when the thoracotomy extends posteriorly. This maneuver is particularly useful in the elderly patient with osteoporotic fragile ribs who is at greater risk for rib fractures. The Finnichietto retractor is inserted and slowly opened. Gradual opening of this retractor during the dissection helps to prevent rib fractures that contribute to postoperative pain and subsequent morbidity.

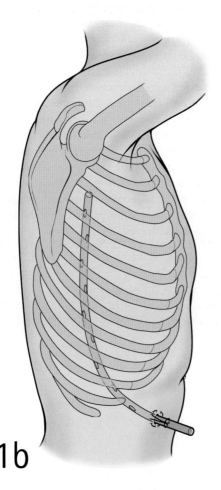

1b

1b After performing the procedure, we place a single chest tube through a lateral tunnel. This chest tube is modified by cutting additional drainage holes. By placing the tube in this fashion, the chest tube courses along the sulcus between the diaphragm and chest wall, then curves posteriorly with the tip resting at the apex. This position allows for complete drainage of the thoracic cavity with a single tube.

1c,d
After unflexing the table, the ribs are reapproximated with a large absorbable suture. We do not overapproximate the ribs but bring them to their normal anatomical position. The muscle layers are closed meticulously, especially posteriorly where the trapezius and rhomboids may have been divided. If a rib has been removed, we approximate the intercostal muscles with an absorbable suture. The various layers are irrigated as they are closed. The fascia is reapproximated, and the skin is closed.

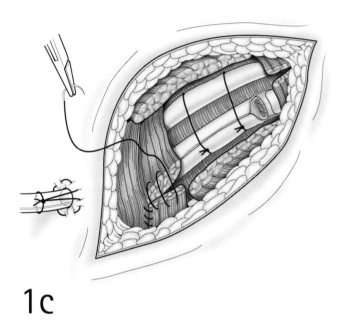

1c

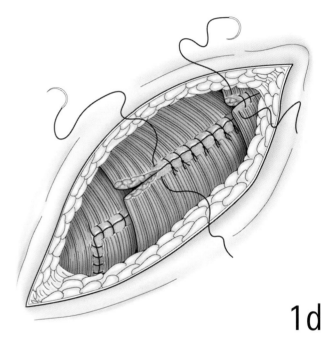

1d

Muscle-sparing thoracotomy

VERTICAL AXILLARY INCISION

The posterolateral thoracotomy is the incision of choice for many thoracic surgeons; however, we frequently reserve this incision for extensive resections and more commonly use a vertical axillary muscle-sparing thoracotomy. For an uncomplicated lobectomy or other intrathoracic procedures, this incision has the advantage that none of the muscles are divided, it ensures excellent exposure, less postoperative pain, and improved cosmesis. Also, because only the intercostal muscles are divided and because it is much shorter, this incision can be closed more rapidly.

2 The patient is positioned as for a posterolateral thoraco-tomy except the axilla is opened slightly by rotating the shoulder slightly posteriorly to expose the axilla. In women we usually place the incision along the lateral breast crease. Care should be taken not to make the incision too far posteriorly because injury to the long thoracic nerve may occur.

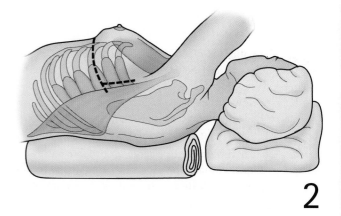

2

The subcutaneous tissues are divided exposing the serratus anterior and the lateral margin of the pectoralis major. Usually, one cannot count the ribs posteriorly as in a postero-lateral thoracotomy so they must be counted anteriorly. The best landmark for doing this is the tubercle of the first rib. The surgeon's hand is placed up through the axillary space in order to palpate this tubercle. When proceeding with this aspect of the incision, it is best to elevate the insertion of the serratus from the ribs initially; this maneuver defines the plane between the intercostal muscles and the serratus. Proceeding in this fashion will allow for easier exposure of this plane. Once the serratus has been mobilized from the third to the fifth rib, enough laxity of this muscle exists to proceed with the thoracotomy. The intercostal muscles are divided along the superior aspect of the fifth rib in the fourth intercostal space. Using an army/navy retractor to elevate the serratus exposes the intercostal muscle for division. A small rib spreader is used to separate the ribs, and then a Balfour retractor is placed perpendicular to this to hold the serratus and other soft tissues out of the field.

MUSCLE-SPARING POSTEROLATERAL THORACOTOMY

The patient is positioned as for a regular posterolateral thoraco-tomy. The skin incision is made along the standard skin incision for a posterolateral thoracotomy, centered on the posterior axillary line. The subcutaneous tissue is divided, and the lateral margin of the latissimus is mobilized initially. The anterior margin of the serratus is mobilized by dividing the areolar tissue as in the posterolateral thoracotomy. Once this step is done, the thoracotomy is made through the fifth intercostal space as in the standard posterolateral thoraco-tomy.

Thoracoabdominal incision

This incision is most commonly used for thoracoabdominal aortic operations, gastroesophageal junction tumors, or other procedures where combined access to the chest and abdomen is necessary. The incision may vary according to the intent of the operation, i.e. whether it is necessary to come midline on the abdomen or how high to make the thoracotomy for exposure of the distal arch.

The patient is placed on a beanbag in a right lateral decubitus position with the left hip rotated to provide exposure of the abdomen and groin. The thoracic incision extends from the posterior axillary line, across the costal margin, and continues on the abdomen in either a paramedian or median fashion. The thoracotomy is made through the sixth to the ninth interspace depending on how high in the chest exposure is required. The incision comes across the costal arch and then is extended onto the abdomen. The diaphragm is divided circumferentially leaving enough muscle along the chest wall to hold sutures. While dividing the diaphragm, we place sutures of alternating color on either side of the cut diaphragm to facilitate reapproximation at the end of the procedure.

Following the procedure, the diaphragm is reapproximated, and chest tubes are placed. We usually resect a margin of cartilage at the costochondral junction. Because the junction usually heals poorly, resecting a margin prevents postoperative pain from a nonunion. We place the paracostal sutures but do not tie them. The abdominal fascia is closed, and then the paracostal sutures are tied.

Median sternotomy

This incision may be used to access the mediastinum and both pleural spaces. Thoracic surgeons have found this particular incision useful for bilateral metastectomy, volume reduction surgery, and resection of anterior mediastinal tumors. Anatomical resections may be performed through this incision but can be a more challenging operation than that performed through a thoracotomy. The position of the heart makes a left lower lobectomy particularly difficult.

3a The patient is placed in the supine position. A rolled sheet is placed behind the shoulders. The patient is prepped from the neck to abdomen. The skin incision is made just below the sternal notch down to the xyphoid. The fascia is divided, and the ligament at the sternal notch is divided with electrocautery.

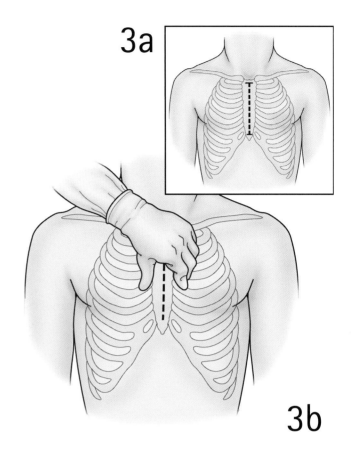

3a

3b The midline is determined by palpating the intercostal spaces on either side of the sternum. We usually mark this point with electrocautery to use as a guide for the sternal saw. This step is to avoid an uneven cut through the sternum.

3b

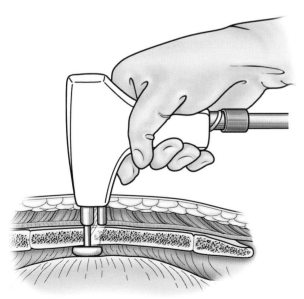

3c The reciprocating sternal saw is placed with the bottom blade hugging the deep border of the sternum, and the sternotomy is made. Once this step is done, each half of the sternum is elevated, and periosteal bleeders are identified and cauterized. If continued bleeding ensues from the sternal marrow, bone wax may be used to stop this. However, we do not use bone wax routinely. A sternal or hemisternal retractor is positioned and slowly opened. A brachial plexus injury can occur if the sternum is opened too widely. For pulmonary parenchymal procedures, the hemisternal retractor is useful. Also, when working posteriorly, placing laparotomy packs can aid in bringing the lung up toward the operative field.

3c

3d Once the procedure has been completed, thoracostomy tubes are placed. The sternum is reapproximated with sternal wires, and the fascia overlying the sternum is closed with a running absorbable suture. One should be aware of the location of the internal mammary vessels to avoid their inadvertent injury at the time of chest closure.

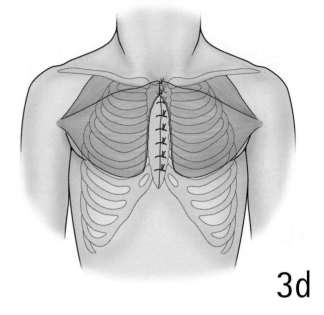

3d

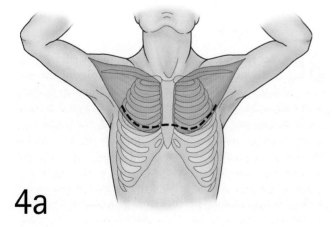

4a

Bilateral thoracosternotomy

4a This approach to the chest has been used most frequently for bilateral sequential lung transplantation. It provides excellent exposure of the hilum as well as the heart and great vessels. Initially, a bilateral submammary incision is made. The subcutaneous tissues and pectoralis muscles are divided exposing the ribs. The fourth intercostal space is opened lateral to medial. The mammary vessels are located approximately 1 cm lateral to the sternal edge. They are identified and ligated.

4b,c

Blunt dissection is used to free the sternum from the underlying mediastinum, and a Lebsche knife is used to divide the sternum horizontally. The anterior chest wall is lifted superiorly and anteriorly by placing two Finnichietto retractors in each intercostal space.

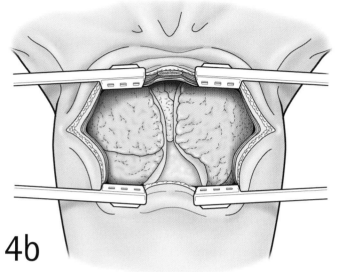

4b

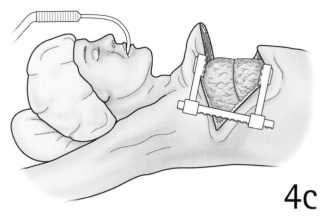

4c

Once the procedure has been performed, bilateral pleural thoracostomy tubes are placed with additional mediastinal tubes as needed. The ribs are reapproximated with heavy paracostal sutures. These sutures are placed but not tied. Two sternal wires are used to bring the sternal edges together, and then the paracostal sutures are tied. The muscles and soft tissues are reapproximated.

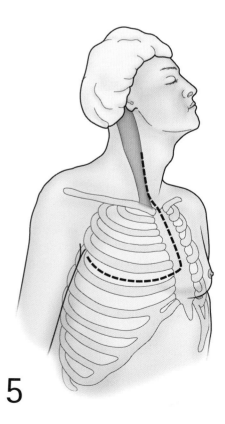

5

Thoracosternotomy

5

A thoracosternotomy is usually performed in the operative management of anterior mediastinal tumors. The incision is carried along the ipsilateral sternocleidomastoid to the sternal notch down to the level of the inframammary fold. It then follows the contour of the inframammary fold across to the anterior axillary line. The incision is then deepened with cautery through the fascia down to the middle of the sternum. Inferiorly, the fascia is divided below the breast. The pectoralis muscle overlying the fourth ICS is divided exposing the underlying chest wall. The fourth intercostal space is entered laterally and the incision continued medially. Usually, it is necessary to divide the mammary vessels. Next, the sternal saw is used to divide the sternum to the level of the fourth intercostal space and is then brought across the remaining sternum. A Ruhltract retractor is used to elevate the chest wall and provide exposure of the anterior mediastinum and thoracic cavity.

After performing the procedure, the sternum is reapproximated with number 5 wires, and the ribs are reapproximated with a large absorbable suture. Again, the paracostal sutures are placed but not tied. The sternal wires are placed. The muscle and soft tissues are closed in the usual fashion.

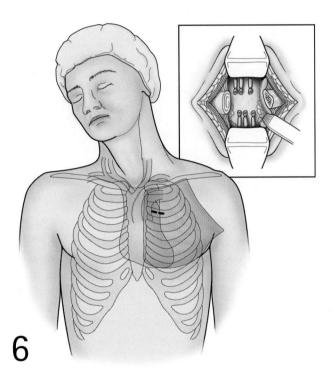

6

Anterior mediastinotomy

6 This incision is used to biopsy nodes or masses in the superior mediastinum. A 2-cm incision is made overlying the second costal cartilage, and the subcutaneous tissues are divided. The muscle fibers of the pectoralis major are divided exposing the periosteum overlying the second rib. The periosteum is incised and dissected away from the rib. Once it has been circumferentially dissected, a portion of the costal margin is resected. The posterior perichondrium is divided, and the underlying pleura is reflected laterally if not previously displaced. The mammary vessels may be retracted medially or ligated if hindering exposure.

The mass is palpated, and biopsies are taken. We usually use a biopsy forceps. During this procedure, one must work closely with the pathologist in order to determine when an adequate amount of tissue has been taken to obtain a diagnosis. For lymphomas, at times at least a gram of tissue may be necessary. If a mass is not readily palpable, the deeper space can be explored with the aid of a mediastinoscope.

This procedure may also be performed through the second intercostal space. One must work medially to stay out of the pleural space. If the pleural space is inadvertently entered, the residual air may be evacuated at the time of closure by reapproximating the tissues over a red rubber catheter.

Transcervical approach

This incision is used for a transcervical thymectomy or to biopsy or resect small anterior mediastinal masses. The patient is placed on an inflatable pillow, and the head is fully extended as if performing a mediastinoscopy. The chest is prepped and draped from the chin to the umbilicus in case of

the need for a sternotomy. Initially, a curvilinear incision is made just above the heads of the clavicle. The platysma is divided with electrocautery. The strap muscles are incised along the midline and retracted laterally. The sternal ligament is divided, and the substernal space is bluntly dissected.

Details of the transcervical thymectomy are found in Chapter 5 on thymectomy. If proceeding with a biopsy, the polytrac retractor is positioned under the sternum, and the inflatable pillow is decompressed. Anterior mediastinal masses can be palpated and biopsied or resected. After performing the procedure, the strap muscles and platysma are reapproximated. The skin is closed with a running subcuticular suture.

Cervicothoracic approach to the apex

Currently, this incision is preferred for the operative management of apical lung tumors. It can also be used for high posterior neurogenic tumors, as well as exposure to the upper thoracic vertebrae or arterial reconstructions.

7 The patient is placed in the supine position with a shoulder roll behind the scapulae and the head turned to the contralateral side. An "L" shaped skin incision is made, coursing along the edge of the inferior border of the sternocleidomastoid, to the sternal notch, and then gently curving infraclavicularly out to the deltopectoral groove. The subcutaneous tissues are divided. The pectoralis and subclavius are dissected away from the clavicle. The superior border of the medial clavicle is dissected by dividing its attachment to the sternocleidomastoid. The head of the clavicle is divided in a horizontal fashion with the oscillating saw. This maneuver allows for a more stable reapproximation of the clavicle at the end of the procedure. The Ruhltract retractor is inserted to elevate the clavicle, and the sternocleidomastoid is further mobilized. This step exposes the distal brachiocephalic, internal jugular, and subclavian veins. Once this has been done, the chest is entered by incising the intercostal muscle along the superior aspect of the rib, one rib below the level of chest wall involvement. After the procedure, the clavicle is reapproximated with number 5 sternal wires, and the soft tissues and skin are closed.

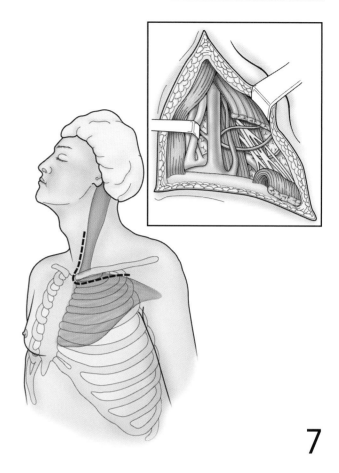

7

If this approach is being used for operations where one does not anticipate resection of chest wall, as in neurogenic tumors, approaches to the upper thoracic spine, or vascular reconstructions, then we usually lower the inferior border of the skin incision and use the Lebsche knife to divide the manubrium into the second intercostal space. We then elevate this segment of chest wall with a Ruhltract retractor.

Reoperative thoracotomy

For reoperative procedures in the chest, we tend to either vary the approach, i.e perform an anterior muscle-sparing thoracotomy though the fourth ICS when a posterolateral thoracotomy has previously been performed, and vice versa. This approach can facilitate lysis of adhesions which are usually most dense at the site of previous thoracotomy. If using the same thoracotomy, resecting a rib facilitates exposure.

FURTHER READING

Ginsberg RJ. Alternative (muscle-sparing) incisions in thoracic surgery. *Annals of Thoracic Surgery* 1993; **56**: 752–4.

Heitmiller RF. The left thoracoabdominal incision. *Annals of Thoracic Surgery* 1988; **46**: 250–3.

Mitchell RL. The lateral limited thoracotomy incision: standard for pulmonary operations. *Journal of Thoracic and Cardiovascular Surgery* 1990; **91**: 1259–64.

Pasque ML, Cooper JD, Kaiser LR, et al. Improved technique for bilateral lung transplantation: rationale and initial clinical experience. *Annals of Thoracic Surgery* 1990; **49**: 785–91.

Urschel HC Jr, Razzuk MA. Median sternotomy as a standard approach for pulmonary resection. *Annals of Thoracic Surgery* 1986; **41**: 130–4.

24

Bronchoplastic procedures

LARRY R. KAISER, MD
The John Rhea Barton Professor and Chairman, Department of Surgery, University of Pennsylvania; Surgeon-in-Chief, University of Pennsylvania Health System, Philadelphia, Pennsylvania, USA

HISTORY

The first sleeve lobectomy was performed by Price-Thomas in 1947 for an endobronchial adenoma. Five years later, Allison reported a sleeve lobectomy for carcinoma. Shaw and Paulson, however, popularized sleeve resection with their 1955 paper entitled "Bronchial anastomosis and bronchoplastic procedures in the interest of preservation of lung tissue." The use of their techniques allows the modern thoracic surgeon to perform parenchymal sparing procedures on patients who would not tolerate a pneumonectomy. In the case of malignancy, sleeve resections are performed without compromise of oncological principles.

PRINCIPLES AND JUSTIFICATION

Pneumonectomy is associated with an increased morbidity and mortality when compared to lobectomy and sleeve lobectomy. Thus, in our practice, we make every effort to avoid pneumonectomy. This strategy includes complex bronchoplastic and bronchovascular reconstructions when required. The justification of this approach is simply that by avoiding pneumonectomy we avoid its attendant risks while providing an equivalent cancer operation. In addition, lung-sparing procedures allow us to offer curative operations to patients with poor pulmonary function who would otherwise not tolerate an operation.

PREOPERATIVE ASSESSMENT AND PREPARATION

Our preoperative evaluation includes a complete history and physical examination. Special attention is focused on previous thoracic procedures and chest irradiation. Systemic illnesses or use of high-dose steroids which might interfere with bronchial anastomotic healing are noted. All patients have a chest X-ray, a chest computerized tomographic (CT) scan, and pulmonary function testing with diffusion capacity. Patients with a diagnosis or suspicion of malignancy also have an extent of disease workup which includes a bone scan and magnetic resonance imaging (MRI) of the brain when indicated.

We perform selected mediastinoscopy in patients with malignant disease. Patients who have mediastinal adenopathy of greater than 1.0 cm on CT scan undergo mediastinoscopy prior to thoracotomy. If the mediastinoscopy is negative, we proceed with the thoracotomy. If the mediastinoscopy reveals ipsilateral N2 disease, the patient is referred for preoperative chemo/radiation therapy and returns later for resection. Those patients with contralateral N3 disease are referred for chemo/radiation therapy and are not offered surgical resection.

ANESTHESIA

1 Following the induction of general anesthesia, all patients undergoing sleeve resection require bronchoscopy by the operating surgeon. This procedure can be done with either a rigid or flexible bronchoscope. Bronchoscopy allows visualization of the lesion and planning of the resection. Following bronchoscopy, the surgeon should have a complete discussion with the anesthesiologist regarding the operative plan. If a right-sided sleeve is being performed, a left-sided double lumen tube should be placed. If a left-sided sleeve is being entertained, a right-sided tube is placed. For sleeve pneumonectomy or a carinal sleeve resection, a sterile anesthesia circuit is required to allow direct ventilation from the surgical field.

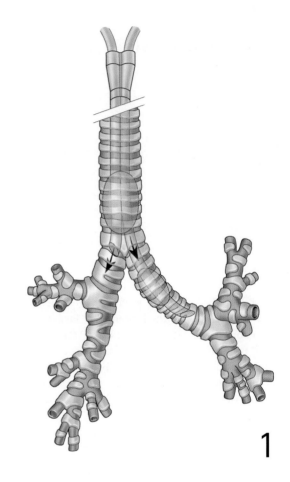

1

OPERATIONS

We have performed sleeve resections through standard posterior lateral incisions, serratus muscle-sparing posterior lateral incisions, and vertically oriented serratus and latissimus muscle-sparing incisions. The surgeon should choose an incision which provides complete exposure and he/she is comfortable working through; for most this choice will likely be the posterior lateral approach.

Following entry into the chest, complete exploration is made to rule out disseminated disease. On both the right and left side we begin our dissection in the anterior hilum and completely dissect out the main pulmonary artery. Special care must be taken on the left side to avoid damage to the short left main pulmonary artery. If bulky disease exists or any difficulty is encountered with dissection, we do not hesitate to open the pericardium on either side to obtain proximal control. Next, we encircle the main pulmonary artery with an umbilical tape and snare it with a Rumel tourniquet in the event that proximal arterial control is needed. The remaining steps are specific to the sleeve being performed, and each will be described independently below.

Right-sided resections

RIGHT UPPER LOBECTOMY SLEEVE RESECTION – THE PROTOTYPE BRONCHOPLASTIC PROCEDURE

2 After proximal arterial control has been obtained, we continue our dissection superiorly and enter the plane of the right upper lobe bronchus. The lung is retracted anteriorly, and we continue our dissection in the crotch between the right upper lobe bronchus and the bronchus intermedius. A "crotch" lymph node is a consistent finding in this location. This node is elevated away from the crotch to reveal the pulmonary arterial branch to the superior segment of the right lower lobe. Once this branch is identified, the posterior portion of the fissure is completed with a linear stapler. This approach avoids extensive parenchymal dissection in the fissure. Up to this point, we have not made any irreversible maneuvers. A complete inspection is carried out to ensure that all disease including nodal disease can be removed. Once complete resectability is confirmed, we begin by ligating and dividing the pulmonary arterial branches to the right upper lobe.

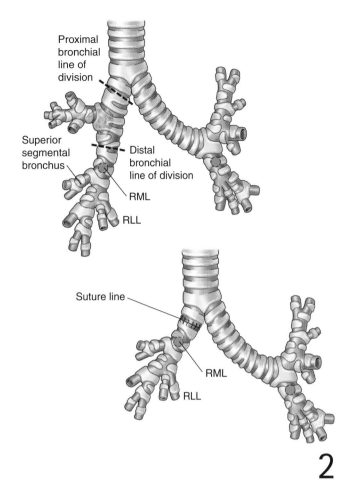

2

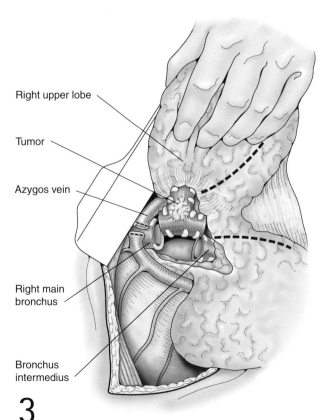

3

3 Likewise, the venous drainage is divided with a vascular stapler taking care to preserve the middle lobe venous drainage. The anterior portion of the fissure is completed with a linear stapler. At this juncture, the only point of attachment is the bronchus. We divide the mainstem bronchus with a fresh number 15 blade just proximal to the right upper lobe take off. Similarly, the bronchus intermedius is divided just distal to the right upper lobe take off. For upper lobe sleeve resections, these cuts must be perpendicular to the long axis of the airway; a "sciving" cut is to be avoided. The proximal and distal airway margins are cut from the specimen and inked by the surgeon. They are then taken to the pathologist for a frozen section examination. Once the margins have been cleared, the reconstruction is started. A positive margin requires additional resection of the involved area. We perform our bronchial sleeve anastomosis in either a running or interrupted fashion. The key to a successful bronchial sleeve anastomosis is a precise tension-free repair which is pneumostatic. When required, tension can be relieved by incising the inferior pulmonary ligament or performing other release maneuvers.

4 When performing an interrupted anastomosis, we use 4.0 oiled vicryl suture. The first suture is placed in an "outside to in" fashion at the junction of the cartilaginous and membranous bronchi. The suture is not tied but is secured to a suture guide. Additional sutures are placed at 2-mm intervals to complete the first half of the cartilaginous anastomosis. Once the midpoint of the cartilaginous bronchi is reached, we begin tying the sutures starting at the corner. The surgeon "crosses" the next suture in the series to relieve tension while the assistant ties. The cartilaginous anastomosis is completed from the midpoint down to the opposite corner in a similar fashion. The lung is retracted anteriorly to reveal the membranous portion of the bronchus. The membranous portion of the anastomosis is completed with interrupted sutures. The chest is filled with saline, and the anastomosis is tested to 20 cm water pressure. Needle hole air leaks are ignored; however, air leaks between the cut edges of the bronchus are reinforced with simple interrupted sutures.

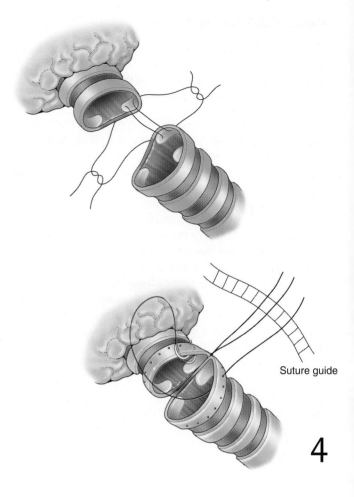

Suture guide

4

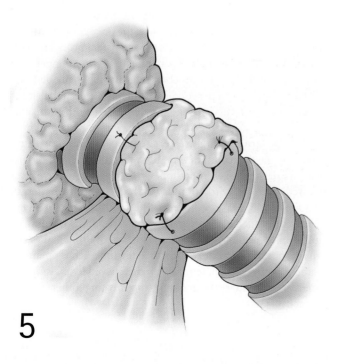

5

5 We wrap all anastomoses with either a pleural flap or pericardial fat. We avoid the use of intercostal muscle which has been reported to calcify and cause anastomotic stricture. When performing a running anastomosis, we use a 4.0 absorbable monofilament suture (Maxon). The anastomosis is started at the midpoint of the cartilaginous bronchi with the knot placed on the outside. The suture is brought inside on the mainstem bronchus, and the surgeon runs the first half of the cartilaginous anastomosis away from himself up to the corner, at the junction of the cartilaginous and membranous portion of the bronchi. The suture is brought to the outside, and tension is kept on the suture by securing it to the drape with a rubber-shodded clamp. The surgeon now sews from the midpoint towards himself to the opposite corner. The assistant follows the suture to maintain tension. Sutures are placed with precision so that alignment is perfect at the corner. The lung is retracted anteriorly, and the membranous portion of the anastomosis is completed by running each suture from the corner to the midpoint of the membranous bronchus. The suture is tied, and the anastomosis checked for pneumostasis and wrapped with pericardial fat.

MIDDLE LOBE SLEEVE RESECTION

6 The middle lobe sleeve resection is an infrequently performed operation. Following proximal arterial control, the middle lobe vein is identified, isolated, and divided. The bronchus to the middle lobe lies immediately posterior to the middle lobe vein. The bronchus is followed back to its origin. A right angled clamp is placed around the bronchus intermedius, and it is divided at a location proximal to the middle lobe orifice. The division is slightly angled. The distal division is also angled to preserve the orifice to the superior segment of the lower lobe. The pulmonary artery lies directly behind the bronchus, and care must be taken to avoid injury when dividing the bronchus. After division of the airway, the middle lobe arterial branch is easily visualized. The branch is ligated and divided. Next, the fissures are completed with firings of a linear stapler.

Following confirmation of negative margins, the airway anastomosis is performed. This step can be done in either a running or interrupted manner as described above for the right upper lobectomy sleeve resection. Special considerations in performing a middle lobe sleeve resection must be given to the superior segmental orifice of the lower lobe. This orifice should not be narrowed or occluded when creating an anastomosis. Pericardial fat is used to wrap the anastomosis and separate it from the pulmonary artery.

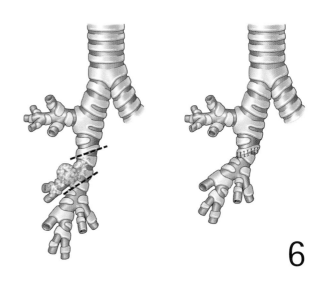

6

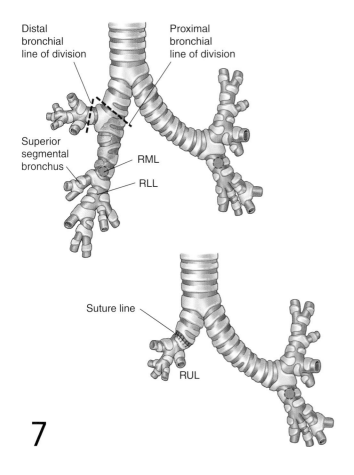

Distal bronchial line of division

Proximal bronchial line of division

Superior segmental bronchus

RML

RLL

Suture line

RUL

7

BILOBECTOMY SLEEVE RESECTION

7 Bilobectomy sleeve resection is performed for endobronchial lesions in the bronchus intermedius. The basic principles of proximal arterial control, microscopic negative margins, and a precise tension free anastomosis apply. Due to the reorientation of the upper lobe bronchus after removal of the middle and lower lobe, special care must be taken to avoid torsion of the bronchus at the anastomosis.

Left-sided resections

LEFT UPPER LOBE SLEEVE RESECTION

8 Proximal arterial control is obtained with care to avoid injury to the short apical segmental branch of the left pulmonary artery. An umbilical tape is passed around the proximal pulmonary artery and secured with a Rumel tourniquet. The tourniquet is not tightened unless proximal arterial control is needed. We continue our dissection along the plane of the artery and identify the superior segmental branch to the lower lobe. At this point we complete the posterior fissure with a linear stapler. The anterior segmental artery is ligated and divided. The lingular branches of the pulmonary artery are identified, ligated, and divided. The lung is retracted posteriorly, and the upper lobe venous drainage is divided with a vascular stapler. The anterior portion of the fissure is completed with a linear stapler. The only remaining attachment to the specimen is the bronchus. Two 2.0 silk stay sutures are placed in the proximal left mainstem and used for retraction. The airway is divided with a fresh number 15 blade proximal and distal to the left upper lobe take off. These cuts should be perpendicular to the longitudinal axis of the airway. The margins are inked and a frozen section examination performed. Once the margins are confirmed to be microscopically negative, the reconstruction is begun. We use either a running or interrupted technique as described above for the right upper lobe sleeve.

Because the left mainstem is long, extensive proximal resections can be performed. This situation can create a technically challenging anastomosis because proximal exposure is obscured by the aortic arch. If required, the arch can be mobilized and carefully retracted to provide additional exposure. As greater amounts of proximal airway are removed, increased tension on the anastomosis can become a problem. Usually, the tension is relieved by simply incising the inferior pulmonary ligament. If additional release is required, the pericardium can be incised in a U-shaped manner beneath the inferior pulmonary vein to effect an infrahilar pericardial release.

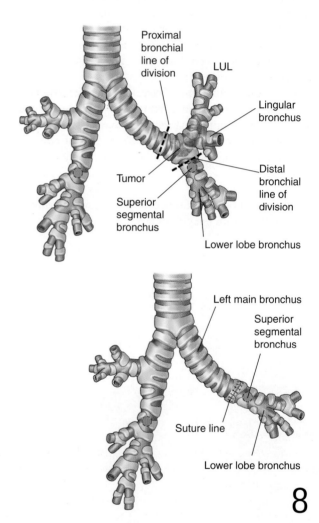

8

LEFT LOWER LOBECTOMY SLEEVE RESECTION

9 For lesions involving the left lower lobe orifice without extension into the upper lobe orifice, a lower lobectomy with sleeve of the left upper lobe bronchus can be performed. The arterial and venous connections to the lower lobe are divided, and the fissures are completed. We dissect out and pass an umbilical tape around the left mainstem and left upper lobe bronchus. Two 0 silk stay sutures are placed in the mainstem and used for retraction. The left upper lobe bronchus is divided first with a fresh number 15 blade. It is important for the division to be perpendicular to the long axis of the airway. Next, the mainstem is divided proximal to the extent of the tumor. The specimen is removed from the field, and frozen section examination of the airway margins is performed. Once the margins are confirmed to be microscopically negative, the reconstruction is completed.

The anastomosis can be performed in an interrupted or running fashion as described above for the right upper lobe sleeve resection. Often, a large size discrepancy exists between upper lobe bronchus and the mainstem. This situation requires precise placement of sutures so that the discrepancy is distributed over the entire circumference of the anastomosis.

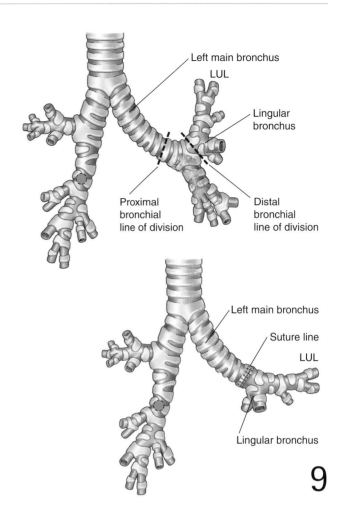

9

POSTOPERATIVE CARE

Following sleeve resection, the patient is extubated in the operating room. Postoperative pain relief is guaranteed by a functioning thoracic epidural. We utilize patient-controlled epidurals which provide a basal as well as demand epidural dose. Pain control is re-evaluated every shift by the nursing staff and adjusted by the anesthesia pain service. The epidural remains in place until the chest tubes are removed. Atelectasis and subsequent pneumonia in the lung distal to the anastomosis must be avoided. This goal is accomplished by good pain relief and aggressive pulmonary toilet. We start incentive spirometry as soon as the patient is awake and begin ambulation on postoperative day 1. The chest tube remains in place until no air leak exists, and the drainage is less than 200 ml/day. This situation usually occurs by postoperative day 5. The epidural is capped 12 hours after the chest tube is removed, and oral narcotics are started. If adequate pain relief is obtained on an oral regimen, the epidural is removed. Awake flexible bronchoscopy is performed prior to discharge to inspect the anastomosis.

OUTCOME

Major complications following sleeve resection include: anastomotic dehiscence, empyema, and bronchovascular fistula. Fortunately, the incidence of these complications is low. We maintain a low threshold for bronchoscopy in the postoperative period. Persistent or evolving atelectasis in the lung distal to the bronchial anastomosis mandates bronchoscopy. A small partial anastomotic dehiscence (<30%) with a good pericardial fat wrap and no bronchopleural fistula can be treated conservatively. A complete dehiscence is caused by anastomotic tension. This problem requires reoperation and usually a completion pneumonectomy. An empyema can occur with or without a bronchopleural fistula. When it occurs without a bronchopleural fistula, an empyema is handled with drainage, antibiotics, and ablation of any residual space with muscle transposition. In this case it is related to preoperative pneumonia and soilage of a reisidual pleural space during the operation. When empyema occurs with a bronchopleural fistula from the anastomosis, a completion pneumonectomy is required, and management of the infected pneumonectomy space is problematic.

Bronchovascular fistula may present with massive hemoptysis. This complication occurs when an anastomotic breakdown occurs with peribronchial abscess formation which invades into the adjacent pulmonary artery. Under these circumstances, completion pneumonectomy is performed. As expected, the mortality of this complication is very high.

The mortality rate for sleeve lobectomy should be equivalent to lobectomy alone (3–5%). The most frequent respiratory complication is pneumonia which can be avoided by aggressive postoperative pulmonary toilet and adequate pain control. Local recurrence rates following bronchoplastic procedures are low (<5%) as long as the resection margins are free of disease. This situation illustrates the importance of frozen section examination of the bronchial margins prior to completing the airway anastomosis. Late strictures occasionally occur and are related either to ischemia or a healed partial anastomotic dehiscence. Strictures can be handled with dilation and silastic bronchial stent placement.

25

Resection of posterior mediastinal masses

JOSEPH B. SHRAGER MD

Associate Professor of Surgery; Chief, Thoracic Surgery, Hospital of the University of Pennsylvania and Pennsylvania Hospital, University of Pennsylvania School of Medicine, Philadelphia, Pennsylvania, USA

The vast majority of posterior mediastinal masses in adults are benign tumors or cysts. The solid masses among these most frequently represent slow-growing neurogenic tumors such as schwannomas (neurilemmomas), neurofibromas, or ganglioneuromas, and less frequently leiomyomata of the esophagus. The cysts generally represent congenital bronchogenic or esophageal duplication cysts. Certainly, esophageal carcinoma, esophageal diverticulum, diaphragmatic hernia, and descending aortic aneurysm must always be considered, but these lesions are commonly suggested by standard radiological studies (contrast esophagogram, computed tomography (CT)), and one is typically left with a differential diagnosis including the various benign, neoplastic, or congenital processes listed above.

Often, these masses present as asymptomatic radiographic abnormalities on a study obtained for unrelated reasons. Respiratory symptoms, dysphagia, chest pain, or symptoms related to cyst infection, however, do occur in some patients – usually those with larger masses and more often in children than in adults.

1 Radiographs generally demonstrate a smoothly marginated cystic or solid mass which is quite characteristic. The CT demonstrates the classic appearance of a posterior mediastinal schwannoma in the costovertebral sulcus.

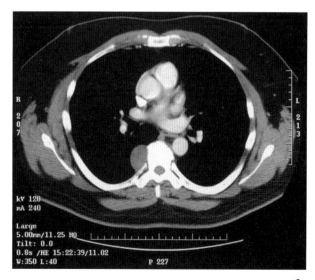

PRINCIPLES AND JUSTIFICATION

Because of the almost uniformly benign nature of these masses, surgical treatment has evolved rapidly in the past decade from an approach mandating traditional thoracotomy to one in which video-assisted thoracoscopic (VATS) approaches have become equally acceptable if not preferable. Certainly, VATS approaches, which have been demonstrated to result in reduced pain and more rapid functional recovery versus thoracotomy, find their most appropriate application in benign diseases such as these. By either approach – VATS or thoracotomy – exactly the same operation is performed. The goal is complete resection, and this can almost always be achieved. However, the potential negative consequences of a grossly complete, but perhaps microscopically incomplete, resection are minimal when dealing with many of these posterior mediastinal tumors, thus rendering the VATS approach ideal for these entities.

In addition, controversy continues to exist as to whether many of these masses require resection *at all*. A number of studies have addressed the issue of whether the incidence of an asymptomatic posterior mediastinal cyst progressing to symptoms is sufficiently high to merit its resection at an asymptomatic stage, and whether a measurable incidence of malignant degeneration exists in the benign neurogenic tumors. Although these studies have reached conflicting conclusions, it is fair to say that most thoracic surgeons, including the author, feel that these lesions should be resected upon discovery in most patients. This aggressive approach is rendered more palatable by the availability of VATS excision. It is reasonable, however, to follow small, asymptomatic lesions in the elderly or those with significant comorbidities.

The VATS approach is, in the author's practice, offered for solid masses or cysts that are relatively small, usually asymptomatic, without signs of invasion of surrounding structures on CT, and occurring in patients without prior surgery in that hemithorax or another reason to suspect that major adhesions may be present. This description would include most posterior mediastinal masses in adults. For patients who present with infected cysts, which create a surrounding inflammatory process obscuring normal tissue planes, or signs of invasion, thoracotomy is most prudent. Similarly, large masses (over 5–6 cm) are also best approached by thoracotomy because they too are likely to be more difficult to dissect safely from surrounding structures and may be difficult to remove via small VATS port sites. Although a number of different techniques have been described for combined anterior/posterior approaches to tumors invading the neural foramen ("dumbbell tumors"), these also are amenable to having the anterior portion of the operation performed by VATS in most cases. For suspected esophageal duplication cysts, in the rare event that any suggestion of a communication exists between the native and cyst lumens (demonstration of fistula on esophagogram or air within the cyst), the author favors thoracotomy to facilitate perfect mucosal repair. Otherwise, duplication cysts may be resected by VATS.

Major morbidity and mortality are rare after these procedures. The entities most likely to lead to significant complications are the esophageal duplication cysts, resection of which are associated with a small but real risk of postoperative esophageal leak, and the "dumbbell" tumors, where one must discuss preoperatively with the patient the occasional occurrence of cerebrospinal fluid (CSF) leak into the pleural space. Additionally, if great care is not taken during resection of any tumor that encroaches upon the neural foramen, hematoma within the spinal canal with cord compression may occur. The small risk of prolonged incisional pain following VATS or thoracotomy must also be discussed with the patient, as before any thoracic procedure. Since the intercostal nerve is commonly resected along with neurogenic tumors, the patient should be told to expect an area of numbness in the associated dermatome following these procedures. Resection of tumors associated with the upper thoracic vertebrae at the apex of the chest may require resection of the stellate ganglion, resulting in Horner's syndrome; and if these tumors are on the right side, recurrent laryngeal nerve injury is also a possibility that is rare but should be mentioned. Finally, every patient who undergoes a VATS approach to one of these lesions must understand and consent to the possibility of a thoracotomy if it becomes necessary.

PREOPERATIVE ASSESSMENT AND PREPARATION

Although preoperative studies often suggest that one is dealing with one of the benign posterior mediastinal processes listed above, it is neither necessary nor simple to differentiate among the various cystic or solid lesions preoperatively. A needle biopsy of a discrete, posterior mediastinal mass with smooth margins is unnecessary and unlikely to provide any useful information. After CT delineates whether the mass is cystic or solid, certain features may, however, dictate additional studies.

A cystic mass that abuts the esophagus should be evaluated for a communication with the esophagus, as the presence of such a communication suggests the need for thoracotomy rather than VATS (see above). This situation can be ruled out by preoperative barium esophagogram and confirmed by esophagoscopy performed by the surgeon immediately prior to surgery. Although leiomyomata have a fairly characteristic CT appearance, a solid mass in association with the esophagus should also prompt preoperative esophagoscopy to confirm that normal mucosa overlies the mass and that it may not, in fact, represent an esophageal malignancy. Endoscopic ultrasound (EUS) can provide the strongest evidence short of excision that one is dealing with a leiomyoma, and EUS may also be useful in the occasional case where cyst fluid is of sufficiently high density that the cystic versus solid nature of a mass is in doubt.

A solid mass in the costovertebral sulcus must be evaluated carefully for invasion of the neural foramen. A magnetic resonance imaging (MRI) study should be performed if it is not entirely clear by CT that the foramen is clear. Identification of foramenal invasion is critical and should be identified preoperatively for appropriate planning of a combined anterior-posterior approach. Patients with solid masses and a history of hypertension should have serum catecholamine levels and 24-hour urine levels of homovanillic acid and vanillylmandelic acid determined given the rare occurrence of functional pheochromocytomas in this location.

ANESTHESIA

Since more manipulation at the port sites is performed during these operations than during simpler VATS procedures such as lung biopsy, epidural catheters for postoperative analgesia should be placed in these patients regardless of whether a VATS or a thoracotomy approach is planned. General anesthesia is provided through a double-lumen endotracheal tube with the distal cuff in the left mainstem bronchus, allowing reliable, complete collapse of the lung in the hemithorax of interest. The patient is placed in a full, lateral decubitus thoracotomy position. Of particular importance for these cases,

the patient should be securely held in this position. This positioning allows the operating table to be tilted as far as 45 degrees to either side without any risk of patient slippage. Tilting in this way often allows the lung to fall sufficiently away from the mediastinum by virtue of gravity alone, so that an additional port site for passage of a lung retractor is not necessary.

OPERATION

Figures 2–6 illustrate the resection of a benign neurogenic tumor of the costovertebral sulcus. The arrangement of incisions for resection of all posterior mediastinal masses is similar but, of course, must be varied slightly depending on the craniad-caudad level of the tumor. For resection of bronchogenic cysts of the posterior mediastinum, the procedure is essentially identical to that described for neurogenic tumors, with the exception of a few technical details described in the text following Figure 6. Technical details that are different for esophageal-associated posterior mediastinal masses such as duplication cysts and leiomyomata are demonstrated in Figures 7 and 8.

Skin incision placement

2 The author has found the illustrated placement of 2–3 cm port incisions to be optimal for the resection of most posterior mediastinal masses. If the camera port is placed much more anteriorly than the midaxillary line, the view of the mass is often obscured by the lung despite rotation of the operating table anteriorly. If one does place the port more anteriorly, a fourth port site for a lung retractor may become necessary, and this maneuver only creates an additional chance for intercostal nerve injury and increased postoperative pain. A 0 degree telescope is preferred, but this decision is purely surgeon's preference, and a 30 degree telescope may be equally effective.

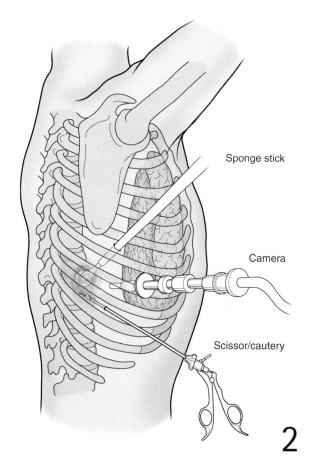

Sponge stick

Camera

Scissor/cautery

2

The two working ports are placed at approximately the posterior–axillary line, as far craniad and caudad as possible, and approximately equidistant from the mass on this axis. The main working instruments are an endoscopic scissors-cautery, a ring clamp used both with and without a gauze sponge-ball ("sponge-stick"), an endoscopic peanut dissector, a long right-angle clamp, and an endoscopic clip applier.

Pleural incision

3 Initial exposure involves circumferentially incising the pleura overlying the tumor. The pleura is incised with a margin of about 2 cm around the tumor in all directions. Gentle traction on the mass can be established with the sponge-stick, which stretches the pleura sufficiently to allow safe initial incision with the cautery scissors in the most accessible area.

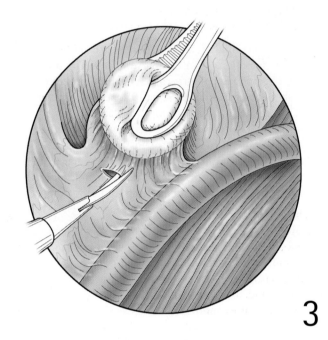

3

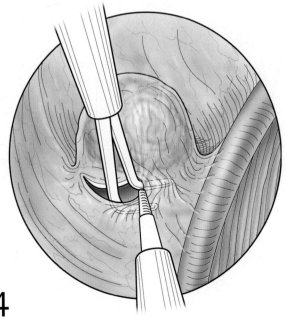

4

Extension of pleural incision

4 As one proceeds circumferentially around the tumor, the pleura is easily tented up on a standard right-angle clamp to separate it from underlying critical structures. This separation allows one to use the cautery while incising, without fear of damage to structures such as the esophagus and azygos. Since the pleura can sometimes be somewhat vascular, it is advantageous to use the cautery in this manner.

Further mobilization from attachments

5 Once the pleura has been incised circumferentially, soft tissue attachments with differing degrees of vascularity and density must now be mobilized off of the mass. Much of this portion of the dissection can be done bluntly, using the sponge-stick, or, more often, as pictured here, the peanut dissector. Bands of tissue that are more vascular in appearance are clipped or cauterized, taking care to stay away from the azygous vein, esophagus, and vagus nerve.

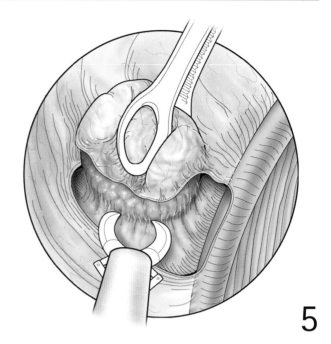

5

The degree of traction one exerts on the tumor becomes an important issue as the dissection proceeds towards the nerve (usually an intercostal) to which the tumor is attached. A certain amount of gentle traction is necessary to provide counter-tension to allow the blunt dissection to proceed. On the other hand, overly zealous traction can result in tearing of vascular structures and/or the nerve root at the neural foramen. The latter may result in a CSF leak, while the former may result in the disastrous complication of intraspinal hematoma with possible cord compression.

The author exerts this gentle traction by one of several means. In most cases, simply pulling on the tumor gently with the sponge-stick, as shown here, is sufficient. Sometimes, the pleural covering which has been incised is sufficiently adherent to the mass that this pleural overlay itself can be grasped and manipulated to provide traction. For smaller tumors, the mass itself can be completely encompassed in the jaws of the ring-clamp as the base is approached, allowing the desired level of traction to be created.

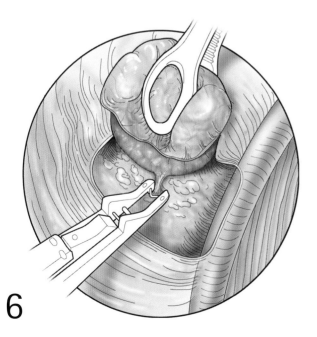

6

6 The intercostal bundle lateral to the tumor is mobilized, doubly clipped, and ligated lateral to the tumor (not shown) after the other soft tissue attachments have been taken down. This maneuver leaves the nerve root and associated vessels emerging from the neural foramen as the only remaining attachment, as shown here. These structures are now similarly doubly clipped, and the specimen is completely free and may be removed. Care is taken again, at this step, not to exert too much tension on the nerve root as these clips are applied, for fear of causing a CSF leak or paraspinal hematoma. The tumor is placed in an endoscopic bag for removal through the anterior-most port site (where the intercostal space is naturally widest). A 24 French chest tube is left in place.

If the tumor arises from the sympathetic chain, the intercostal bundles can generally be spared and the sympathetic chain clipped and divided above and below the mass in the final step of freeing it.

If at any time during the VATS procedure described above, unexpected pleural studding or pleural effusion, or invasion of the spine, head of rib, or esophagus is identified, these findings suggest that the tumor is malignant, and conversion to thoracotomy is appropriate. Similarly, any concern about incompleteness of resection or, certainly, safety, should result in immediate conversion to thoracotomy.

In the case of tumors identified as "dumbbell" tumors preoperatively, the operation should be performed by a combined posterior neurosurgical and anterior thoracic approach. A detailed description of the neurosurgical component of this procedure is beyond the scope of this chapter, but involves laminectomy and intervertebral foraminotomy performed with the patient in a prone position. The patient is subsequently repositioned, and the VATS procedure is carried out exactly as described above. In the rare case that unexpected invasion of the neural foramen is identified while performing attempted primary VATS excision, one should consult intraoperatively with a neurosurgeon. If possible, the patient should be repositioned for an immediate posterior approach by the neurosurgeon, followed by completion of the resection by VATS.

If after resection of a tumor approaching the foramen one finds persistent oozing of blood from this area, one should never pack hemostatic agents into the area. This maneuver may block the path of egress of blood from the spinal canal and create a closed space in which a disastrous spinal hematoma may form. If oozing at the foramen does not stop with careful use of bipolar cautery at the bony margins of the foramen or watchful waiting with temporary use of a collagen hemostatic agent, then neurosurgical consultation should be obtained.

Resection of neurogenic tumors arising from the posterior mediastinum at the *apex* of the chest poses more complex challenges than those at lower levels, and in most cases a VATS approach to these tumors is inappropriate.

Bronchogenic cysts also occur not infrequently near the costovertebral sulcus. For these, the dissection is essentially the same as for the neurogenic tumors illustrated above. The author has found that it is helpful to dissect these, initially, with the cyst intact. Once one has gone as far as possible in this manner, the cyst is drained by needle aspiration. This fluid is sent for culture and cytological examination. The deepest recesses of the cyst cavity can be seen from within the cyst if it is subsequently opened widely. This step generally allows the final stages of dissection and resection. If a small portion of the cyst wall is densely adherent to a critical structure, it may be left in place and cauterized. If a large portion of the cyst is adherent and is difficult to safely dissect at VATS, thoracotomy should be performed. Figures 7 and 8 illustrate the approach to *esophagus-associated* posterior mediastinal masses such as leiomyomata and duplication cysts (a leiomyoma is pictured).

7 Although the procedure is very similar in most respects to that described above for the more posteriorly located masses in the costovertebral sulcus, a few differences bear discussion. These masses are located beneath the longitudinal muscle of the esophageal wall, but depending upon the size of the tumor, this muscle may be so thinned out that its normal, striated texture is hard to identify. The first step after incising the pleura, then, is to incise this muscle layer directly over the mass and to extend this incision approximately 1 cm proximal and distal to the mass. As shown here, this step is often best accomplished with a blunt, right angle clamp used to carefully dissect the muscularis off of the underlying esophageal mucosa. The muscle is then tented up off of the mucosa and divided.

It should be noted that if a mass is associated with a portion of the esophagus that is obscured by the azygous arch, this vessel can be easily sacrificed to improve exposure. This step is accomplished with an endoscopic gastrointestinal anastomosis (GIA) stapling device with a vascular cartridge.

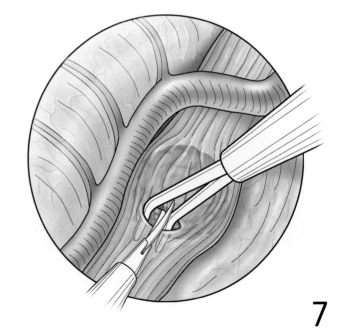

7

8 After bluntly dissecting the tumor from surrounding adhesions as described in Figure 5, one eventually reaches the critical plane where the tumor meets the mucosa directly. Leiomyomata usually are not densely adherent to the mucosa, and with patience this plane can almost always be bluntly dissected completely with the endoscopic peanut while exerting gentle traction on the mass. This dissection can be facilitated by introducing an endoscope from above and transilluminating the mucosa, allowing clearer identification of the interface between mucosa and mass.

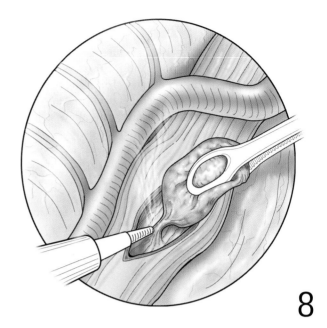

8

In contrast to leiomyomata, the author has found that duplication cysts are often so densely adherent in this plane with the mucosa that it is impossible to safely separate the deep wall of the cyst from the mucosa (in fact, the two may share a common wall). Two options are available in this circumstance. One option is conversion to a thoracotomy for incision and precise repair of the mucosa, leaving no doubt that one has achieved complete excision of the cyst wall. The author has generally chosen the second option, which is leaving up to 25% of the cyst wall intact against the esophageal mucosa and gently cauterizing the epithelial lining of the residual cyst.

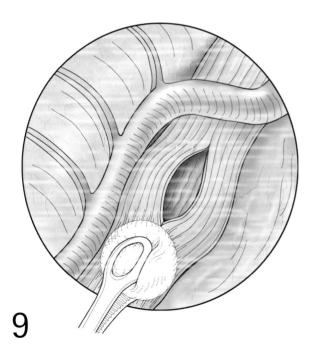

9

9 Once the tumor or cyst has been removed, the esophageal mucosa is tested for integrity by insufflating air via the endoscope with the area of dissection submerged in saline while simultaneously occluding the distal esophageal lumen with a sponge-stick. Any mucosal leak would be identified as a stream of bubbles emanating from the area of exposed mucosa. A leak identified at this point mandates precise suture closure, which may be done endoscopically by a surgeon experienced in endoscopic suturing or, more likely, by conversion to thoracotomy. The author has not found it necessary to reclose the muscularis of the esophagus, although this goal could certainly be achieved via VATS if felt to be necessary.

POSTOPERATIVE CARE

The typical hospital stay is 1–2 days after a VATS resection and 4 days after a thoracotomy, and the usual postoperative course is smooth and uncomplicated. Following resection of tumors in the costovertebral sulcus, patients undergo regular neurological examinations of the lower extremities so that the rare occurrence of a compressing spinal hematoma would be rapidly identified and relieved. The chest tube in these patients is removed on the first postoperative day if the volume of drainage is low.

High output of clear or serosanguinous fluid would raise the suspicion of a CSF leak. This suspicion, if the diagnosis is not clear, can be confirmed by documenting beta-2 transferrin in the fluid – this protein is present in CSF but not pleural fluid. The presence of a CSF leak mandates reoperation by a neurosurgeon; the leak is repaired and generally buttressed with vascularized tissue.

Following resection of esophageal leiomyomata and duplication cysts, a contrast esophagogram is obtained on postoperative day 1. If this study shows no leak, the patient's diet is advanced, and the chest tube is removed.

OUTCOME

The author's experience includes 23 posterior mediastinal masses removed by the VATS approaches described herein. Primary thoracotomy was employed for several larger or invasive masses during the same time period, but in only one case did a procedure begun thoracoscopically require conversion to a thoracotomy. This case involved an esophageal leiomyoma near the gastroesophageal junction that proved to be multilobulated and far more extensive than anticipated from preoperative studies, wrapping itself around the esophagus in a horseshoe fashion. It must be emphasized, however, that absolutely no hesitation should exist to convert a VATS procedure to thoracotomy if required.

The principles described above have allowed these cases to be performed without a complicating CSF leak, spinal hematoma, or esophageal leak. One patient with a schwannoma did suffer persistent, painful dysesthesia postoperatively in the dermatome of the resected nerve. In no case where a portion of a bronchogenic or esophageal duplication cyst wall was left intact has there been a known recurrence. Further, following resection of leiomyomata or duplication cysts, we have not identified any diverticula at the surgical site despite leaving the muscularis incision open. It must be admitted, however, in presenting these results, that the patients are followed only by history, physical examination, and chest radiogram, not by chest CT. It should be mentioned, also, that isolated case reports of recurrences following incomplete cyst wall excision have been published, so complete excision must remain the goal when possible, until studies with longer follow-up are published.

FURTHER READING

Demmy TL, Krasna MJ, Detterbeck FC, Kline GG, Kohman LJ, DeCamp MM Jr, Wain JC. Multicenter VATS experience with mediastinal tumors. *Annals of Thoracic Surgery* 1998; **66**: 187–92.

Vallieres E, Findlay JM, Fraser RE. Combined microneurosurgical and thoracoscopic removal of neurogenic dumbbell tumors. *Annals of Thoracic Surgery* 1995; **59**: 469–72.

26

Lung transplantation

JOHN DARK
Professor, Regional Cardiothoracic Centre, Freeman Hospital, Newcastle upon Tyne, UK

HISTORY

Clinical success in isolated lung transplantation was first achieved by Cooper and the Toronto group in 1983. They built on three decades of laboratory work through which had evolved most of the technical steps, for instance the need for cuff for the venous anastomosis and various approaches to bronchial healing.

PRINCIPLES AND JUSTIFICATION

Indications were clearly defined; initially restrictive or fibrotic disease, expanding to include obstructive (principally emphysematous) conditions after 1988. Emphysema is now the commonest pretransplant diagnosis. In the early 1990s the single lung option was not used, particularly in the USA, for patients with pulmonary hypertension.

Recipients with septic lung disease require removal of all the infected tissues – invariably both lungs. This goal was initially achieved with combined heart–lung transplantation, but such patients received an unnecessary cardiac graft. However, once safe techniques for bronchial anastomoses had evolved, the advantage of the very reliable tracheal healing in the heart–lung operation evaporated.

The first alternative approach was the *en bloc* double lung transplantation. Considerable morbidity, including the need for cardiopulmonary bypass and cardioplegic arrest, the extensive mediastinal dissection, and a 20% tracheal dehiscence rate prevented widespread popularity. Placing the bronchial anastomoses close to the lung parenchyma, and performing all of the vascular suture lines at the hilar rather than the mediastinal level, was the approach originally described by Pasque and colleagues from St Louis and is the basis of our standard bilateral lung transplantation. In the original description a bilateral anterior thoracotomy, linking across the sternum (the clam shell incision), was an essential part, giving excellent access to the pleural space often obliterated by dense vascular adhesions. Subsequently, access through a sternotomy or limited bilateral anterior thoracotomies, keeping the sternum intact, have both been described, particularly for patients with obstructive as opposed to septic lung disease.

For the very earliest lung transplantations, the donor was taken to an operating room adjacent to the recipient; distant procurement was described in the late 1980s. A fairly standard approach has evolved; the lung and heart are simultaneously flushed *in situ* with a cold crystalloid preservation solution. The heart and then the lungs may be extracted separately, or (the norm in Europe) as a single block and then separated. The tissue can safely be preserved for 6–8 hours using current techniques although a 10–20% primary organ dysfunction rate remains.

PREOPERATIVE ASSESSMENT AND PREPARATION

Donor lung procurement

Less than 20% of solid organ donors yield usable lungs. In addition to damage from trauma, aspiration, and ventilator-related infection, brainstem death itself may precipitate lung injury. A combination of hydrostatic stress and inflammatory activation result in endothelial damage and increased alveolar permeability. "Neurogenic pulmonary edema" is the most extreme form, but a degree of injury, with some features of early stages of adult respiratory distress syndrome (ARDS), is probably present in every donor lung. The decision about suitability for donation is based on assessment of the chest X-ray, the arterial blood gases, the findings at bronchoscopy, and finally the texture and appearances of the lungs themselves. Areas of actelectasis that re-expand, patchy contusion, and purulent endobronchial secretions (in the absence of an inflamed mycosis) are not of themselves contraindications to use of the lungs. The presence of extensive consolidated areas that will not re-aerate or the appearance of airway inflammation that might be associated with established infection or significant aspiration, suggest that the lung is not useful. The function of each lung can be assessed separately by measuring blood gas samples taken directly from the pulmonary veins. This technique may identify a perfectly usable single lung in situations where one lung has poor function; and as a result, arterial blood gases are misleadingly poor.

OPERATION

Donor lung procurement

If not already done by the team retrieving the intra-abdominal organs, the chest is opened via a median sternotomy. The heart is exposed and examined, and then both pleurae are incised just behind the sternum. The pleural spaces are explored and all lobes of the lungs examined. Posterobasal segments are often atelectatic and should be re-expanded by a combination of bronchoscopy and vigorous hand-bagging via the endotracheal tube.

After heparinization, a standard cardioplegia cannula is placed in the ascending aorta, and a 14-mm bullet-tipped cannula in the proximal main pulmonary artery. The brachiocephalic vein is ligated and divided, thus allowing access through the posterior pericardial reflections to the lower trachea. This tissue should be separated off the esophagus and encircled by a nylon tape.

1 To initiate organ retrieval, the superior vena cava (SVC) is doubly ligated just below the azygos vein and the inferior vena cava (IVC) clamped intrapericardially. Cardioplegia delivery is begun, and this step should satisfactorily drain out of the divided IVC. Inflow of lung preservation solution is begun while the main pulmonary artery is palpated to ensure that high pressure is not generated. The tip of the left atrial appendage should be removed so as to allow a generous orifice for drainage of the pulmonary effluent. Ventilation of the lungs continues during this phase, but both pleural cavities are flooded with ice-cold saline. Care should be taken to avoid overdistension of either side of the heart. This problem can easily occur on the left if the drainage via the left atrial appendage is impeded.

Toward the end of pulmonary flushing, the effluent should run almost clear. It may be more convenient to remove the heart at this stage, and this maneuver certainly shortens the overall ischemic time for that organ. The aorta is divided just proximal to the clamp and dissected off the right pulmonary artery. The main pulmonary artery can then be divided, opening up the transverse sinus. The SVC is divided and again dissected off the right pulmonary artery. At this stage, only the left atrium connects the heart to the lungs.

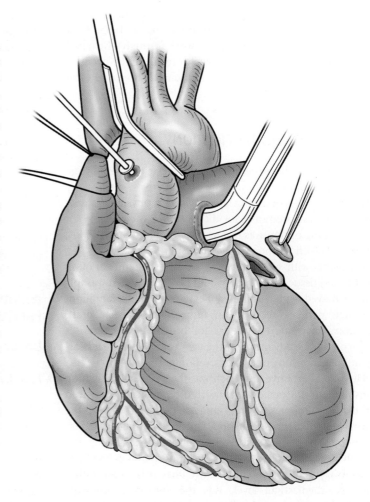

1

2 An incision is made on the left-hand side, midway between the origin of the pulmonary veins and the atrioventricular groove and well posterior to the base of the left atrial appendage. This incision is extended over the roof of the left atrium (i.e. the floor of the transfer sinus), again skirting well to the posterior aspect of the left atrial appendage and running around to behind the SVC. Inferiorly, the incision is continued parallel with the coronary sinus until only a strip of tissue running adjacent to the intra-atrial septum is left connecting the heart to the lungs. This strip is carefully divided, taking care not to buttonhole the intra-atrial septum. In practice, a thin ribbon of tissue is left attached to the lungs, and the heart can be removed intact.

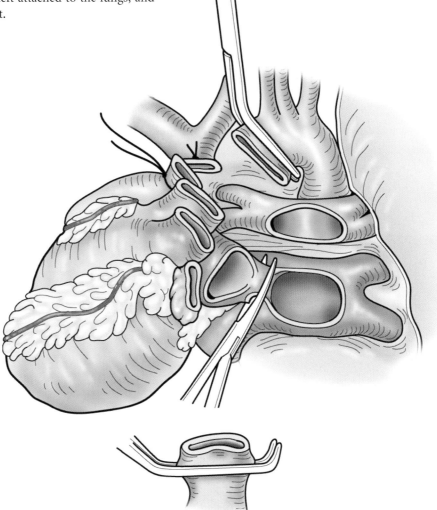

2

Stopping ventilation at this stage is reasonable, but the endotracheal tube should be left in place. The pericardium is incised vertically on both sides parallel to and just above the diaphragm, a dissection that leads backwards towards the inferior pulmonary ligaments. These tissues can easily be divided under direct vision, and then the two pericardial incisions are joined inferiorly. An obvious plane exists immediately in front of the esophagus and is revealed with division of the inferior ligaments; dissection continues up this plane. The scissors are used to divide the pleural reflexions on each side. On the right, this dissection comes up behind the main bronchus and is then brought in front of the azygos vein, eventually linking up with the tape around the trachea. On the left, dissection is taken up at the level of the aortic arch which may often be included with the lung block, dividing the arch branches superiorly and again linking up with the tape around the trachea.

3 At this stage the anesthetist should be instructed to reinflate the lungs to approximately three quarters of total lung capacity; a stapling instrument is placed around the trachea which is now the only structure holding the lung block into the chest. The endotracheal tube is pulled back a little and the trachea stapled. The trachea is divided above the staple line and the donor lung block removed from the chest.

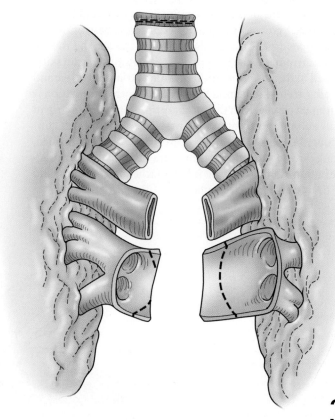

3

Splitting of the donor lung block

If bilateral lung transplantation is to be performed, the donor lung block can be transported, inflated and wrapped in appropriately sealed sterile bags containing lung preservation fluid, to the recipient. If two separate single lung recipients in different institutions are to be transplanted, the block must be split at the donor hospital.

The wall of the left atrium is divided in the midline thus generating two separate donor atrial cuffs. Prior to this step, the pulmonary artery can be divided in the line of its bifurcation. An ample amount of pulmonary artery is always present. The posterior part of the pericardium is now divided from below with an incision which leads up towards the tracheal bifurcation. Care is taken to stay away from the origin of the right main bronchus, and the proximal left main bronchus is isolated. Two stapling devices are then used to divide the proximal left main bronchus such that the trachea remains attached to the right main bronchus. With division of the left bronchus, the two lungs can be completely separated, packaged, and dispatched to their recipients.

PREOPERATIVE ASSESSMENT AND PREPARATION

Single lung transplantation

The majority of candidates will have end-stage respiratory disease as a result of either emphysema (smoking induced or subsequent alpha 1 antitrypsin deficiency) or pulmonary fibrosis. The timing of referral for transplantation, as well as the investigation of the individual condition, has been well set out in the international consensus document.

Potential candidates must be thoroughly screened to exclude other organ dysfunction, particularly cardiovascular and renal. Patients with obstructive lung disease, who often have a history of heavy cigarette consumption, should be appropriately screened for cardiovascular disease. Left ventricular function must be normal, and any coronary disease should be dealt with by appropriate angioplasty and stenting. Before acceptance, suitable recipients should have shown at least the potential for rehabilitation. Bed-bound or moribund patients are no longer accepted for lung transplantation.

Lung perfusion scanning is used to identify the "worse" lung, and this lung will usually be the side selected for transplantation. On the other hand, a site of any extensive previous surgery, for instance pleurodesis, should be avoided. Many patients with fibrotic disease may have had an open or video-assisted thoracoscopy (VAT) lung biopsy. This procedure is of little or no consequence and can be ignored when selecting the site for surgery.

ANESTHESIA

Single lung transplantations, other than those done for pulmonary hypertension, do not usually require cardiopulmonary bypass. The first essential is reliable one-lung ventilation with a double-lumen endotracheal tube placed to the contralateral side. Standard monitoring includes a radial artery line for blood pressure and blood gas estimation together with central venous access. Continuous monitoring of end-tidal CO_2 should be regarded as essential. Additional measurements, in the form of a pulmonary artery catheter or transesophageal echo for the observation of right ventricular function, may be helpful in borderline patients. We have found that simple measures, in particular blood gases, safely predict patients who will require cardiopulmonary bypass. No advantage is obtained in struggling with an acidotic, hypoxic, or hypotensive patient merely for the sake of avoiding bypass. We, and others, have shown that the use of bypass does not disadvantage the patient.

The hemodynamic behavior during one-lung ventilation is determined by the underlying pathology. In restrictive disease, oxygenation can usually be maintained, but very high inflation pressures are required for adequate minute ventilation, and an inexorable rise in arterial or end-tidal P_{CO_2} may occur. This problem, or hypotension during trial pulmonary artery (PA) clamping (see below), indicates right ventricle (RV) embarrassment and the need for bypass. On the other hand, those patients with restrictive disease can almost always be managed conservatively as long as the effects of air trapping or the occasional occult contralateral pneumothorax are detected and dealt with appropriately.

The problems, and solutions, are similar for the patient undergoing bilateral lung transplantation. Monitoring of the patient is as for a single lung transplantation. A left-sided double-lumen tube is placed – only rarely does it interfere with the left bronchial anastomosis. If the situation is such that bypass would inevitably be required, i.e. in a pulmonary hypertensive patient, or where it is local habit, only a single-lumen tube is required.

Bronchial toilet is essential for the patient with septic lung disease; loss of function of a segment or lobe because of failure to clear secretions and maintain ventilation may precipitate major problems in borderline patients. The most difficult periods are: (i) after the completion of the removal of the first lung; (ii) then during the second pneumonectomy; and (iii) when the patient is entirely dependent upon the newly implanted and recently reperfused transplant lung. Function of this first lung is often precarious as it is literally squeezed between the vigorous right ventricle often found in these patients and intermittent elevations of left atrial pressure as access to the posterior part of the hilum is sought. In this situation and analogous to the patient undergoing single lung transplantation, avoiding cardiopulmonary bypass at the cost of a compromised recipient circulation is not wise.

Primary lung dysfunction occurs in up to 20% of recipients and is manifest by a noncardiogenic pulmonary edema, often with proteinaceous fluid appearing in the airway. Management is supportive although inhaled nitric oxide (20–30 parts/million) appears to have had a considerable impact on the management of these patients.

OPERATION

Single lung transplantation

After induction of anesthesia, and in particular the demonstration of reliable one-lung ventilation, the patient is placed in the fully lateral position. The chest is opened through a standard thoracotomy along the upper border of the sixth rib. Patients with fibrotic disease have a shrunken chest, and the surgeon should be aware of entering the pleura an interspace too low. This problem greatly increases the difficulties of what is already an awkward operation.

Intrapleural adhesions are unusual and can be easily dealt with. The anesthetist is instructed to deflate the nonoperated lung whilst the hilar structures are identified. A tape should be passed around the pulmonary artery at an early stage. Even in the most stable patient, the PA should be clamped for a trial period of 10–15 minutes to ensure that ventilation and perfusion of the dependent lung only can be tolerated. This situation will be the case for almost all patients with obstructive disease and for the majority with restrictive physiology, although maintaining their stability is always a challenge to the anesthetist.

4a,b A straightforward pneumonectomy is then performed. Our habit is to ligate and divide pulmonary artery branches first to avoid at this stage having a clamp in the operative field. Similarly the pulmonary veins are ligated and divided outside the pericardial cavity, and the inferior pulmonary ligament is divided with cautery, staying clear of the vagus nerve. On the right, the phrenic nerve runs close to the hilar structures, and damage must be avoided at all costs. The bronchus is simply divided at the level of this first branch and any bleeding bronchial artery controlled with metal clips. By dividing the bronchus so far distally, the vagus nerve can be protected.

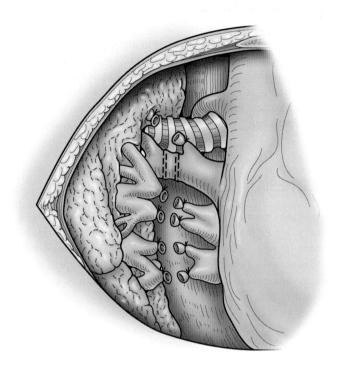

4a

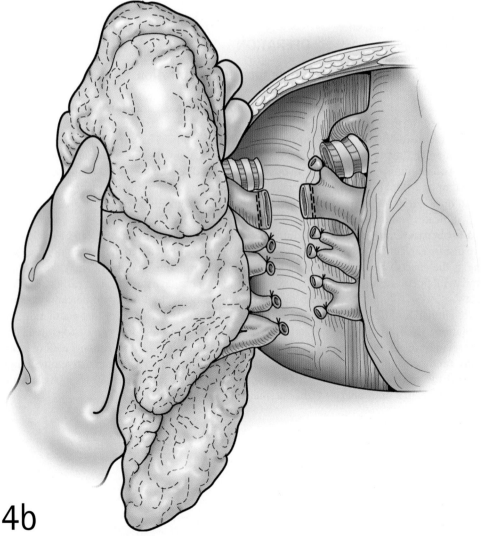

4b

PREPARATION OF THE HILUM

The pulmonary artery is mobilized off adjacent structures, particularly the bronchus, in order to produce a length suitable for subsequent clamping. On the right, the dissection is carried under the SVC. On the left, it is rarely necessary to divide the ligamentum; and indeed, the area around the recurrent laryngeal nerve can be avoided.

The pericardium is opened in front of the pulmonary veins which are then mobilized completely off the pericardial reflexions. This maneuver may be awkward posteriorly, but it is important to stay within the pericardium and not to develop the plane between the bronchus and the pericardium which may threaten the blood supply to the recipient's bronchial stump. The complete mobilization of the pulmonary veins is important to allow comfortable placement of a side-biting clamp. Finally, the bronchus is trimmed back so that it is flush with the mediastinal tissues and in particular is not devascularized. 4/0 polypropylene sutures are placed at each junction of the membranous and cartilaginous portions of the bronchus.

In the donor lung, the vascular structures are prepared, and the bronchus is trimmed with a knife as close as possible to the origin of the first (upper lobe) branch. Peribronchial tissues are preserved, so as not to disturb the blood supply from pulmonary to bronchial collaterals. The lung is placed in the posterior part of the chest (i.e. the costo-vertebral angle). The emphysematous patient with very large total lung capacity has a great deal of room, and the access is straightforward. In the small chest cavity of the patient with restricted disease, access may be exceedingly difficult. Problems with vascular anastomoses are much commoner in recipients, particularly females, with fibrotic disease.

5 Implantation is begun along the posterior part of the bronchus joining the two membranous portions with a continuous suture. The anterior part is performed with intra-figure-of-eight sutures. The completed suture line is then buried by the peribronchial tissues tacked in place with a handful of interrupted sutures.

The most important steps in the bronchial anastomosis are to ensure that there is a short donor bronchus so that the suture line is placed as close as possible to the lung parenchyma. End-to-end apposition of the donor lung, and the separate components should be achieved, particularly avoiding telescoping or overlapping. Suture material (absorbable or nonabsorbable) or technique (interrupted, figure-of-eight or continuous suture) are probably unimportant compared with the principles of short donor bronchus and accurate tissue apposition. This approach can easily result in a complication rate of less than 2%. Once the bronchial anastomosis has been completed, the chest cavity can be flooded with ice-cold saline to ensure the continued cooling of the still-ischemic lung.

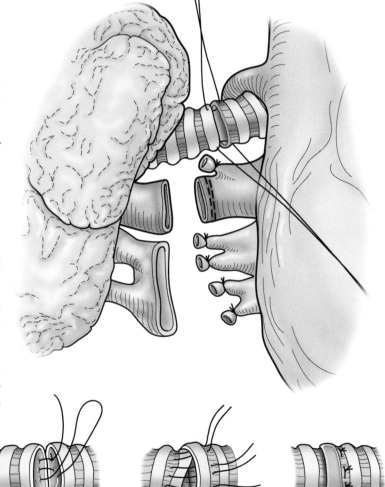

5

6 A side-biting clamp is placed on the recipient atrial cuff, and the two ligated pulmonary veins are joined together into a single orifice. This vessel is then anastomosed easily to the donor atrial cuff using continuous 4/0 polypropylene. It is important to ensure that this anastomosis is widely patent. The two ends of the stitch are left untied so as to allow for subsequent de-airing of the lung.

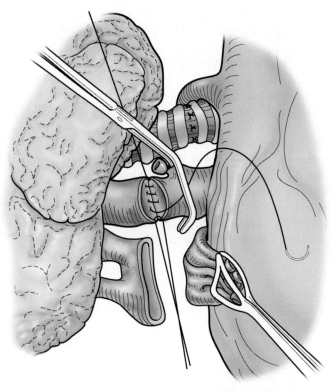

6

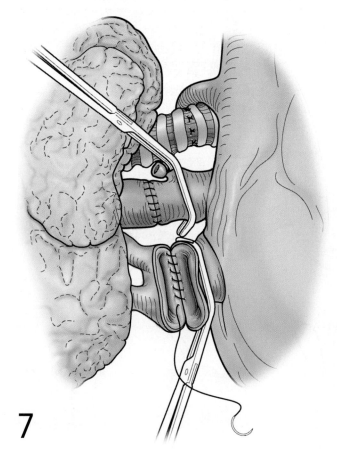

7

7 The transplantation is completed by simply trimming and then anastomosing two ends of the pulmonary artery using 5/0 polypropylene sutures. Orientation is relatively straightforward. The position of the ligamentum relative to the side-biting clamp on the pulmonary artery can be reconciled with the position of the ligamentum on the donor.

Prior to reventilation, the anesthetist should suction all the secretions out of the newly implanted lung, ideally under direct vision with a bronchoscope. The lung now needs to be de-aired and then reperfused in a controlled fashion.

The pulmonary artery clamp is eased open in a very gradual fashion so as to gently fill the pulmonary artery and its branches. The previously pale lung will be seen to gradually turn pink, and blood and a few bubbles of air appear at the still untied atrial suture line. These should be allowed to exit from the atrial cuff in an obstructed fashion. The anesthetist should inflate the lung gently just a couple of times at this stage. When a flow of blood with no residual bubbles is seen coming from the atrial suture line, two ends of the suture can be tied and the atrial clamp removed.

A monitoring cannula, usually tipped with a fine needle, is introduced into the pulmonary artery beyond the clamp. Avoidance of high pressure reperfusion is important; and indeed, events during the first 10 or 15 minutes are vital. The clamp is gradually removed so as to produce a very damp pulmonary artery flow pattern with a mean pressure no higher than 20 mmHg and a peak pressure no higher than 25 mmHg. So-called controlled pressure reperfusion is continued for a period of 10 minutes. Abrupt release of the clamp can expose the ischemic endothelium to a hydrostatic stress injury. The lung is gently inflated during this reperfusion phase and then regularly ventilated. At the end of 10 or 15 minutes the pulmonary artery clamp can be completely removed. Lung function is good; pulmonary artery pressure hardly rises any further upon fully removing the clamp.

The suture line should be checked for hemostasis. A little bit of bleeding is always present on the cut edges of the donor lung collecting flow from pulmonary artery to bronchial artery collaterals. This bleeding can usually be ignored. Apical and basal chest drains are placed, and the chest is closed in routine fashion. Suture lines should again be examined via bronchoscopy at the completion of the procedure to ensure that no secretions or in particular blood clots are within the major airways.

PREOPERATIVE PREPARATION AND ASSESSMENT

Bilateral lung transplantation

Patients with septic lung disease require removal of all the infected material, to all intents and purposes both lungs. They are classically those patients with bronchiectasis, predominantly as a result of cystic fibrosis. These patients are the prime group for whom the procedure was developed. Its hallmark features such as access through a clam shell incision and minimal mediastinal dissection have particular advantages in the setting of inflammatory lung disease. Pleural adhesions are often dense and vascular in these patients and can easily be taken out under direct access through the trans-sternal bilateral anterior thoracotomy incision. The very vascular and enlarged lymph glands found at the hilum can easily be dissected and any hemorrhage controlled while at the same time minimizing the risk of damage to vital structures such as the phrenic and the vagus nerve.

A large number of bilateral lung transplantations are also performed for patients with obstructive, emphysematous disease. Such patients gain an improved exercise tolerance and probably have an advantage in terms of long-term quality of life and survival for having two rather than one units of lung tissue transplanted. The risks of occult sepsis in a residual native lung together with the problem of overexpansion are also avoided. Suboptimal donor lungs may possibly be used in the bilateral lung transplantation with a lower risk than would be the case if a single transplantation was performed.

The procedure is also attractive for pulmonary hypertensive conditions where the heart is either anatomically normal or easily repaired. The transplantation of a very large area of pulmonary vascular bed in the two lungs results in greater offloading of the right ventricle and less risk of persistent pulmonary hypertension in the postoperative period. In children, this approach has been linked with repair of intracardiac malformations up to and including pulmonary atresia, to avoid the need for a combined heart and lung transplantation.

OPERATION

Bilateral lung transplantation

POSITION

The patient is supine with the arms abducted slightly from the side. In the original description the arms are elevated over the face, but we no longer find this necessary. The chest should be draped as far as the posterior axillary line.

INCISION

8a,b The bilateral trans-sternal anterior thoracotomy is made at the fourth or the fifth interspace. The former is advantageous in patients with cystic fibrosis where particularly good access to the apices of the chest is required. The internal mammary arteries are ligated and divided prior to sternal division to minimize bleeding. Once both pleural cavities have been opened, twin child's Finnochetto retractors are placed, and the chest is easily opened.

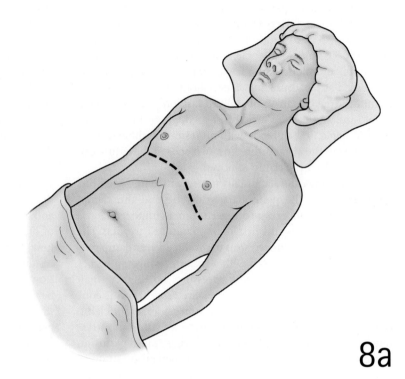

8a

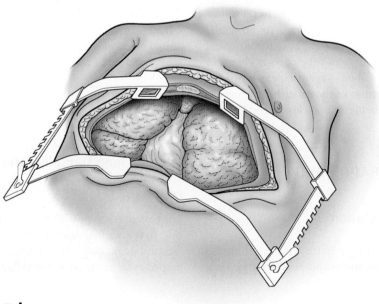

8b

9 Alternatively bilateral anterior thoracotomies without transverse sternal division may be performed. This approach eliminates the potential problems with sternal healing but does not provide as good an exposure as is obtained with sternal division.

A thorough examination should be made of both pleural spaces and adhesions divided as far as possible. For children or small adults, patients with pulmonary hypertension or where it is local custom, cardiopulmonary bypass can be adopted at this stage. Cannulation is via the ascending aorta and two separate caval cannulae. If a single atrial cannula is used, intermittent and troublesome SVC obstruction may occur, while retracting the structures at the right hilum.

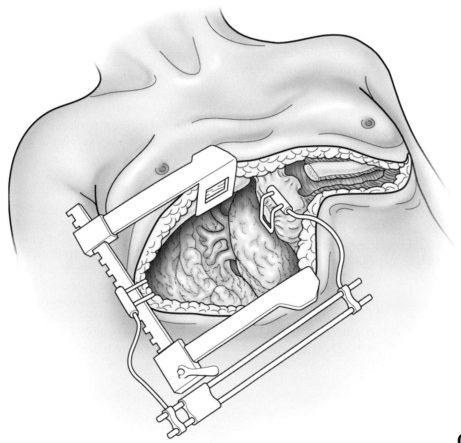

9

Assuming the patient is stable and recourse to cardiopulmonary bypass is not anticipated, the right lung is deflated and ventilation continued on the left side only. Structures of the hilum are exposed and then divided; it is important to ligate the vessels relatively long so as to leave good sized stumps. Intrapericardial dissection is avoided at this stage. The patient can be tilted fairly steeply to the left side to improve access to the right hilum. The inferior pulmonary ligament can be divided by cautery, taking care to avoid the vagus nerve. The bronchus is stapled some way out from the hilum to avoid incorporation of the vagus nerve. Once the lung has been removed, the hilum is prepared as for a single lung transplantation.

IMPLANTATION OF THE FIRST LUNG

The right donor lung is placed in the field, lying posteriorly and surrounded in ice-cold saline-soaked swabs. After suitable suctioning by the anesthetist, the staple line on the right main bronchus is amputated and hemostasis resecured. Access to the back of the hilum after completing the anastomosis is awkward so there should be a meticulous search for bleeding points at this stage.

The bronchus is anastomosed in a standard end-to-end fashion as for a single lung transplantation. Side-biting clamps are placed on the intrapericardial pulmonary veins and on the pulmonary artery to allow appropriate anastomosis to be performed. After de-airing the lung (again as for the single lung transplantation), the lung is cautiously reperfused. Ventilation of the transplanted site is commenced. The bronchus is checked for air leaks and the rest of the hilum for bleeding points. If donor lung selection has been careful and preservation successful, the newly implanted lung readily takes over the function when right-sided one-lung ventilation is adopted.

IMPLANTATION OF THE SECOND LUNG

The patient is rolled steeply over on to the right side and the pericardium retracted within the limits of hemodynamic stability. A similar left-sided pneumonectomy is performed, ligating and dividing the vascular structures and stapling the bronchus at a convenient point. The left lung is removed from the field; and again, great care is taken to avoid spilling infected secretions. The pleural space is again irrigated with an antiseptic solution. Left lung implantation is performed as for the single lung transplantation starting with a bronchial anastomosis, followed by pulmonary venous anastomosis with a side-biting clamp on the pulmonary veins on the left-hand side and ending with the pulmonary artery anastomosis. Hemodynamic embarrassment is not uncommon during the pulmonary venous anastomosis, and it may be necessary to carry out the suture line in a series of stages, resting the heart and the circulation after every few stitches. When the implantation is complete, de-airing and reperfusion is performed as before, and both lungs can be ventilated.

Apical and basal chest drains are placed and the chest closed in a standard fashion with three stainless steel wires to the sternum, absorbable pericostal wires for pulling anterior ribs together, and muscle and overlying skin closed with continuous absorbable sutures.

POSTOPERATIVE CARE

This care is broadly similar for the two types of transplantation although each can provide particular problems. After returning to the intensive care unit, ventilation is continued for at least several hours. Primary lung dysfunction, which occurs in 10–20% of patients, may be evident even on the operating table with frothy, proteinaceous secretions or over the first few hours with the appearance of a pulmonary edema picture on chest X-ray, increasing hypoxia, and decreased compliance. Management is with the application of positive end expiratory pressure and use of inhaled nitric oxide doses up to 40 parts/million. The problem is more easily contained in the bilateral lung transplantation recipient. Management is much more difficult in the setting of a single lung and obstructive disease because of the difficulty of applying positive end expiratory pressure without causing air trapping and overdistension of the residual native lung. It may be necessary to resort to split lung ventilation with a double-lumen tube, ventilating the transplant vigorously and often leaving the contralateral lung completely unventilated, merely insufflating oxygen to prevent a shunt.

Pain control is a major problem, and in bilateral lung transplantation we use an opiate epidural for a minimum of 5 days. Epidural analgesia is also useful in the natural thoracotomy of a single lung transplantation although a paravertebral catheter, carefully placed before the chest is closed, can give equivalent and excellent analgesia. Chest drains are left for several days as a leak of fluid from the newly implanted lung is always present at least partly because lymphatics have been divided. Any air leak at this stage is almost invariably from the lung parenchyma and should not cause concern over integrity of the bronchial anastomosis.

Antibiotics are continued but for only a few days in the "clean" setting of transplantation for obstructive or restrictive disease. Patients with septic lung disease will require broader spectrum and appropriately selected antibiotics. Information from some of the donor airways' secretions may prompt a change of antibiotics and particularly the addition of antifungals if *Candida* species are present in the donor.

Immunosuppressants are obviously essential for the newly implanted lungs. A standard regimen incorporates a calcineurin inhibitor such as cyclosporin or tacrolimus given intravenously for 4 or 5 days together with a second line of attack such as azathioprine or mycophenolate and supplemented by high dose steroids. This triple drug regimen has toxicities to both the kidneys and the bone marrow; the former is a particular problem. A conflict exists between the need to avoid overhydration in the setting of an invariably damaged lung endothelium and combating overtoxicity with good renal perfusion. A compromise is often achieved by giving relatively low dose calcineurin inhibitors and use induction therapy with either a polyclonal antithymal cytoglobulin (ATG) or one of the modern monoclonal IL2 receptor antagonists.

FURTHER READING

Cooper JD, Pearson FG, Patterson GA, et al. Technique of successful lung transplantation in humans. *Journal of Thoracic and Cardiovascular Surgery* 1987; **93**: 173–81.

ISHLT International Guidelines for the selection of lung transplant candidates. *Journal of Heart and Lung Transplantation* 1998; **17**:703–9.

Patterson GA, Cooper JD, Dark JH, et al. Experimental and clinical double lung transplantation. *Journal of Thoracic and Cardiovascular Surgery* 1988; **95**: 70–4.

Pasque MK, Cooper JD, Kaiser LR, Haydock DA, Triantafillou A, Trulock EP. Improved technique for bilateral lung transplantation: rationale and initial clinical experience. *Annals of Thoracic Surgery* 1990; **49**: 785–91.

Sundaresan S, Trachiotis GD, Aoe M, Patterson GA, Cooper JD. Donor lung procurement: assessment and operative technique. *Annals of Thoracic Surgery* 1993; **56**: 1409–13.

Wilson IC, Hasan A, Healy M, et al. Healing of the bronchus in pulmonary transplantation. *European Journal of Cardiothoracic Surgery* 1996; **10**: 521–7.

27

Thoracic outlet syndromes

HAROLD CLIFTON URSCHEL, JR. MD
Chair; Cardiovascular and Thoracic Surgical Research, Education and Clinical Excellence, Baylor University Medical Center, Professor of Cardiothoracic Surgery (Clinical), University of Texas Southwestern Medical Center at Dallas Southwestern Medical School, Dallas, Texas, USA

HISTORY

Clinical manifestations of thoracic outlet syndromes have afflicted humankind since prerecorded history. One of the first cases is described in Genesis 22:1. Abraham was planning to sacrifice his son Isaac to prove his devotion to God. As Abraham raised the knife, an angel of the Lord came to him and with omnipotent compassion created an 'acute thoracic outlet syndrome,' causing Abraham's arm to become numb and weak. He dropped the knife, thus sparing Isaac and forever ending human sacrifice in the Judeo-Christian religions.

The earliest recorded reference to thoracic outlet syndrome was the anatomical recognition of cervical ribs by Galen and Vesalius. The first scientific study reported in the modern literature was in 1740 by the German anatomist Hunauld. Sir Astley Cooper in 1821 was the first to describe symptoms of vascular compression from a cervical rib.

Paget in 1875 in London and von Schrötter in Vienna in 1874 independently described thrombosis of the axillary subclavian vein in the area of the thoracic outlet. The occlusion of the vein today is called the *Paget-von Schrötter syndrome* or *effort thrombosis*.

The term *thoracic outlet syndrome* was first used by Peet in 1956. The purpose of using a single term to encompass the various anatomical abnormalities such as the scalenus anticus, costoclavicular, and neurovascular compression syndromes was to promote simplification, particularly when the abnormalities produced similar symptoms. The first rib was recognized as the 'common denominator' against which the axillary subclavian artery and vein or brachial plexus was compressed by a variety of muscles, ligaments, or bone structures.

In 1962, O. T. Claggett in his presidential address to the American Association of Thoracic Surgery presented the posterior high thoracoplasty approach for removal of the first rib

in thoracic outlet syndrome. In 1966, Roos described the transaxillary approach following the technique of Atkins and Palumbo for transaxillary sympathectomy. Neurophysiological testing was initiated by Caldwell, Krusen, and Crane in the 1960s and reported in 1968. They measured nerve conduction velocities across the outlet in the median, ulnar, and musculocutaneous nerves. To perform reoperations for recurrent thoracic outlet syndrome, Urschel and Razzuk recommended the posterior 'high thoracoplasty' approach. Thoracic outlet syndrome masquerading as coronary artery disease ('pseudo' angina) was described by Urschel *et al.* in 1973.

A 50-year experience of over 5000 cases of thoracic outlet syndrome coming to surgery was presented by Dr. Urschel to the American Surgical Association in 1998, summarizing the changes in diagnosis and management of that disease process over half a century.

PRINCIPLES AND JUSTIFICATION

Indications for surgery include the failure of conservative measures to attenuate the symptoms caused by nerve compression after a 3-month period and the presence of prolonged conduction velocities in the ulnar or median nerve. Other surgical indications include (1) the presence of atypical chest pain unrelieved by conservative management (not related to coronary artery, esophageal, or pulmonary pathological conditions); (2) the presence of hypersympathetic activity; (3) the narrowing or occlusion of the axillary subclavian artery with or without peripheral emboli; and (4) thrombosis of the axillary subclavian vein (Paget-von Schrötter syndrome, effort thrombosis).

For nerve compression, the preferred initial surgical procedure is the transaxillary approach for first rib resection, with decompression of the axillary subclavian artery and vein as well as the brachial plexus. In contrast to the supraclavicular approach, the transaxillary approach allows the first rib to be removed, the scalene muscles divided and resected if necessary, and the outlet decompressed with minimal risk to the critical neurovascular structures that lie away from the first rib. Removing the rib completely is particularly important to minimize recurrence of the symptom complex as a result of regeneration of bone or fibrocartilage from an incompletely removed stump or rib remnant. To remove the first rib completely using a supraclavicular approach, the brachial plexus and neurovascular structures must be retracted, which is a situation that results in a higher complication rate.

For recurrent thoracic outlet syndrome after either primary transaxillary or supraclavicular operations, the posterior 'thoracoplasty' operation provides a safer approach and better access for removing bone remnants and scar from the brachial plexus and subclavian vessels. This approach also allows dorsal sympathectomy to be performed for causalgia and sympathetic maintained pain syndrome.

For arterial reconstruction, the combined supraclavicular-infraclavicular approach is often used when bypass grafts are necessary for either occlusion or aneurysm. For venous occlusion (Paget-von Schrötter syndrome), the ideal management combines clot lysis with administration of urokinase through a catheter, followed by prompt decompression of the thoracic outlet by transaxillary resection of the first rib. Prolonged delay of clot lysis markedly increases morbidity, and failure to perform prompt first rib resection and thoracic outlet decompression leads to extremely high rates of recurrence. Compression and sympathetic nerve hyperactivity not relieved by medical therapy should be treated by dorsal sympathectomy, usually performed in conjunction with resection of the fist rib through the same exposure.

OPERATION

First rib resection: transaxillary approach

1a The incision is transaxillary below the hairline and transverse between the pectoralis major muscle anteriorly and the latissimus dorsi muscle posteriorly. The incision is carried directly to the chest wall without angling up toward the first rib. When the chest wall is encountered, the dissection is carried superiorly to the first rib, with identification of the intercostal brachial nerve that exits between the first and second ribs. This nerve is preserved by retracting it anteriorly or posteriorly. Division produces 6 months to 1 year of paresthesia on the inner surface of the upper arm. The first rib is dissected subperiosteally with a Shaw-Paulson periosteal elevator, and the scalenus anticus muscle is identified. A right-angle clamp is placed behind the muscle, with care taken not to injure the subclavian artery or vein. The scalenus anticus muscle is divided near its insertion on the first rib. This step avoids injury to the phrenic nerve, which courses away from the muscle at this level.

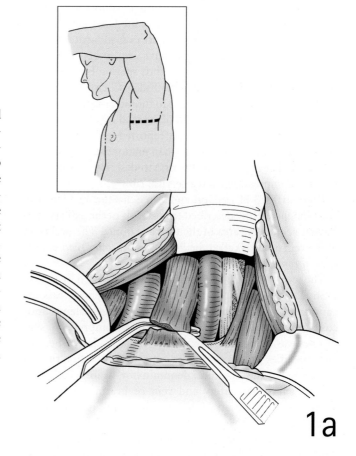

1a

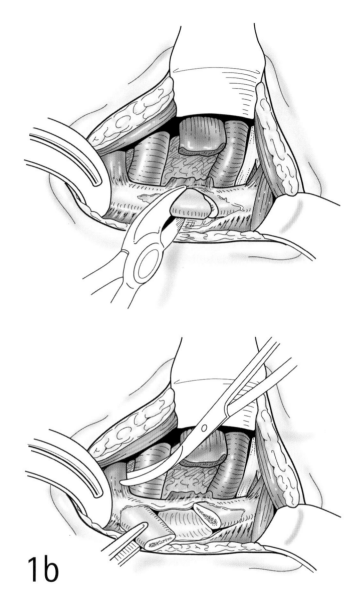

1b After the scalenus anticus muscle is divided, the first rib is dissected free subperiosteally and separated from the pleura. A triangular piece of the rib is removed in the avascular plane. The apex of the triangle removed is at the scalene tubercle. The anterior part of the rib is removed by dividing the costoclavicular ligament and resecting the rib subperiosteally back to the costicartilage of the sternum.

1b

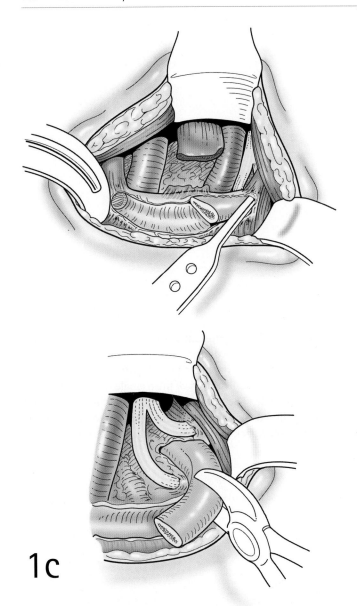

1c The posterior part of the rib is dissected sub-periosteally to the transverse process, where it is divided by a pair of rib shears. The rib may be resected posteriorly with an Urschel-Leksell reinforced rongeur. Care is taken to avoid injury to the C8 and T1 nerve roots as the scalenus medius muscle is dissected from the rib.

1c

1d After the transverse process articulation is visualized, the head and neck of the rib are removed with an Urschel reinforced pituitary rongeur. Removing the complete head and neck of the rib is important to minimize regeneration. Care is taken not to injure the T1 nerve root below nor the C8 nerve root above. After the complete removal of the first rib, neurolysis of the C7, C8, and T1 nerve roots as well as the middle and lower trunks of the brachial plexus is performed. A video thoracoscope is used for this purpose because of its magnification and light. The scalenus medius and scalenus anticus muscles are resected up into the neck so that they will not reattach to the Sibson's fascia or the pleura. Bands and adhesions are removed from the axillary-subclavian artery and the axillary-subclavian vein so that they are completely free. Hemostasis is secured.

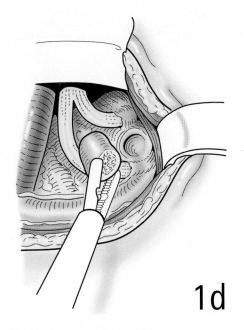

1d

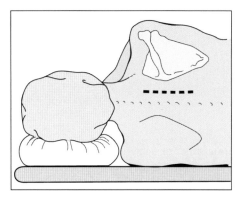

First rib resection: posterior approach

2a In the posterior approach, the patient is placed in the lateral position with an axillary roll under the 'down' side. The upper arm is placed as for a thoracotomy. An incision of approximately 6 cm is made with the midpoint at the angle of the scapulae halfway between the scapula and the spinous process. The incision is carried through the skin and subcutaneous tissue down to the trapezius muscle. The trapezius and rhomboid muscles are split.

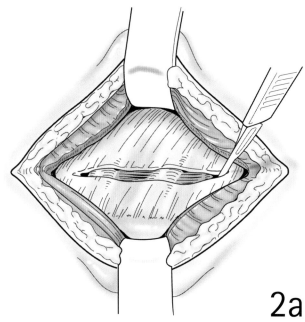

2a

2b The posterior superior serratus muscle is resected, and the first rib stump is identified by retracting the sacrospinalis muscle medially. Cautery is used to expose the first rib remnant (stump) and to open the periosteum. A periosteal elevator, or joker, is used to remove the stump sub-periosteally. The head and the neck of the rib usually have not been removed in the initial operation. The rib shears are used to divide the rib remnant, and the Urschel-Leksell reinforced and Urschel pituitary rongeurs are used carefully to remove the head and neck of the rib. The T1 nerve root is identified grossly or with the nerve stimulator.

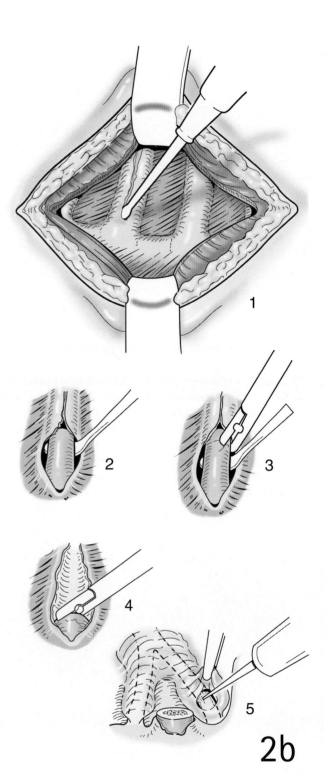

2b

2c Once the T1 nerve root is identified, neurolysis is carried out using a right-angle clamp, magnification, a knife, and special microscissors. A nerve stimulator may be helpful if extensive scarring is present. Neurolysis is extended to the C7 and C8 nerve roots and to the brachial plexus. All the scar is removed as far forward as necessary so that the nerve roots as well as the upper, middle, and lower trunks of the brachial plexus lie free. Care is taken not to injure the long thoracic nerve or any other brachial plexus branch. The axillary subclavian artery and vein are decompressed through the same incision.

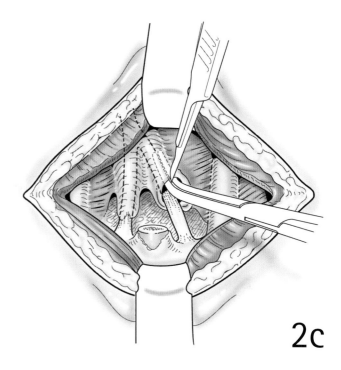

2c

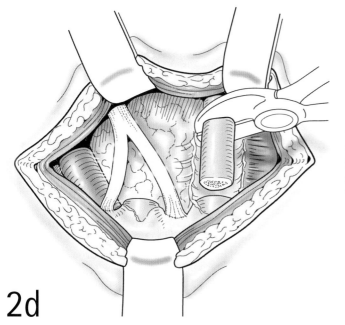

2d

2d The second rib is dissected free, and the cautery is used to open the periosteum linearly. A 2-cm segment of the rib is resected posteriorly, medial to the sacrospinalis muscle, to perform the dorsal sympathectomy. This exposure may also help identify the T1 nerve root.

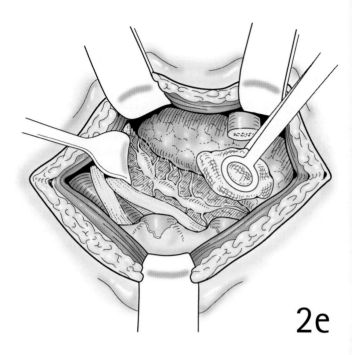

2e After the head and neck of the second rib are removed, the sympathetic chain is identified on the vertebra, or it may have been separated and lie on the pleura. The stellate ganglion lies in an almost transverse rather than vertical position.

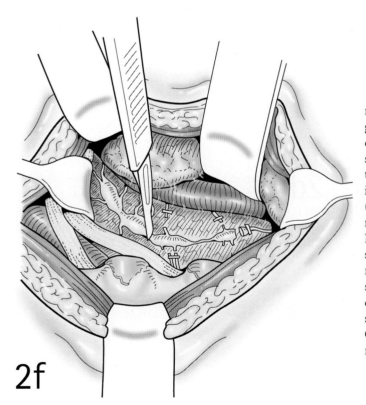

2f The lower third of the stellate ganglion is incised sharply (T1), and the gray and white rami communicantes are clipped and divided. The T1, T2, and T3 ganglia are removed along with the sympathetic chain using clips on all of the branches. Cautery is used to effect hemostasis and to char the area so that sprouting and regeneration of the sympathetic chain are discouraged. After irrigation with antibiotic solution, methylprednisolone (Depo-Medrol) and Sepra Film are left on the areas of neurolysis. The wound is closed in layers with interrupted No. 1 Nurolon in a figure-of-eight fashion (Tom Jones stitch) in each of the muscle layers. Running and interrupted 2/0 Vicryl sutures are used in the subcutaneous tissue and skin clips in the skin. A large round Jackson-Pratt drain is placed in the area of neurolysis through a separate stab wound 2 cm below the inferior part of the incision. Care is taken not to incorporate the drain while closing the muscle layers over the top.

OUTCOME

No deaths occurred in a series of 3914 primary and 1221 reoperative thoracic outlet syndrome decompressive procedures. The major complication observed was the leaving of a rib remnant by the initial surgeon from which fibrocartilage and new bone regenerated, producing a high incidence of recurrence. More retractor help (two arm holders) and increased light improved the technique and facilitated the initial operation. These maneuvers minimized the time of anesthesia, surgery, retractor use, and arm holding.

FURTHER READING

Roos DB. Transaxillary approach for first rib resection to relieve thoracic outlet compression syndrome. *Annals of Surgery* 1966; **163:** 354–8.

Urschel HC, Cooper JD. Atlas of Thoracic Surgery. Churchill Livingstone, New York 1995.

Urschel HC Jr, Razzuk MA. Neurovascular compression in the thoracic outlet: changing management over 50 years. *Annals of Surgery* 1998; **228**(4): 609–17.

Urschel HC Jr, Razzuk MA. The failed operation for thoracic outlet syndrome: the difficulty of diagnosis and management. *Annals of Thoracic Surgery* 1986; **42:** 523–8.

Urschel HC Jr, Razzuk MA, Ryland JW, *et al.* Thoracic outlet syndrome masquerading as coronary artery disease. *Annals of Thoracic Surgery* 1973; **16:** 239–48.

28

Mediastinal lymph node dissection

PAOLO MACCHIARINI MD, PHD

Professor of Surgery, University of Barcelona Medical School; Chairman, Department of General Thoracic Surgery, Hospital Clinic of Barcelona, Spain

HISTORY

Although mediastinal lymph node dissection was first mentioned in the 1940s, its optimal extent remains controversial. Trends have evolved from procedures with virtually no lymph node sampling to more radical operations including minimal or more extensive hilar and mediastinal lymph node sampling, complete ipsilateral mediastinal dissection, and extended lymph node dissection.

Proponents of the sampling of multiple lymph node stations argue that sampling results in improved staging and less perioperative morbidity than lymph node dissection. Conversely, proponents of mediastinal lymph node dissection claim that, without a complete removal of all ipsilateral mediastinal lymph nodes, patients would be understaged, and their cure rates worsened. The operative procedure of extended nodal dissection includes the ipsilateral and contralateral mediastinal nodes and the supraclavicular lymph nodes, but the magnitude of the operation and the fact that non-small cell lung cancer (NSCLC) will recur in distant locations has reduced its popularity except for patients enrolled into clinical trials.

PRINCIPLES AND JUSTIFICATION

The normal patterns of intrathoracic lymphatic drainage are as follows: On the right, the apical and posterior segments of the upper lobe drain into the ipsilateral scalene nodes via the hilar nodes, tracheobronchial angle nodes, and upper paratracheal lymph nodes. The anterior segment of the right upper lobe drains either as previously described (50% of cases) or into the right scalene nodes via the subcarinal and pretracheal lymph nodes, or the anterior mediastinal lymph nodes. Drainage to the left paratracheal nodes seldom occurs and proceeds along the left innominate vein, left anterior mediastinal nodes, and into the left scalene nodes. The middle lobe and superior segment of the lower lobe usually drain to the ipsilateral scalene nodes via the two paths described earlier. However, drainage from the middle lobe to the left scalene nodes through the subcarinal and left paratracheal nodes also may occur. Drainage from the basal segments of the lower lobes reaches the subcarinal nodes via the hilar nodes. Further drainage may reach the right scalene nodes by way of the right paratracheal lymph nodes. On the left, the apical and posterior segment of the left upper lobe drain primarily via the subcarinal lymph nodes and then either along the left vagus nerve to the left scalene nodes or along the recurrent laryngeal nerve to the mediastinal lymph nodes. The anterior and lingular segments drain along the phrenic nerve through the para-aortic nodes to the ipsilateral scalene lymph nodes. Lymph from the basilar segments flows via the subcarinal nodes to the pretracheal and contralateral paratracheal lymphatics to the right scalene nodes. Drainage along the ipsilateral region to high mediastinal lymph nodes also may occur. Drainage from the superior segment occurs via all of these paths.

The patterns of intra- and extrapulmonary lymph node metastasis in patients with NSCLC are as follows: Disease in all right lung lobes commonly metastasizes to the lymph nodes along the bronchus intermedius between the origins of the upper and middle lobe bronchi, whereas tumors in both left lobes commonly metastasizes to the lymph nodes located between the origins of the lobar bronchi. Among right upper lobe tumors, ipsilateral mediastinal lymph nodes represent the most common metastatic site, whereas spread to the subcarinal, contralateral mediastinal, and scalene nodes is uncommon. Conversely, left upper lobe tumors spread more frequently to the contralateral mediastinal and scalene lymph nodes. Right lower lobe tumors spread frequently in the subcarinal and ipsilateral mediastinal regions and less rarely in the contralateral mediastinal or scalene nodes. Left lower lobe tumors spread mostly to the contralateral scalene and contralateral mediastinal nodes. Watanabe *et al.* showed, however, that right upper lobe tumors may spread to the subcarinal lymph nodes, whereas right middle and right lower lobe tumors commonly spread to the ipsilateral paratracheal lymph nodes. They also found that subcarinal metastases commonly arise from left upper lobe and left lower lobe tumors.

This predictable sequence of metastases beginning in the intrapulmonary lymph nodes and progressing to the mediastinal and finally to the scalene lymph nodes is not always observed, however. The absence of intrapulmonary lymph node metastases may be documented in almost one-third of patients with resected NSCLC, and right upper lobe tumors may commonly skip to the ipsilateral paratracheal lymph nodes, left upper lobe tumors to the aortopulmonary window lymph nodes, and lower lobe tumors to the subcarinal region.

The prognosis of NSCLC is directly related to the completeness of resection and the status of the regional lymph nodes. The 50–80% cure rate of patients without lymph node involvement (N0 disease) drops to 30–50% if the N1 (hilar) lymph nodes are involved, and falls further to 10–30% if the lymph nodes in the mediastinum (N2) are involved. N2 disease can be divided into 'minimal' disease, with involvement of only one node by microscopic foci of tumor, or 'advanced', bulky disease. Only 20% of all cases of N2 disease are technically resectable, and most of them are discovered only at thoracotomy. The challenge is to identify correctly patients with N0, N1, or minimal N2 disease who are candidates for curative resection and to avoid inappropriate surgery in patients with advanced N2 or N3 disease. Moreover, patients presumed to have N0 or nonhilar N1 disease at the time of resection have a frequent (10–15%) occurrence of occult mediastinal lymph node metastases. The principles cited earlier make it evident that the status of the mediastinal lymph nodes must be known before surgery and that, without this assessment, a pulmonary resection must be considered as an incomplete procedure.

PREOPERATIVE ASSESSMENT AND PREPARATION

A growing body of evidence indicates that positron-emission tomography (PET) with fluorine-18-fluorodeoxyglucose is more accurate than computed tomography (CT) in the mediastinal staging of NSCLC, and that no significant improvement in accuracy is seen when the CT data are added to the PET result. The recommendation has been that patients with a positive result on PET study for mediastinal disease undergo confirmatory surgical mediastinal exploration, so that no patient is denied potentially curative resection. By contrast, the high negative predictive value of a negative PET

result should provide the surgeon with the impetus to proceed directly to thoracotomy without invasive mediastinal staging. Such a philosophy is certainly followed in North America, where Medicare and many third-party insurers reimburse the costs of PET.

This algorithm is not yet the case in Europe, where CT and invasive mediastinal investigation still represent the reimbursed staging tools. Except in patients with hilar and mediastinal nodes measuring less than 1 cm in the short-axis diameter on preoperative CT scan, mediastinoscopy should be routinely performed preoperatively, especially for left-sided tumors for which the exposure of the left paratracheal nodes is restrained anatomically. Mediastinoscopy should not replace a lymph node dissection, however, but represents the essential tool to obtain a histological and anatomical description of the mediastinal lymph node status.

ANESTHESIA

The anesthetic management mirrors that for the other major pulmonary resections. In our experience, however, the avoidance of perioperative fluid overload reduces the postoperative risks of mechanical noncariogenic edema of the residual lobes. Special care should be given to those patients who have had neoadjuvant chemotherapy and/or radiation therapy in whom mediastinal lymph node dissection is likely to result in additional fluid imbalances in the residual lung tissues.

OPERATIONS

Three approaches can be taken to the intraoperative assessment of the extrapulmonary lymph nodes:

1 Systematic sampling
2 Complete lymph node dissection
3 Extended lymph node dissection

Whichever technique is used, it is mandatory to uniformly label the intrathoracic lymph nodes according to a regional mediastinal lymph node classification (**Table 28.1**), such as that adapted from Mountain *et al.*, which is the one used in my institution. To ensure accuracy and consistency, intraoperative labeling of the level of all harvested lymph nodes must be correct and reproducible, and having the lymph node map in the operative room is very helpful. Although mediastinal lymph node sampling or dissection can be accomplished either before or after the planned lung resection, the wiser course is to determine the lymph node status first to see whether this factor will alter the nature of the operative procedure. Metallic clips are used only to delineate the proximal and distal margins of the dissection to guide postoperative radiation planning; hemostasis is usually obtained with absorbable ligatures.

Table 28.1 *Lymph node classification*[a]

N class	Nodal station[b]	Designation	Anatomical landmarks
N2	1	Highest mediastinal nodes	Nodes lying above a horizontal line at the upper rim of the brachiocephalic (left innominate) vein where it ascends to the left, crossing in front of the trachea at its midline.
N2	2	Upper paratracheal nodes	Nodes lying above a horizontal line drawn tangential to the upper margin of the aortic arch and below the inferior boundary of No. 1 nodes.
N2	3	Prevascular and retrotracheal	Prevascular and retrotracheal nodes may be designated 3A and 3P; midline nodes are considered to be ipsilateral.
N2	4	Lower paratracheal nodes	The lower paratracheal nodes on the right of the midline of the trachea between a horizontal line drawn tangential to the upper margin of the aortic arch and a line extending across the right main bronchus at the upper margin of the upper lobe bronchus, and contained within the mediastinal pleural envelope. The lower paratracheal nodes on the left lie to the left of the midline of the trachea between a horizontal line drawn tangential to the upper margin of the aortic arch and a line extending across the left main bronchus at the level of the upper margin of the left upper lobe bronchus, medial to the ligamentum arteriosum and contained within the mediastinal pleural envelope.
N2	5	Subaortic (aortopulmonary window)	Subaortic nodes are lateral to the ligamentum arteriosum or the aorta or left pulmonary artery and proximal to the first branch of the left pulmonary artery, and lie within the mediastinal pleural envelope.
N2	6	Para-aortic nodes (ascending aorta or phrenic)	Nodes lying anterior and lateral to the ascending aorta and the aortic arch or the innominate artery, beneath a line tangential to the upper margin of the aortic arch.
N2	7	Subcarinal nodes	Nodes lying caudal to the carina of the trachea but not associated with the lower lobe bronchi or arteries within the lung.
N2	8	Paraesophageal nodes (below carina)	Nodes lying adjacent to the wall of the esophagus and to the right or left of the midline, excluding subcarinal nodes.
N2	9	Pulmonary ligament nodes	Nodes lying within the pulmonary ligament, including those in the posterior wall and lower part of the inferior pulmonary vein.
N1	10	Hilar nodes	The proximal lobar nodes distal to the mediastinal pleural reflection and the nodes adjacent to the bronchus intermedius on the right.
N1	11	Interlobar nodes	Nodes lying between the lobar bronchi.
N1	12	Lobar nodes bronchi	Nodes adjacent to the distal lobar bronchi.
N1	13	Segmental nodes	Nodes adjacent to the segmental bronchi.
N1	14	Subsegmental nodes	Nodes around the subsegmental bronchi.

[a]All N2 nodes lie within the mediastinal pleural envelope on the ipsilateral side. All N1 nodes lie distal to the mediastinal pleural reflection and within the visceral pleura.
[b]The American College of Surgical Oncologists suggests designating the lower paratracheal nodes as No. 4s (superior) and No. 4i (inferior) subsets for study purposes; the No. 4s nodes may be defined by a horizontal line extending across the trachea and drawn tangential to the cephalic border of the of the azygos vein; the No. 4i nodes may be defined by the lower boundary of No. 4s and the lower boundary of No. 4, as described earlier.
Adapted with permission from Mountain and Dresler.

Systematic sampling

1 Systematic sampling refers to visual and tactile examination of each of the mediastinal lymph node levels followed by biopsy of selected lymph nodes, whether or not they have been exposed by opening the mediastinal pleura. On the right side (the regional nodal station locations), sampling should include one or two lymph nodes from stations 2, 4, 7, and 10. Levels 2 and 4 may not be resampled at thoracotomy if a mediastinoscopy had shown negative lymph nodes. The numbers in this figure and Figure 2 correspond with those explained in detail in Table 28.1.

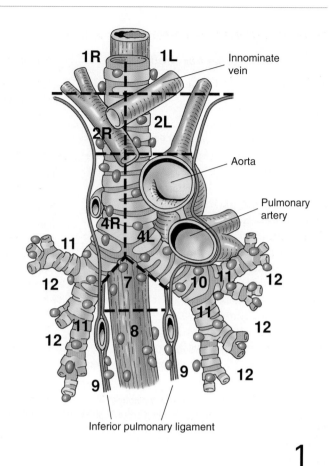

1

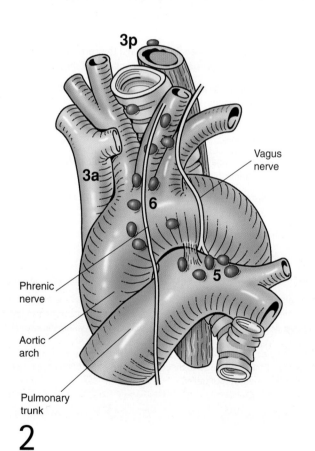

2

2 For left-sided tumors (the regional nodal stations in the left hemithorax), sampling consists of removing one or two lymph nodes from stations 5, 6, 7, and 10. This approach may be inaccurate, especially when the *in situ* lymph nodes assessment (level and number) is made through an intact pleura, because it relies on the personal experience of the operating surgeon as to which and how many nodes are sampled.

Complete mediastinal lymph node dissection

Complete mediastinal lymph node dissection refers to the removal of all the mediastinal nodes found at the common nodal sites within the ipsilateral hemithorax. This procedure, which I prefer, is usually best performed through an ipsilat-

eral posterolateral thoracotomy or a muscle-sparing incision in the fifth intercostal space. Patients with contralateral lymph nodes involvement (N3 disease) are usually approached through a median vertical sternotomy, and this approach represents my preference for all N3 left-sided tumors.

COMPLETE LYMPH NODE DISSECTION FOR A RIGHT THORACOTOMY

SUPERIOR MEDIASTINAL DISSECTION

3 Dissection of the superior mediastinum (view is as by a right posterolateral thoracotomy) removes all tissue lying in an area bounded inferiorly by the takeoff of the right upper lobe, superiorly by the innominate artery, ventrally by the superior vena cava (SVC), and dorsally by the trachea. The mediastinal pleura is elevated and opened with a cautery midway between the trachea and SVC. The dissection is continued to the cephalic border of the azygos vein caudally and the innominate artery cephalad. Ligation of the azygos vein is unnecessary. Several small vessels may be present near the innominate artery that need to be ligated. The right recurrent nerve should be identified. The fat pad containing the lymph nodes is bluntly dissected away from the anterolateral borders of the trachea and posterior aspects of the SVC, grasped *in situ*, and then elevated from the medially located posterior pericardium and aortic arch. Before transection, ligatures or clips are applied at the most cephalad aspect of the fat pad. The specimen is removed and labeled as 2R (above aortic arch) or 4R (below aortic arch). When present, lymph nodes in front of the SVC and in the retrotracheal area are removed and labeled as 3A and 3P, respectively (Figure 2). A warm gauze pad can be placed in the dissection root to enhance hemostasis.

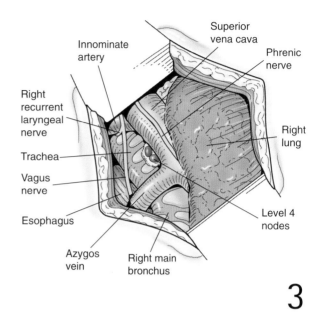

3

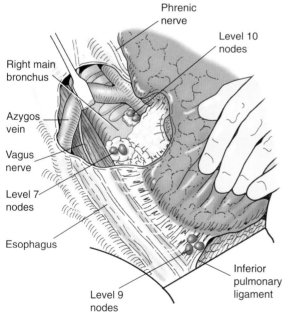

4

HILAR DISSECTION

4 The azygos vein is slightly elevated with a vein retractor, and the nodes located between the right upper lobe takeoff and the origin of the right main stem anteriorly beyond the reflection of the pleura (in the pleural cavity) are grasped away and removed and labeled as 10R (N1 lymph nodes). Care should be taken to avoid injury of the phrenic nerve and pulmonary artery. This figure depicts the hilar (level 10) and subcarinal nodal (level 7) right mediastinal lymphadenectomy. The view is as by a right posterolateral thoracotomy. The numbers correspond with those explained in detail in Table 28.1.

SUBCARINAL DISSECTION

The subcarinal dissection is begun by retracting the lung anteriorly. The pleura is opened in the posterior hilum in a caudal direction midway between the anterior border of the esophagus and the medial border of the bronchus intermedius beginning at the caudal margin of the azygos vein (Figure 4). The pleural edge overlying the esophagus is grasped and retracted posteriorly. After ligation and division of small branches of the vagus nerve and bronchial arteries crossing the subcarinal area, the right and left main stem, upper lobe, and bronchus intermedius are exposed with blunt dissection. The floor of the dissection is the posterior pericardium, and it is carried superiorly until the carina is reached. Posteriorly, the lymph nodes are dissected off the esophagus. Care should be taken to preserve the vagus nerves. At the apex of the subcarinal triangle are several nourishing blood vessels of the subcarinal lymph nodes that need to be identified to ensure hemostasis before removing the subcarinal lymph node packet. I usually ligate these vessels rather than clipping them. These lymph nodes are labeled as level 7. A warm gauze pad can be placed in the subcarinal space to enhance hemostasis.

INFERIOR PULMONARY LIGAMENT DISSECTION

5 Lymph nodes along the length of the esophagus (paraesophageal nodes) from the level of the azygos vein to the diaphragm are removed and labeled as level 8. Removal is accomplished by opening the overlying pleura. The inferior pulmonary ligament should be divided close to the lung, and any lymph tissue in the ligament should be removed and labeled as level 9. Level 11 (interlobar) and level 12 (lobar) lymph nodes are excised with the specimen and should be identified by the pathologist. This figure depicts the paraesophageal (level 8), inferior pulmonary ligament (level 9), and nonhilar (levels 11 and 12) mediastinal lymphadenectomy. The view is as by a right posterolateral thoracotomy. The numbers correspond with those explained in detail in Table 28.1.

The previously placed packs are removed, and hemostasis is double-checked. At the completion of the procedure, the lymph node dissection sites should be inspected again.

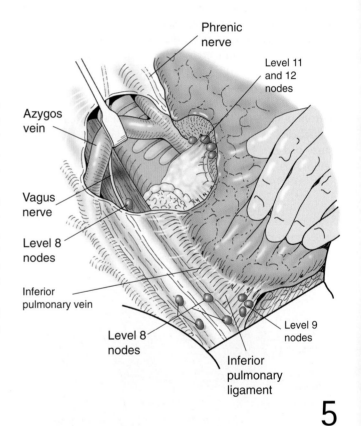

5

COMPLETE LYMPH NODE DISSECTION FOR A LEFT THORACOTOMY

SUPERIOR MEDIASTINAL DISSECTION

The dissection is begun by incising the mediastinal pleura between the phrenic and vagus nerves. Lymph nodes between the phrenic and vagus nerves, anterior to the ascending aorta or the innominate artery, are removed and labeled level 6. For patients with documented tumors at stations 2L and 4L, the operation is usually best performed through a median vertical sternotomy being the floor of dissection of the interaorticocaval groove. This strategy permits a complete exenteration of the anterosuperior mediastinum and the enclosed lymph node stations, as well as the resection of stations 2R and 4R and the subcarinal lymph nodes. Although they are more technically demanding, all major pulmonary resections can be safely made through the same incision except for resection of lower lobe tumors, for which a separate anterolateral thoracotomy in the fifth space can be made.

AORTOPULMONARY WINDOW DISSECTION

6 Dissection is continued into the aortopulmonary window. The compartment between the aorta and the pulmonary artery should be cleared of lymph tissue and labeled as level 5. These lymph nodes are lateral to the ligamentum arteriosum and proximal to the first branch of the left pulmonary artery. The recurrent laryngeal nerve is identified and preserved. Cautery should be avoided to prevent thermal injury to all these nerves. This figure depicts the aortopulmonary window (level 5), para-aortic (level 6), subcarinal (level 7), and paraesophageal (level 8) mediastinal lymphadenectomy in the left hemithorax.

Resection of stations 2L and 4L requires mobilization of the aortic arch and left tracheobronchial angle. Numbers correspond with those explained in detail in Table 28.1.

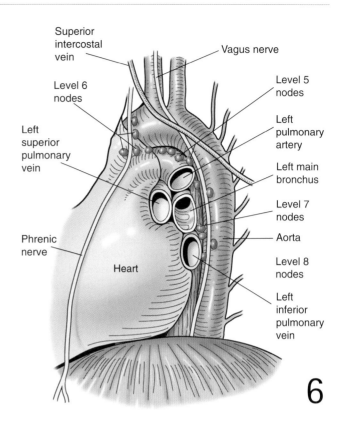

SUBCARINAL DISSECTION

The entire lymph node packet underneath the left main stem bronchus, down to the right main stem bronchus, should be removed and labeled as 7 (subcarinal lymph nodes). In the subcarinal area, the dissection is begun by retracting the lung anteriorly and opening the pleura lying between the esophagus and the main bronchus. The only difference from the right side dissection is that the subcarinal space lies deeper on the left than on the right, which renders the access more laborious. A warm gauze pad can be placed in the subcarinal space to enhance hemostasis.

HILAR DISSECTION

Anteriorly, along the left main stem bronchus, between the carina and the left upper lobe bronchus, lymph nodes that are within the left pleural cavity are removed and labeled 10L. These are intrapleural lymph nodes (N1) medial to the ligamentum. Dissection should be continued proximally along the left main bronchus to the tracheobronchial angle, and after division of the ligamentum arteriosum; these mediastinal nodes are removed and labeled 4L.

INFERIOR PULMONARY LIGAMENT DISSECTION

The inferior pulmonary ligament is divided, and all lymph nodes included in it are completely removed and labeled as level 9L. All lymph nodes along the esophagus (para-esophageal nodes) from the aortic arch to the diaphragm are removed and labeled as level 8. Care should be taken to carefully dissect the overlying pleura between the esophagus and aorta, especially when the normal anatomical relations are distorted by concurrent inflammation or tumor modifications. The previously placed packs are removed and hemostasis is double-checked. At the completion of the procedure, the lymph node dissection sites should be inspected again.

Extended lymph node dissection

The extended lymph node dissection includes the following in addition to the steps described for the radical lymphadenectomy. On the right, all soft tissue lying in the superior mediastinum and in front of the SVC up to both brachiocephalic veins is removed; the right subclavian artery, right recurrent nerve, and ascending aorta are skeletonized; and the thoracic ductus is ligated. On the left, stations 2 and 4 are removed after dissection and division of the ligamentum arteriosum and mobilization of the aortic arch. Supraclavicular lymphadenectomy is performed.

POSTOPERATIVE CARE

Although complications can potentially occur after a complete mediastinal dissection, with careful attention to all technical details, the morbidity of the procedure is minimal and is not significantly different from that observed after systematic node sampling. The only major complications observable in patients who have neoadjuvant therapy before surgery is the likelihood of developing lung edema after removal of all ipsilateral and contralateral lymph node draining stations. Adequate intra- and postoperative fluid restriction, however, can minimize this problem.

OUTCOME

A multicenter randomized trial has shown that, mediastinal systematic sampling was as efficacious as complete mediastinal lymph node dissection in staging patients with NSCLC. However, complete mediastinal lymph node dissection identified significantly more levels of N2 disease, and complete mediastinal lymph node dissection was associated with improved survival with right NSCLC when compared with systematic sampling in patients with stage II and IIIa tumors. Whether complete mediastinal lymph node dissection is superior to node sampling for patients with N0 or N1 (less than hilar) disease is currently being investigated in an open randomized trial sponsored by the American College of Surgeons Oncology Group.

FURTHER READING

Berlangieri SU, Scott AM. Metabolic staging of lung cancer. *New England Journal of Medicine* 2000; **343**: 290–2.

Hata E, Hayakawa K, Miyamoto H, *et al*. Rationale for extended lymphadenectomy for lung cancer. *Thoracic Surgery* 1990; **5**: 19–25.

Keller S, Adak S, Wagner H, Johnson D. Mediastinal lymph node dissection improves survival in patients with stages II and IIIa non-small lung cancer. *Annals of Thoracic Surgery* 2000; **70**: 358–65.

Lung Cancer Study Group. Randomized trial of lobectomy versus limited resection for T1 N0 non-small cell lung cancer. *Annals of Thoracic Surgery* 1995; **60**: 615–23.

Mountain CF, Dresler CM. Regional lymph node classification for lung cancer staging. *Chest* 1997; **111**: 1718–23

Naruke T. Significance of lymph node metastases in lung cancer. *Seminars in Thoracic and Cardiovascular Surgery* 1993; **5**: 510–18.

Watanabe Y, Shimizu J, Tsubota M, Iwa T. Mediastinal spread of metastatic lymph nodes in bronchogenic carcinoma. *Chest* 1990; **97**: 1059–63.

29

The pericardium

JOHN C. KUCHARCZUK MD

Assistant Professor of Surgery, Division of Cardiothoracic Surgery, Hospital of the University of Pennsylvania, Philadelphia, PA, USA

HISTORY

Throughout antiquity, the pericardium and heart were considered "off limits" by physicians. In 1766 Morgagni described the entity we now refer to as cardiac tamponade. This condition was recognized as usually fatal, and no interventions were attempted. In 1801, Francisco Romero performed the first pericardial procedure for "hydropericardio." Romero did not report his experience until 1815 when he presented two pericardial drainage procedures and five open pleural drainage procedures to the Society of the School of Medicine in Paris. Baron Dominique-Jean Larrey, Napolean's chief surgeon, is credited with performing and reporting the first surgical procedure on the pericardium in 1810, 5 years prior to Romero's presentation in Paris. The American surgeon Claude Schaeffer Beck recognized the clinical triad of high venous pressure, hypotension, and distant heart sounds associated with cardiac tamponade in 1935. This constellation of findings is referred to as Beck's triad.

Modern surgeons are presented with a number of diagnostic and therapeutic options in dealing with pericardial effusions, pericardial tamponade, and constrictive pericardial processes. This chapter will review the surgical approaches to the pericardium including subxiphoid pericardial window, thoracoscopic-assisted pericardial window, and transsternal pericardial resection. Special attention will be directed towards the indications for selecting one approach over another.

PRINCIPLES AND JUSTIFICATION

The goals of performing the pericardial window are: to relieve impending tamponade; to determine the underlying cause for fluid in the pericardium; and to prevent the re-accumulation of fluid. Thus, a surgical pericardial window can be diagnostic, therapeutic, or both. In the setting of penetrating trauma to the chest with subsequent concern for cardiac injury, the presence of blood in the pericardium during the performance of a pericardial window confirms the diagnosis of cardiac injury and the need for cardiac repair. In patients with advanced malignancy, relief of impending cardiac tamponade due to a malignant pericardial effusion can be life saving, and obliteration of the pericardial space can result in significant palliation. In patients with infected pericardial collections, drainage can result in isolation of the offending pathogen and guide antimicrobial therapy.

The pericardium is composed of fibrous tissue and a serosal surface. A potential space exists between the serosal surface of the pericardium and the epicardium of the heart. Accumulation of fluid within this potential space causes increasing intrapericardial pressure and results in compression of the lower pressure right heart with overall decreased cardiac filling. This pathophysiology accounts for the clinically observed pulsus paradoxus consisting of a fall in arterial pressure of greater than 10 mmHg during inspiration. The diagnosis of impending cardiac tamponade can be made on clinical grounds (Beck's triad), although imaging studies are almost always obtained for confirmation prior to surgery. The echocardiogram has become the standard for diagnosis of pericardial fluid and impending pericardial tamponade. A confirmatory study includes: diastolic compression or collapse of the right atrial or ventricular wall, leftward shift of the ventricular septum during inspiration, and an inspiratory decrease in left ventricular size. Small pericardial effusions which accumulate rapidly are often symptomatic. This situation occurs when the elastic limit of the pericardium is exceeded, and the intrapericardial pressure rises quickly. By contrast, effusions that accumulate slowly over long periods of time, such as those with renal failure, may reach very large sizes without symptoms. This scenario occurs because the pericardium slowly stretches, thus minimizing the increase in intrapericardial pressure and the hemodynamic effects of the effusion.

Constrictive pericarditis results from chronic inflammation with fibrosis of the pericardium. Often, the serosal surface of the pericardium fuses to the epicardium of the heart and calcifies. This fusion results in compression of the ventricles with impaired diastolic filling. Patients are usually symptomatic with shortness of breath, hepatomegaly, abdominal ascites, and lower extremity edema. In advanced cases myocardial atrophy and fibrosis occurs. Differentiating constrictive pericarditis from restrictive myocardial fibrosis can be difficult. Nevertheless, the distinction is of paramount importance as patients with restrictive myocardial fibrosis will not benefit from pericardial resection.

ANESTHESIA

The safe induction of anesthesia in patients with impending tamponade can be challenging for the patient, surgeon, and anesthesiologist. When required, the subxiphoid pericardial window can be performed under local anesthesia with light sedation; the alternative approaches to the pericardium require a general anesthetic. The hypotension associated with the induction of traditional anesthetics can result in complete cardiovascular collapse and death. For patients with impending tamponade, we select a subxiphoid approach. The patient is prepared for surgery awake with the head of the bed elevated 45 degrees. The operating surgeon is scrubbed, and a pericardiocentesis needle is available for emergency use prior to the administration of any anesthesia. Induction agents such as etomidate are selected for their minimal hemodynamic effects. Once the patient is anesthetized, the airway is secured and the procedure completed. Performing a pericardial window for impending tamponade requires cooperation and communication between the anesthesiologist and operating surgeon.

For patients without impending tamponade, alternative surgical approaches may be chosen. A video-assisted thoracoscopic procedure may be indicated in patients with a concomitant pleural effusion or those with a failed prior subxiphoid window. This approach requires a general anesthetic and placement of either a double-lumen endotracheal tube or bronchial blocker for isolated lung ventilation. Following induction of anesthesia and control of the airway, the patient must be repositioned into the lateral decubitus position for the procedure.

Those patients with constrictive pericardium are approached via a median sternotomy under general anesthesia. Most pericardectomies are performed without the aide of cardiopulmonary bypass; nevertheless, it should be immediately available should a coronary artery or significant myocardial injury occur.

OPERATION

Subxiphoid pericardial window

1 The patient is positioned in a supine manner with both arms tucked. The procedure can be performed under local anesthesia if needed, though most are performed under a general anesthetic. A 4 cm incision is centered over the xiphoid process. Electrocautery is used to achieve hemostasis in the subcutaneous tissues and dissect down directly onto the xiphoid. Care is taken to avoid inadvertent entry into the peritoneal cavity.

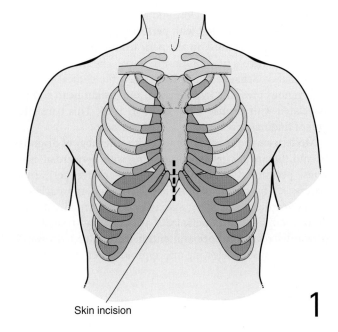

Skin incision

1

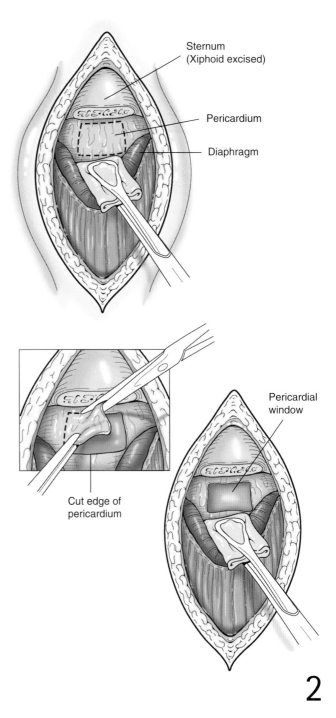

Sternum
(Xiphoid excised)

Pericardium

Diaphragm

Cut edge of
pericardium

Pericardial
window

2 Exposure is improved by the routine removal of the xiphoid process. The tip of the xiphoid is grasped with a Kocher clamp, mobilized completely with electrocautery, and removed with heavy scissors. A small self-retaining retractor is used to retract the subcutaneous tissues. The pericardium is often covered with a layer of adipose tissue. Dissection is continued until the pericardial membrane is visualized. Exposure is aided by downward traction applied by a "sponge on a stick." In patients with significant pericardial effusions the membrane appears tense and bulging. The pericardium is grasped, and a 1 cm incision is made with a scalpel. The cut edge is grasped, and a large rectangular portion of the pericardium is removed with a scissors. The pericardial tissue and pericardial fluid samples are sent to pathology and to microbiology for further analysis. A finger is introduced into the pericardium to assess for tumor implants and to break up any loculation.

2

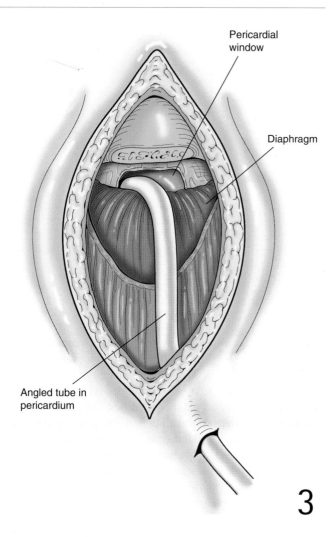

Pericardial window

Diaphragm

Angled tube in pericardium

3

3 A 28 French right angled chest tube is placed through a separate stab incision and directed into the pericardium. The wound is closed in layers with special attention to closure of the linea alba to avoid future epigastric hernia formation. The tube is placed to suction and remains in place for 4–5 days to effect obliteration of the pericardial space by sclerosis. Adjuvant use of sclerosing agents is not required.

In patients with penetrating thoracic trauma, a blue pericardial membrane confirms the presence of pericardial blood and should prompt conversion to median sternotomy.

Video-assisted thoracoscopic pericardial window

Patients selected for a video-assisted thoracoscopic pericardial window should be hemodynamically stable and must be able to tolerate single lung ventilation. As the initial approach to a symptomatic pericardial effusion, the thoracoscopic approach has no role. The value of a thoracoscopic approach is the ability to examine, biopsy, and treat associated pleural or parenchymal lung processes. A thoracoscopic approach is also of benefit in patients who recur with loculated posterior pericardial effusions following a subxiphoid approach and echocardiographic evidence of obliteration of the anterior pericardial space.

The patient is positioned supine, and general anesthesia is induced. A double-lumen endotracheal tube or bronchial blocker is positioned for isolated lung ventilation during the procedure. Once the airway is secured, the patient is placed in a lateral decubitus position, and the table is flexed. Thoracoscopic pericardial window creation has been described from both the right and left chest. In our experience, visualization is much better and the procedure much easier when performed from the right side. Ultimately, the side for thoracoscopic approach is dictated by the associated pathology, for example an associated pleural effusion which needs to be drained.

A 3 cm incision is made overlying the eighth intercostal space in line with the anterior superior iliac spine. Electrocautery is used to achieve hemostasis in the subcutaneous tissues. Isolated lung ventilation is begun, and the airway on the operative side is opened to atmospheric pressure. The pleural cavity is entered with a dissecting finger to avoid lung injury. The thoracoscope is introduced and pleural examination carried out. Two additional working port sites are made, one in the fifth intercostal space just below the tip of the scapula and one more anteriorly in the third intercostal space. The thoracoscope is moved to the fifth intercostal space site.

4 The lung is allowed to fall posteriorly by slightly rotating the table. The phrenic nerve is identified and protected throughout its course. A location anterior to the phrenic nerve is selected; the pericardium is grasped and incised. The cut edge is grasped, and fluid samples are obtained. A large rectangular portion of the pericardium is removed with an endoscopic shear. A chest tube is placed through the camera port site and directed across the pleural cavity and into the pericardial window. Alternatively, separate pericardial and pleural tubes can be placed. Bilateral lung ventilation is resumed, and the port sites are closed. The pericardial tube remains in place for 4–5 days on suction and then is removed. As with the subxiphoid approach, the success of this procedure relies on drainage of the pericardium with subsequent obliteration of the pericardial space by sclerosis.

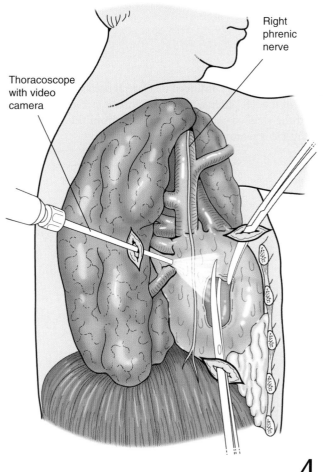

Right phrenic nerve

Thoracoscope with video camera

4

Transsternal pericardiectomy for constrictive pericarditis

The patient is positioned in a supine manner with both arms tucked. A roll is placed under the shoulders. A median sternotomy incision is made, and the thymus gland is resected. Cardiopulmonary bypass is not routinely used but is immediately available should a malignant arrhythmia occur or if a coronary artery is injured.

A small incision is made in the pericardium with a scalpel to the left of the anterior descending coronary artery. The incision is very carefully deepened to the level of the myocardium, and a dissection plane is established. Release of the left heart prior to the right ventricle is important to avoid pulmonary edema.

5 Dissection is continued in a lateral fashion to the border of the left phrenic nerve; the phrenic nerve is preserved; and the strip of pericardium elevated from the anterior left ventricle is removed.

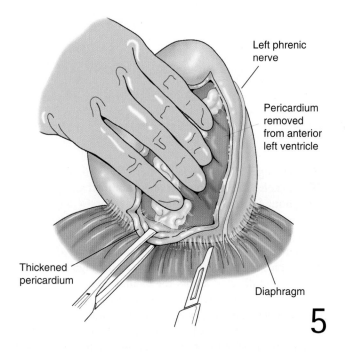

Left phrenic nerve

Pericardium removed from anterior left ventricle

Thickened pericardium

Diaphragm

5

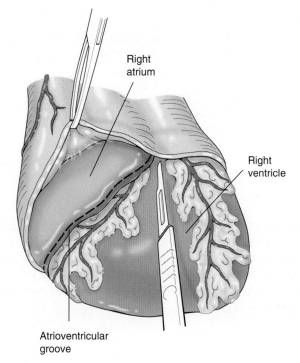

Right atrium

Right ventricle

Atrioventricular groove

6

6 Next, the inferior portion of the left ventricle is released by establishing a plane between the myocardium and diaphragm. Following this maneuver, the right ventricle is released up past the atrioventricular groove.

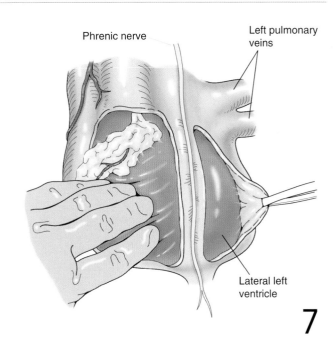

Phrenic nerve

Left pulmonary veins

Lateral left ventricle

7 The operation is completed by retracting the heart to the right and releasing the pericardium overlying the lateral left ventricle posterior to the left phrenic nerve and down to the level of the pulmonary veins. Hemostasis is confirmed, and the sternotomy is closed over drains.

7

POSTOPERATIVE CARE

The postoperative care of patients following a pericardial window is straightforward. A pericardial tube is left in place and on suction for 5 days. It is then removed. The majority of patients have dramatic improvement in their hemodynamics and symptoms immediately following surgery. A failure to respond immediately to drainage should raise concerns over the validity of the preoperative diagnosis and prompt a search for alternative explanations.

The postoperative care of patients following pericardial resection for constrictive pericarditis revolves around hemodynamic stabilization. This procedure often results in significant blood loss, and intraoperative as well as postoperative blood transfusions may be required. Mediastinal drains are monitored closely for ongoing bleeding and the need for re-exploration.

OUTCOME

A subxiphoid pericardial window is highly sensitive in ruling out occult cardiac injury in patients with penetrating chest trauma. Although many patients with penetrating cardiac trauma die prior to reaching the hospital, up to 20% of those arriving in the emergency room hemodynamically stable with a high risk trajectory will have an occult cardiac injury. The subxiphoid pericardial window can be performed quickly with high predictive value. If intrapericardial blood is present, the incision can easily be extended to a median sternotomy for definitive repair of the cardiac injury.

In patients with malignant pericardial effusions, the subxiphoid approach is preferred. The procedure is performed quickly with the patient in a supine position and without the need for isolated lung ventilation as required for the thoracoscopic approach. When required, this procedure can be performed under local anesthesia. This approach provides durable palliation of symptoms in greater than 90% of patients with malignant effusions.

Transsternal pericardial resection is a highly effective treatment for relief of symptoms in patients with constrictive pericarditis. Nevertheless, the procedure does carry significant perioperative mortality rates of about 5%. Long-term results are mixed depending on the etiology of the constrictive process. The long-term outcome is predicted by age, NYHA classification at presentation, and previous chest radiation. Patients with radiation-induced disease have the worst long-term outcome.

FURTHER READING

Andrade-Alegre R. Mon L. Subxiphoid pericardial window in the diagnosis of penetrating cardiac trauma. *Annals of Thoracic Surgery* 1994; **58:** 1139–41

Aris A. Francisco Romero, the first heart surgeon. *Annals of Thoracic Surgery* 1997; **64:** 870–1.

Hancock WE. Differential diagnosis of restrictive cardiomyopathy and constrictive pericarditis. *Heart* 2001; **86:** 343–9.

Johnson SB, Nielsen JL, Sako EY, Calhoon JH, Trinkle JK, Miller OL. Penetrating intrapericardial wounds: clinical experience with a surgical protocol. *Annals of Thoracic Surgery* 1995; **60:** 117–201

Ling LH, Oh JK, Schaff HV, Danielson GK, Mahoney DW, Seward JB, Tajik AJ. Constrictive pericarditis in the modern era: evolving clinical spectrum and impact on outcome after pericardiectomy. *Circulation* 1999; **100:** 1380–6.

Shumacker HB Jr. When did cardiac surgery begin? *Journal of Cardiovascular Surgery* 1989; **30:** 246–9.

30

Extrapleural pneumonectomy

JOHN C. KUCHARCZUK, MD
Assistant Professor of Surgery, Division of Cardiothoracic Surgery, Hospital of the University of Pennsylvania, Philadelphia, PA, USA

LARRY R. KAISER, MD
The John Rhea Barton Professor and Chairman, Department of Surgery, University of Pennsylvania; Surgeon-in-Chief, University of Pennsylvania Health System, Philadelphia, PA, USA

HISTORY

The extrapleural pneumonectomy operation was described in 1949 for application in patients with pleural-pulmonary tuberculosis. Today, the procedure is used almost exclusively in carefully selected patients with malignant pleural mesothelioma. The intent of the procedure, although elusive, is cure and as such the procedure is performed as part of a multimodality treatment regimen. Adequate palliation of symptoms can often be obtained in patients who are not candidates for cure by less invasive/aggressive procedures with lower morbidity and mortality rates.

PRINCIPLES AND JUSTIFICATION

The relationship between malignant pleural mesothelioma and asbestos exposure was observed over 45 years ago in South African miners. Unfortunately, asbestos use was widespread in construction and heavy industry worldwide, exposing large numbers of workers. In the 1970s, American government agencies including the Occupational Safety and Health Administration and the Environmental Protection Agency set forth strict regulations for asbestos exposures in the workplace and nonoccupational setting. Because of these regulations, the incidence of malignant pleural mesothelioma, which presents 30–40 years after exposure, has peaked in the United States. Worldwide, however, the incidence of malignant pleural mesothelioma is expected to increase for the next 20–30 years.

Traditionally, malignant pleural mesothelioma has been viewed as a locally aggressive disease; it was thought that metastatic disease occurred late. Largely because of this point of view, the radical operations proposed for the eradication of advanced pleural pulmonary tuberculosis were modified and applied to patients with malignant pleural mesothelioma. Initial results from series published in the 1970s and 1980s revealed only a few long-term survivors with relatively high morbidity and mortality rates. Recently, with improved patient selection and refined surgical techniques, 2-year survival rates have been reported in the 30% range with acceptable morbidity and mortality. Combined multimodality treatments hold out the prospect of even better future outcomes.

PREOPERATIVE EVALUATION AND PATIENT SELECTION

The clinical difficulty in managing patients with malignant pleural mesothelioma begins with diagnosis. Patients usually present with shortness of breath, chest pain, and imaging studies showing a pleural effusion and pleural nodularity. Many will have had thoracentesis and/or closed pleural biopsy which may still be cytologically inconclusive. Needle aspiration of a pleural lesion usually provides inadequate material for a definitive diagnosis. Usually, a video-assisted biopsy with specialized immunohistochemical staining and electron microscopy is required to finalize the diagnosis. Securing an accurate diagnosis is critical. Patients with pleural carcinomatosis will not benefit from extrapleural pneumonectomy; they would be better served by other palliative or experimental treatments. We use a single pulmonary pathologist with special interest and expertise to review and confirm all malignant mesothelioma cases. In institutions without such expertise, outside pathological consultation should be obtained.

In symptomatic patients with large pleural effusions talc pleurodesis is performed at the time of diagnostic thoracoscopy if the lung fully expands. Despite popular notion, effective pleurodesis does not complicate later extrapleural pneumonectomy; it actually makes establishment of the extrapleural plane easier and provides symptomatic relief while evaluation is underway.

An interesting and early observation in malignant pleural mesothelioma was that patients with epithelioid histology had the best outcomes following aggressive surgery. By contrast, patients with mixed or sarcomatoid features had poor outcomes regardless of the treatment selected. In our current practice we consider only patients with pure epithelioid histology for extrapleural pneumonectomy. Patients with mixed or sarcomatoid pathology are encouraged to consider enrolling in experimental treatment trials. This histological selection criterion is particularly important if patients are to be subjected to the potential morbidity and mortality of extrapleural pneumonectomy. The procedure should be confined to those patients with the best chance of long-term survival where the potential benefit justifies the risk.

Once the diagnosis of pure epithelioid mesothelioma is confirmed, the preoperative evaluation focuses on determining the patients' extent of disease and fitness to undergo aggressive surgical resection. Unfortunately, no staging system or preoperative evaluation is universally agreed upon for patients with malignant pleural mesothelioma. Presently, the staging systems used include: the Union International Contre le Cancer Staging System, The New International Staging System proposed by the International Mesothelioma Interest Group, The Brigham and Women's Hospital/Dana Farber Cancer Institute Staging System, and the original Butchart Staging System proposed in the late 1970s. Regardless of the staging system used, patients considered for extrapleural pneumonectomy must have disease confined to a single hemithorax. As previously mentioned, the traditional view of malignant pleural mesothelioma as strictly a local disease is erroneous. We have come to understand that a substantial number of patients have metastatic disease to the mediastinal lymph nodes and/or through the diaphragm into the peritoneal cavity, or into the other pleural space. Our current pre-operative assessment includes cervical mediastinoscopy and diagnostic laparoscopy with biopsy. Often, we perform these procedures separately to allow for complete assessment of the pathological specimens. Patients determined to have mediastinal nodal metastasis and/or peritoneal involvement are not offered extrapleural pneumonectomy.

Physiological evaluation also requires experience and mature surgical judgment. The performance of an extrapleural pneumonectomy puts a significant physiological stress on the patient above and beyond that imposed by a standard pneumonectomy. The intrapericardial procedure and the excision of the hemidiaphragm add to the morbidity of the procedure. All patients undergo preoperative cardiac evaluation and pulmonary function testing. Eligible patients should have a postoperative predicted FEV_1 of greater than 1 liter. Although we do not have strict age criteria, we offer the procedure only rarely in those over age 60. Perhaps this approach is being somewhat conservative, but older patients tend to show their age following this procedure, and the mortality in those over age 60 is considerable.

OPERATION

Right extrapleural pneumonectomy

The patient is brought to the operating room, and a thoracic epidural catheter is placed for intra- and postoperative pain management. Preoperative antibiotics are administered, and pneumatic compression boots are applied to avoid venous stasis in the lower extremities. General anesthesia is induced, and the patient is intubated with a left-sided double-lumen endotracheal tube. A flexible pediatric bronchoscope is used to examine the airway and position the tube for isolated lung ventilation. The tube is secured. A nasogastric tube is placed and used later as a guide when the extrapleural dissection approaches the esophagus. The patient is repositioned in the left lateral decubitus manner.

1 A long skin incision is made along the sixth rib. Electrocautery is used to achieve hemostasis in the subcutaneous tissues. The latissimus dorsi muscle is divided with electrocautery. When possible, we like to mobilize and spare the serratus anterior muscle as this can be used as a pedicled muscle flap later in the procedure if needed.

The sixth rib is identified, and its periosteum is scored. A periosteal elevator is used to completely strip the periosteum from the rib, and then the entire rib is removed with a bone cutter. Removing the sixth rib facilitates the initiation of the extrapleural dissection. We like to begin the dissection sharply by establishing the extrapleural plane under the fifth rib. Once the plane is established the entire lateral dissection is done quickly and bluntly with a dissecting hand. Chest wall bleeding is temporarily controlled with packing sponges. After the lateral extrapleural dissection is done both superiorly and inferiorly, a chest retractor can be placed. The packing sponges are removed, and any ongoing chest wall bleeding is controlled with electrocautery or the argon beam coagulator.

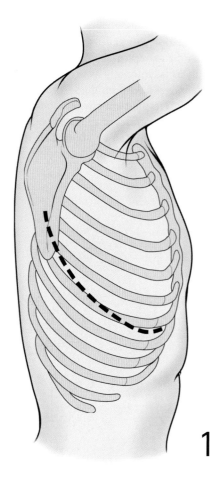

1

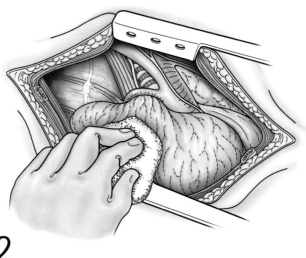

2

2 Dissection proceeds around the apex of the lung in a more controlled manner with sharp scissor dissection. Care must be taken to avoid injury to the subclavian artery and vein. As the dissection moves medially, the internal mammary vessels are identified and allowed to remain on the chest wall. Likewise the pleural envelope is carefully dissected away from the superior vena cava and azygous vein.

3 Attention is directed posteriorly for dissection of the specimen from the esophagus. The nasogastric tube is palpated in the esophagus and used as a guide. The attachments between the extrapleural plane and the esophagus are divided sharply as far inferiorly as possible. Up to this point, no irreversible moves have been made. If the disease is found to be more extensive than anticipated and to involve non-resectable thoracic structures or to have invaded through the chest wall, the procedure can be aborted. If the mass is still deemed resectable, we move onto the diaphragmatic portion of the procedure.

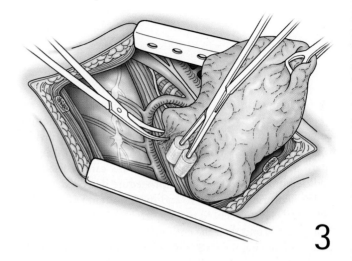

3

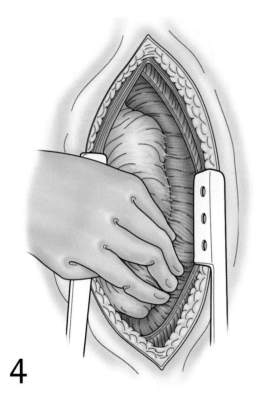

4

4 Several different techniques have been described for facilitating the diaphragmatic dissection, resection, and reconstruction. We have found the most effective technique to be simply making a second intercostal muscle incision two interspaces lower without making any additional skin incisions. A small child chest retractor is used and exposure to the diaphragm is excellent. The diaphragmatic division is begun at the lateral attachment of the diaphragm to the chest wall.

5 A small incision is made, and the underlying peritoneum is swept away with a sponge stick.

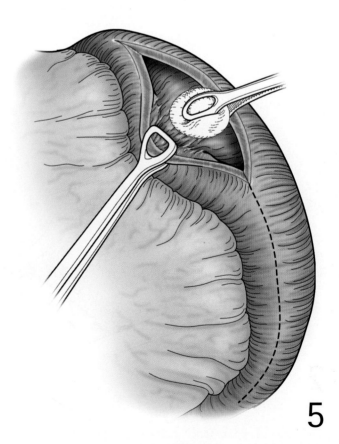

5

6 Once the peritoneum is pushed away with a sponge stick, the lateral diaphragmatic resection is completed with electrocautery.

Moving medially, we switch to sharp dissection with tissue scissors. The pleural envelope is carefully dissected away from the inferior vena cava and distal esophagus. At this juncture we mass ligate all tissue on the spine between the esophagus and the aorta with a 2-0 silk suture as a prophylactic maneuver to decrease the incidence of thoracic duct leak. Dissection continues in a cephalad direction toward the pericardium. The chest retractor is removed and repositioned into the sixth intercostal space incision. The pericardium is opened and removed with the specimen.

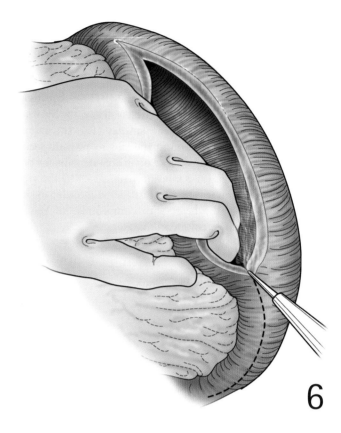

6

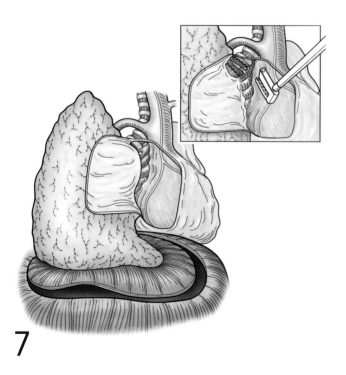

7

7 The right main pulmonary artery is isolated within the pericardium and taken with a single firing of an Endo GIA vascular stapling device. Likewise the pulmonary veins are isolated within the pericardium and divided with a vascular stapling device. Finally, the bronchus is circumferentially dissected, small bronchial vessels are controlled with electrocautery, and the right mainstem bronchus is taken flush with the carina using a TA stapling device. The specimen is removed from the field, oriented, and forwarded to pathology for evaluation.

Meticulous hemostasis is required. Residual chest wall bleeding from the endothoracic fascia is controlled with electrocautery or the argon beam coagulator. When available, the pericardial fat pad is mobilized to cover the bronchial stump. Otherwise, the uncut serratus anterior muscle is mobilized and transposed into the chest to provide a buttress for the bronchial stump. When it is required, the serratus anterior muscle is brought into the chest through the third intercostal space. We reoutinely buttress a right pneumonectomy stump.

8 Next, attention is turned towards diaphragmatic and pericardial reconstruction. The retractor is moved to the lower intercostal incision. The diaphragm is reconstructed with a 2-mm polytetrafluoroethylene (PTFE) soft tissue patch. The patch is secured to the chest wall laterally by placement of interrupted #1 Prolene sutures. The sutures are placed at close intervals around the ribs to provide secure purchase. Medially, an unsecured open area remains for passage of the esophagus and inferior vena cava. On the right side the pericardium must be reconstructed in order to prevent herniation of the heart with compromise of venous return, a potentially lethal situation.

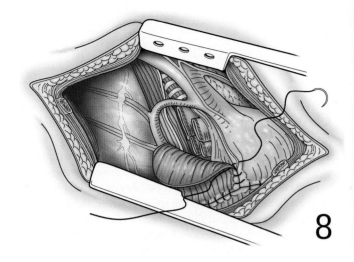

8

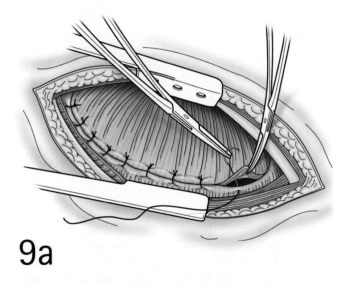

9a

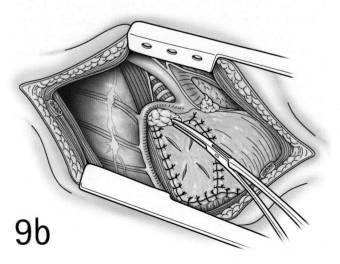

9b

9 The pericardium is reconstructed with a 0.1-mm PTFE pericardial patch. The patch is fenestrated to allow drainage and avoid tamponade. It is secured to the cut edges of the pericardium with 4-0 Prolene suture placed in a running fashion. Inferiorly, the patch is secured to the diaphragmatic patch with several interrupted Prolene sutures.

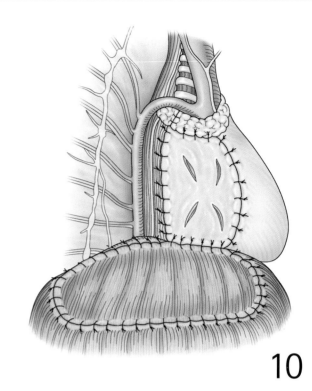

10 The completed repair is shown. The entire chest is irrigated with several liters of sterile saline.

10

A 28 Fr. chest tube is brought through a separate stab incision and directed toward the apex. The chest tube is connected to a balanced drainage system with a safety mechanism that precludes any attachment to suction.

Number 1 braided absorbable sutures are placed in a pericostal position. The ribs are brought together with the aid of a Bailey rib approximator. The pericostal sutures are secured. The incision is irrigated, and the latissimus dorsi muscle is reapproximated with a running number absorbable suture. The subcutaneous tissues are approximated with running absorbable suture, and the skin is closed with a subcuticular suture. The patient is returned to the supine position and allowed to emerge from anesthesia.

Left extrapleural pneumonectomy

Performance of the left extrapleural pneumonectomy is technically easier than the right. Following induction of general anesthesia, a right-sided double-lumen endotracheal tube is placed. The tube is positioned for isolated lung ventilation with a pediatric bronchoscope. The Murphy's eye of the right-sided double-lumen endobronchial tube is aligned with the right upper lobe orifice. Improper placement can result in right upper lobe consolidation with hypoxia during single lung ventilation. The tube also can migrate during patient positioning or extrapleural dissection. The pediatric bronchoscope remains with the anesthesia team during the procedure, and confirmation of tube position should be performed if the patient becomes hypoxic during single lung ventilation.

The patient is repositioned in the right lateral decubitus position. A long posterolateral incision is made along the left sixth rib. The latissimus dorsi muscle is divided with electrocautery. The serratus anterior muscle is mobilized and spared when possible. The periosteum of the sixth rib is stripped, and the entire sixth rib is removed. The dissection is begun by sharply establishing an extrapleural plane under the fifth rib, as was described above for the right-sided pneumonectomy. Once the plane is developed, the entire lateral dissection is performed with a dissecting hand. The space is packed with surgical sponges to control chest wall bleeding, and the chest retractor is placed. The sponges are removed, and chest wall hemostasis is obtained with electrocautery or the argon beam coagulator. As on the right side, careful sharp dissection is used at the apex to avoid injury to the subclavain artery and vein. Likewise medially, the internal mammary vessels are left on the chest wall. As dissection continues along the mediastinum, care is taken to avoid injury to the left vagus and left recurrent laryngeal nerve. Damage to the recurrent laryngeal nerve will lead to postoperative left vocal cord paralysis with susceptibility to aspiration. This complication can be life threatening following pneumonectomy.

Attention now is directed posteriorly. The extrapleural dissection is continued along the aorta with careful scissor dissection. As with right extrapleural pneumonectomy, we make an accessory intercostal incision through the eighth intercostal space and move the rib spreader to this interspace. This maneuver provides excellent exposure to the diaphragm. The extrapleural dissection is continued bluntly well into the costophrenic sulcus. The diaphragmatic dissection is started by incision of the lateral attachments of the diaphragm to the chest wall. The peritoneal membrane is swept away, and the diaphragmatic resection is continued with electrocautery. Occasionally, the peritoneal cavity is entered inadvertently. This situation is not a particular problem since the diaphragm is to be reconstructed. Care is taken medially along the diaphragmatic hiatus to avoid injury to the esophagus and left vagus nerve. Once the inferior dissection is complete, the retractor is moved back to the fifth intercostal space. The pericardium is opened and widely incised to complete the dissection. The left main pulmonary artery is isolated in an intrapericardial location and ligated and divided with an endoscopic linear stapling device. As the intrapericardial portion of the left pulmonary artery is short, care must be taken to avoid injury or encroachment on the main or right pulmonary artery. The upper and lower pulmonary veins are encircled within the pericardium and individually divided with a vascular stapling device. Finally, the left main bronchus is circumferentially dissected back to the carina and taken with a stapling device. The bronchus is divided flush with the carina to avoid an excessively long stump which is susceptible to breakdown. The left-sided stump retracts back into the mediastinum and usually does not require buttressing as is required on the right. Hemostasis is confirmed, and attention is directed toward diaphragmatic reconstruction.

The retractors are moved to the lower intercostal incision. The diaphragm is reconstructed with a 2-mm thick PTFE soft tissue patch. The patch is secured to the chest wall laterally by placement of interrupted #1 sutures in the same fashion as used on the right. Unlike on the right side, pericardial reconstruction is not required on the left since torsion with compromise of venous return is not an issue in the left chest.

The entire chest is irrigated with several liters of sterile saline. A 28Fr. chest tube is brought through a separate stab incision and directed toward the apex. The chest tube is connected to a balanced pneumonectomy drainage device. #1 absorbable sutures are placed in a pericostal position. The rest of the closure proceeds as usual as described above.

The patient is returned to the supine position and allowed to emerge from anesthesia.

POSTOPERATIVE CARE

Our intent is to extubate all patients in the operating room following extrapleural pneumonectomy. After a short stay in the postanesthesia recovery area, they are transferred to the thoracic surgical unit for their postoperative care. The pneumonectomy tube is removed the following morning after a chest X-ray confirms the midline position of the mediastinum. The epidural catheter remains connected to a patient-controlled epidural administration device for 5 days. During this time, patients receive intensive pulmonary physiotherapy. Starting on postoperative day 2, they are ambulated three times per day in the hall with assistance. A chest radiograph is obtained every other day to follow appropriate

filling of the pneumonectomy space. Rapid filling may indicate unrecognized bleeding and the need for re-exploration. The hemoglobin is checked every other day as patients have a tendency to become progressively anemic as the pneumonectomy space fills. Symptomatic patients with a hemoglobin level below 8 mg/dL are transfused. Occasionally, the space fills rapidly with a shift of the mediastinum. This situation requires drainage of the space to prevent hemodynamic embarrassment. Patients with an uncomplicated course are usually discharged on postoperative day 7.

Pitfalls, complications

The most common intraoperative complication is bleeding. Chest wall bleeding should be controlled as the operation progresses to avoid excessive blood loss. This goal is facilitated by use of the argon beam coagulator. Catastrophic bleeding can occur due to injury of major vascular structures during dissection around the apex of the chest or when dissecting around the inferior vena cava. The complication is avoided by careful attention to detail and absolute familiarity with the anatomy.

Transient hypotension in the immediate postoperative period is often related to sympathectomy with vasodilation due to the thoracic epidural administration of narcotic or local anesthesia. The blood pressure is supported with intravenous vasoactive drugs such as neosynephrine. Large fluid boluses are avoided. Profound hypotension with tamponade physiology may be due to acute mediastinal shift. Because of our use of a balanced pneumonectomy drainage system, we have avoided this complication. It must, however, be considered in those units which use only a single catheter with a stopcock to add or remove air to move the mediastinum to a midline position. An overly tight pericardial patch can cause constriction, with tamponade physiology. Finally, if the fenestrations in the pericardial patch are too small to allow free drainage, even a small amount of clot within the reconstructed pericardium can result in tamponade. Early recognition of these potential problems is mandatory if the patient is to be salvaged.

From a pulmonary perspective, the most dangerous complication is development of postpneumonectomy pulmonary edema. Unfortunately, the etiological factors causing this phenomenon remain obscure. When it occurs, the treatment is supportive. In any event, we limit perioperative fluid administration in an attempt to minimize this complication. The complication occurs much more commonly following right extrapleural pneumonectomy than left. This complication usually manifests within the first 96 hours following the resection.

Postoperative space infections are particularly difficult to manage because of the presence of prosthetic material used to reconstruct the diaphragm and the pericardium. In patients without pneumonectomy stump breakdown, early space infection occasionally can be managed with complete drainage, high volume lavage, and antibiotics. Those patients presenting with a pneumonectomy stump breakdown require open window thoracostomy and removal of prosthetic material. If this problem occurs on the right side before the mediastinum is fixed, the prosthetic material must be removed in a staged fashion.

OUTCOME

The outcomes following extrapleural pneumonectomy alone are disappointing. Surgery as a single treatment modality usually does not provide long-term survival. Currently, the best outcomes are in highly selected patients with epithelioid mesothelioma, negative lymph nodes, and negative resection margins receiving trimodality therapy including chemotherapy and radiation therapy. In this small cohort 5-year survival is in the 35–40% range. Clearly, the ideal treatment regimen for malignant pleural mesothelioma has yet to be defined.

FURTHER READING

Butchart EG, Ashcroft T, Barnsley WC, Holden MP. Pleuropneumectomy in the management of diffuse malignant mesothelioma of the pleura. Experience with 29 patients. *Thorax* 1976; **31:** 15–24.

Robinson BW, Lake RA. Advances in malignant mesothelioma. *New England Journal of Medicine* 2005; **353:** 1591–603.

Sugarbaker DJ, Garcia JP. Multimodality therapy for malignant pleural mesothelioma. *Chest* 1997; **112:** 272S–5S.

Sugarbaker DJ, Flores RM, Jaklitsch MT, et al. Resection margins, extrapleural nodal status, and cell type determine postoperative long-term survival in trimodality therapy of malignant pleural mesothelioma: results in 183 patients. *Journal of Thoracic and Cardiovascular Surgery* 1999; **117:** 54–65.

Sugarbaker DJ. Jalkitsch MT, Bueno R et al. Prevention, early detection and management of complication after 328 consecutive extrapleural pneumonectomies. *Journal of Thoracic and Cardiovascular Surgery* 2004; **128:** 138–46.

31

Surgical management of superior sulcus tumors

M. BLAIR MARSHALL MD
Chief, Division of Thoracic Surgery, Georgetown University Medical Center, Washington, District of Columbia, USA

LARRY R. KAISER, MD
The John Rhea Barton Professor and Chairman, Department of Surgery, University of Pennsylvania; Surgeon-in-Chief, University of Pennsylvania Health System, Philadelphia, PA, USA

HISTORY

In 1838 a patient with an apical lung tumor and involvement of the brachial plexus was described. This entity became more widely recognized when Pancoast reported a series of seven patients with apical lung tumors, Horner's syndrome, rib destruction, atrophy of the intrinsic muscles of the hand, and pain. Because of their location, Pancoast tumors involve the neurovascular structures and historically were deemed inoperable.

The current "standard," if one could actually call it a standard, came about serendipitously when a patient who was deemed inoperable underwent radiation therapy. This patient was restudied, found to be resectable, and went on to live for an additional 27 years. This case drove the management of these tumors toward preoperative radiation therapy followed by "curative" resection.

In 1961, Shaw reported results in 18 patients who received preoperative radiation therapy followed by resection. These results set the "standard of care" in these patients for years to follow. Currently, many surgeons continue to treat these patients with preoperative radiation followed by surgical resection, though the dose and schedule of preoperative radiation has not been standardized. Because several clinical trials have suggested a benefit in survival in patients who received neoadjuvant chemoradiotherapy, some centers have added this treatment to their preoperative regimen for Pancoast tumors. Thoracic surgeons should be aware that no randomized prospective trials exist showing a benefit of preoperative radiation and/or chemotherapy in patients with Pancoast tumors. This situation is due mainly to the fact that too few of these tumors are seen to allow for the conduct of a randomized trial that would be complete in our lifetime.

PRINCIPLES AND JUSTIFICATION

Not all apical lung tumors are classical Pancoast tumors. If this term is to be used, it should be reserved for those apical lung tumors involving the chest wall including the first rib with secondary involvement of the brachial plexus and/or vascular structures. From both a therapeutic and prognostic standpoint, this distinction is important. True Pancoast tumors have a poor survival because of the locally advanced nature of these tumors with involvement of the brachial plexus and often the spine. Apical lung tumors that have not invaded the neurovascular structures can usually be completely resected and are associated with a better outcome, especially in the absence of lymph node involvement. These patients are not necessarily treated with preoperative radiotherapy.

PREOPERATIVE ASSESSMENT AND PREPARATION

Apical lung tumors, including those commonly referred to as Pancoast tumors, represent a significant challenge to thoracic surgeons. Patients presenting with Pancoast's syndrome should undergo a meticulous preoperative workup to determine the diagnosis, as other diseases and other tumors have been associated with this syndrome. Bronchoscopy with brushings may obtain a diagnosis in 40%, and needle biopsy results in a diagnosis in about 90% of these lesions.

A complete history and physical examination should be performed, paying close attention to any cardiac or respiratory disease. An extent of disease workup is carried out to determine stage and operability. A complete neurovascular examination is performed. If any question of vascular involvement exists, we perform magnetic resonance imaging (MRI) or angiography preoperatively.

The preoperative chest CT scan is helpful in determining which thoracic outlet structures are involved as well as the extent of chest wall and vertebral body involvement. Mediastinal nodal disease can be assessed. Because patients with mediastinal disease have the poorest survival, we perform a mediastinoscopy on all patients preoperatively. Those patients with a Pancoast tumor and mediastinal disease should be referred for either combined radio/chemotherapy or radiotherapy alone.

ANESTHESIA

In operations being performed through an anterior cervicothoracotomy, we have not found it necessary to place an epidural catheter for postoperative analgesia. This incision is associated with minimal pain when compared with a posterolateral thoracotomy. Epidural analgesia is definitely beneficial for pain management following the posterolateral or combined approach. The patient is placed under general anesthesia, and a double-lumen endotracheal tube is placed. Appropriate electrocardiography (ECG) leads and an arterial line are placed for intraoperative monitoring. Bronchoscopy is performed in the operating room by the surgical team.

OPERATION

1,2 These tumors classically have been approached through a posterolateral thoracotomy. However, more recently, we have begun to approach the majority of these lesions through a cervicothoracic approach. This incision is similar to that described by Dartevelle and his colleagues. Although some discussion exists in the literature about which approach is best for specific locations, anterior versus posterior, we use the cervicothoracic approach for all apical lung tumors involving the thoracic outlet and/or first rib.

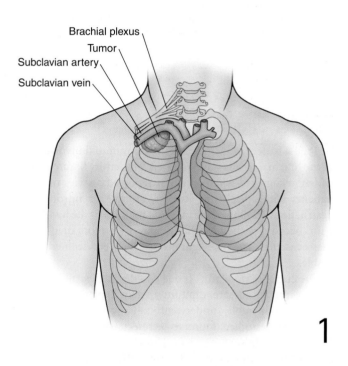

1

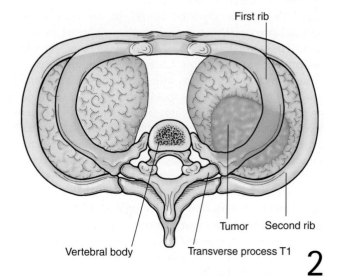

2

Cervicothoracic approach (Dartevelle)

The patient is placed in the supine position, with the arms tucked and either a shoulder roll or inflatable bag beneath the scapulae. The patient is placed under general anesthesia, and a Foley catheter and an arterial line are placed. The arterial line should be on the contralateral side in case of subclavian artery involvement.

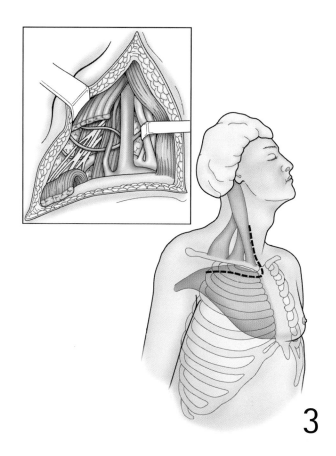

3 An "L" shaped incision is made along the medial border of the sternocleidomastoid down to the sternal notch and then out along the inferior border of the clavicle to the deltopectoral groove. The subcutaneous tissues are divided and the clavicle is circumferentially dissected just above its insertion onto the manubrium.

3

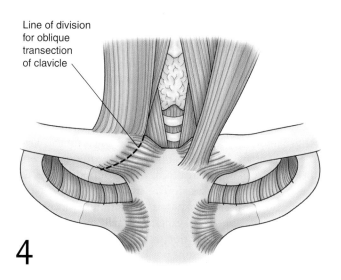

Line of division for oblique transection of clavicle

4 We divide the clavicle obliquely with a Gigli saw, or more recently with an oscillating saw. This maneuver makes reapproximation of the clavicle possible at completion. We have not found it necessary to remove the medial third of the clavicle as described by Dartevelle and colleagues.

4

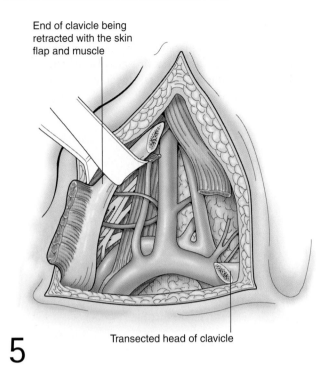

End of clavicle being retracted with the skin flap and muscle

Transected head of clavicle

5

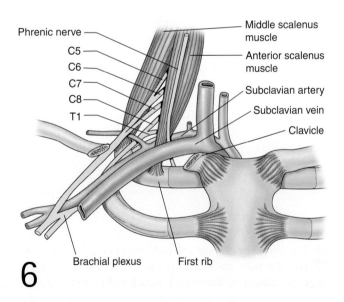

Phrenic nerve

C5
C6
C7
C8
T1

Middle scalenus muscle

Anterior scalenus muscle

Subclavian artery

Subclavian vein

Clavicle

Brachial plexus   First rib

6

5 The sternal attachments of the sternocleidomastoid, sternohyoid, and sternothyroid muscles are divided, and a Ruhltract retractor is used to elevate the clavicle. This maneuver exposes the brachiocephalic, subclavian, and internal jugular veins. The scalene fat pad is dissected and pathologically examined for disease. The veins are dissected, and at this point we usually divide the mammary vessels. The ascending cervical vein is divided. The resectability of the lesion is assessed.

6 The anterior scalene muscle is identified, and the phrenic nerve can be observed coursing along its anterior border. Before the insertion of the anterior scalene onto the first rib, the phrenic nerve turns medially. Thus, when dividing the anterior scalene, it is best to stay close to the rib if possible. The phrenic nerve should be carefully preserved or, if involved, deliberately resected. The subclavian vein may be divided if involved with tumor. If one anticipates involvement of the vessels, proximal and distal control should be obtained early in the dissection. This maneuver is facilitated by the anterior approach and is significantly easier than when attempted from the posterolateral approach. The subclavian artery is dissected in the subadventitial plane. Branches from the subclavian artery may be sacrificed if necessary. The internal mammary, ascending cervical, and vertebral arteries may all be ligated. We divide the vertebral artery only if it is invaded by the tumor. The continuity of the circle of Willis should be established preoperatively if it is anticipated that the vertebral artery will need to be sacrificed. If necessary to obtain a complete resection, the subclavian artery is clamped and divided. The reconstruction may be performed with a direct end-to-end anastomosis or with a polytetrafluoroethylene (PTFE) interposition graft after the tumor has been resected.

The brachial plexus is evaluated. The middle and posterior scalene muscles are divided sharply as the brachial plexus is in close proximity. One should preserve the long thoracic nerve that courses along the posterior border of the middle scalene. If the brachial plexus is involved, most commonly it is the lower trunk that is encased. The upper trunks are rarely involved, but the occasional tumor may infiltrate widely thorough the plexus. The stellate ganglion usually must be divided to achieve a complete resection, recognizing that the patient will have a Horner's syndrome postoperatively. Once the vessels and brachial plexus have been freed from the tumor, the chest wall can be resected. Initially, the first rib is divided anteriorly at the junction of the manubrium.

7 Posteriorly, we incise the ligament between the neck of the first rib and transverse process. An osteotome is placed into this space, and the rib is disarticulated from the transverse process and vertebral body. The C8 and T1 nerve roots can be identified straddling the head of the first rib. The T1 nerve root may be sacrificed with minimal residua, but taking both the C8 and T1 roots results in a significant disability of the hand. The nerve roots must be identified at the level of the neural foramina to assure that only the T1 root is taken as opposed to the entire lower trunk. The head of the second rib may be identified from within the chest and then dissected off the transverse process from an anterior approach. The pleura overlying the costovertebral junction is divided. This step gives access to then use the osteotome to disarticulate the rib from an anterior approach. Any additional posterior rib resections are done in this fashion. Partial vertebrectomy may be done, if necessary recognizing the negative prognostic implications of vertebral involvement.

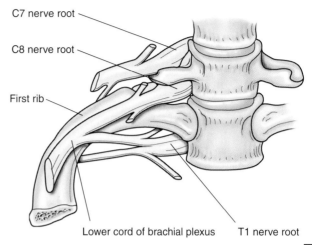

7

The pleura around the lesion and corresponding chest wall is incised, and the lesion with the attached chest wall is left with the underlying lung. The lobectomy is now completed. Usually we are able to complete this procedure through the cervicothoracic approach without an additional thoracotomy.

After the lobectomy and lymph node dissection, the chest is closed as described elsewhere. If the anterior chest wall has been removed, we reconstruct this with methylmethacrylate and polypropylene mesh. If the chest wall resection is limited to the posterior region, prosthetic reconstruction is not needed as the scapula covers the defect.

Posterolateral approach

This approach was popularized by Paulson. It is standard for apical lung lesions; however, exposure and control of the brachiocephalic vessels and the brachial plexus is more difficult, especially with a larger tumor. The cervicothoracic approach, as described above, may be the more versatile approach to these lesions but does require a detailed knowledge of the anatomy of the thoracic inlet.

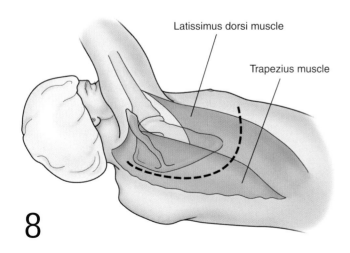

8

8 For the posterolateral approach, the patient is positioned in the standard lateral decubitus position after placement of a double-lumen endotracheal tube as described in Chapter 23 on incisions. The chest is prepped from the C7 prominence to below the costal margin and from the spine to the nipple. A posterolateral thoracotomy is made as described elsewhere.

9 The fifth intercostal space is entered for exploration. If the initial exploration indicates that the lesion is resectable, the incision is extended up to the C7 prominence, and the trapezius muscle and the rhomboids are divided. The Finochietto retractor is positioned with the inferior blade resting on the sixth rib and the superior blade under the tip of the scapula. The retractor is cranked open elevating the scapula off of the chest wall. This maneuver exposes the apex of the chest. The posterior scalene is divided with cautery.

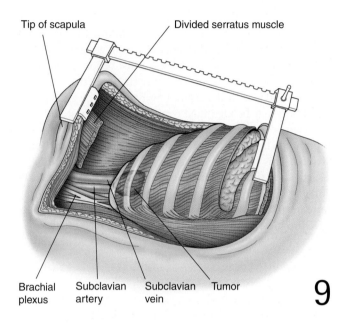

Tip of scapula   Divided serratus muscle

Brachial   Subclavian   Subclavian   Tumor
plexus   artery   vein

9

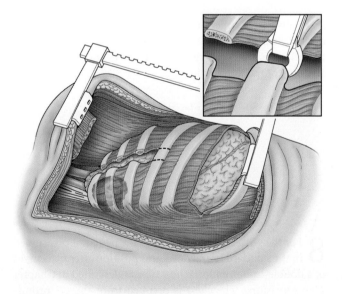

10

10 The middle and anterior scalenes are dissected off the first rib in the subperiosteal plane, recognizing that the brachial plexus and subclavian vessels lie superior to the first rib. Dividing the scalene muscles is made easier by placing the first rib on downward traction. The anterior scalene muscle inserts on the first rib between the subclavian vein and artery. Initially, the first rib is dissected in the subperiosteal plane. This step frees the rib of the medial and anterior scalenes without risking injury to the brachial plexus or phrenic nerve. The exact location to begin the chest wall resection is determined by observing the extent of tumor from within the chest. Usually, a 4-cm margin is necessary. The dissection begins at the inferior margin and progresses superiorly. It is easiest to divide the rib to be taken at the anterior aspect first and then divide posteriorly. The inferior ribs are taken working up toward the first rib.

11 The sacrospinalis and thoracicus iliacus are dissected away from the chest wall. The posterior margin is most commonly obtained by disarticulating the head and neck of the rib away from the transverse process and corresponding vertebral body. The ligament between the neck of the rib and transverse process is incised with electrocautery. A curved osteotome is inserted between these structures, and the rib is disarticulated. This maneuver exposes the nerve roots at the foraminal level where they may be ligated and divided in a controlled fashion. One must be careful to avoid avulsing these roots as the dural sheath may extend beyond the foramen for a variable extent and avulsion may result in a cerebrospinal fluid leak. Sacrificing the T1 nerve root may result in minimal motor weakness but often has no functional consequence, as mentioned above. Sacrifice of both C8 and T1 nerve roots results in a clawed hand with minimal function. Bleeding from the venous plexus at the neural foramen or intercostal vessels should be controlled with sutures or a bipolar cautery. Surgicel or other hemostatics should never be packed against the foramen in an attempt to control bleeding as migration of this material into the canal may result in compression of the spinal cord and paraplegia.

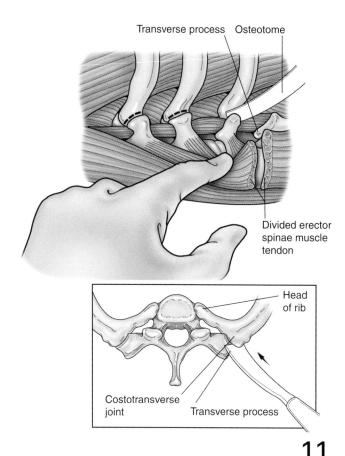

11

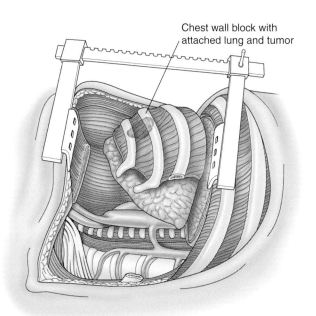

12 Once the chest wall has been divided and freed, it is left in-continuity with the lung, and a formal lobectomy with lymph node dissection is performed.

12

If extensive involvement of the brachial plexus exists above these levels and a complete resection cannot be performed, all of the nerves are left intact, and the patient is referred for postoperative radiotherapy. Prior to dividing any of these structures, the resectability of the lesion should be thoroughly investigated. An incomplete resection is associated with poor long-term survival.

Following the lobectomy and lymph node dissection, a single thoracostomy tube is placed. Posterior defects involving the first to third ribs do not need to be reconstructed. If the fourth rib is resected, we tend to reconstruct these with polypropylene mesh so that the tip of the scapula does not get trapped in the chest wall defect.

POSTOPERATIVE CARE

With the cervicothoracic approach, patients have less pain and limitation of motion in the immediate postoperative period. They are able to ambulate more readily. We put these patients in a sling for comfort. Physical rehabilitation plays an important role in their postoperative care. Patients with extensive apical dissections may have prolonged drainage; however, one must make sure that this situation does not represent a chyle or CSF leak.

Postoperative complications include those associated with lobectomy, bleeding, infection, bronchopleural fistula, and chyle leak. These patients may also have neurological deficits associated with resection of the lower roots of the brachial plexus.

OUTCOME

The outcome for patients with Pancoast tumors has been variable with 5-year survival ranging from 17–40%.

Treatment regimens include preoperative radiation therapy followed by complete resection, resection both complete and incomplete, followed by radiation therapy with or without chemotherapy, and curative radiation therapy alone. Negative prognostic indicators include mediastinal lymph node disease, subclavian artery involvement, and vertebral body involvement, although the latter two remain somewhat controversial. Some controversy exists over whether ipsilateral supraclavicular lymph node involvement (N3) represents "local" spread; and therefore, these patients have a better prognosis than those with supraclavicular lymph node disease in non-Pancoast non-small cell lung carcinoma (NSCLC).

FURTHER READING

Dartevelle P, Chapelier A, Macchiarini P et al. Anterior transcervical approach for radical resection of lung tumors invading the thoracic inlet. *Journal of Thoracic and Cardiovascular Surgery* 1993; **105**: 1025–34.

Ginsberg RJ. Resection of a superior sulcus tumor. *Chest Surgery Clinics of North America* 1995; **5**: 315–31.

Pancoast HK. Superior pulmonary sulcus tumor: tumor characterized by pain, Horner's syndrome, destruction of bone and atrophy of hand muscles. *Journal of the American Medical Association* 1932; **99**: 1391–6.

Paulson DL. The "superior sulcus lesion." In: Delarue N, Echapasse H eds. *International Trends in General Thoracic Surgery*. Vol I. *Lung Cancer*. Philadelphia:WB Saunders, 1985, pp. 121–31.

Shaw RR, Paulson DL, Kee JL. Treatment of the superior sulcus tumor by irradiation followed by resection. *Annals of Surgery* 1961; **154**: 29–40.

SECTION II

Esophageal surgery

32

Rigid esophagoscopy

MICHAEL T. MARRINAN FRCS(ED)
Consultant Cardiothoracic Surgeon, King's College Hospital, London, UK

CLAUDE DESCHAMPS MD
Professor of Surgery, Mayo College of Medicine, Rochester, Minnesota, USA

PRINCIPLES AND JUSTIFICATION

Rigid esophagoscopy is a useful and safe procedure in the evaluation of esophageal disorders. In recent years flexible fiberoptic esophagoscopy has enjoyed widespread use, mainly because general anesthesia is not required, the stomach and duodenum can be examined, and the risk of perforation is lower. Nevertheless, the specific situations outlined later show that a need for rigid esophagoscopy persists, and the technique should remain part of the armamentarium of all esophageal surgeons.

In some circumstances, the relatively cheap cost of a rigid esophagoscope, combined with its greater durability, may make the rigid instrument preferable to the fiberoptic instrument. The greater ease of sterilization of the rigid instrument may also be a factor, particularly where human immunodeficiency virus infection is endemic.

Indications

Removal of ingested foreign bodies is greatly facilitated by the large-bore rigid open tube with appropriately proportioned grasping forceps. When severe esophageal bleeding is encountered, suctioning is far more efficient. To decrease the risk of aspiration, impacted megaesophagus should be treated using the rigid endoscope. This allows for liberal irrigation and more efficient evacuation of debris. This technique also facilitates the evaluation of high lesions at or just beyond the cricopharyngeus, an area poorly examined with the flexible endoscope. Whenever the need dictates, larger biopsy specimens can be obtained through the rigid endoscope.

When an endoesophageal prosthesis is being considered to palliate intrinsic and extrinsic compression of the esophagus or malignant esophagorespiratory fistula, rigid endoscopy is of particular help intraoperatively in dilatation, guide wire positioning, and verification of the position of the prosthesis after insertion.

Although injection sclerotherapy of esophageal varices is preferably performed under sedation using a flexible esophagoscope, it is possible and safe to perform chronic sclerotherapy using a rigid esophagoscope.

Contraindications

Contraindications to the procedure are few, but it should not be performed if the cervical spine is unstable and it may be impossible to perform if severe kyphoscoliosis or restricted jaw opening is present. Great care should be exercised if large cervical osteophytes are seen on radiographs of the cervical spine, if a large thoracic aortic aneurysm is present, or if a pharyngoesophageal or epiphrenic diverticulum is present. A chest radiograph and barium swallow results should be reviewed, and radiographs of the cervical spine may be required if symptoms are present.

PREOPERATIVE ASSESSMENT AND PREPARATION

Patient preparation

The patient should have taken nothing by mouth overnight or for a minimum of 8 hours. This precaution is specifically to decrease the risk of aspiration during the procedure. Dentures should be removed. The esophagus should be empty, which may require consumption of a clear liquid diet for 24 hours before the procedure and aspiration of the esophagus immediately before performing the endoscopy.

Equipment

1 Chevalier Jackson, Negus, or Moersch-type esophagoscopes may be used. At the Mayo Clinic, the preference is for the Moersch esophagoscope modified to carry a fiberoptic light source. This modification uses a fiberoptic light rod to provide illumination directly at the level of the object being examined.

A full range of sizes, up to 20 mm for a man and 16 mm for a woman, should be on hand. An endoscope with magnification is advisable for use in children to compensate for the loss of visual acuity associated with the use of a small-bore open esophagoscope.

Large-bore and small-bore suction devices longer than the overall length of the esophagoscope should be available, as well as a variety of long biopsy forceps and a full range of esophageal dilators and guidewires.

Anesthesia

Premedication consisting of pethidine hydrochloride, 1 mg/kg, and atropine sulphate, 0.4 mg, may be given intramuscularly before the procedure.

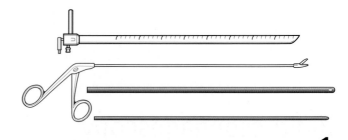

1

General anesthesia is delivered via a cuffed endotracheal tube. Muscle relaxation is helpful for the safe performance of rigid esophagoscopy, as this reduces the risk of perforation. Rigid esophagoscopy can also be performed under neuroleptanalgesia, although the benefits of complete muscle relaxation are lost. Throughout the procedure the patient's eyes are kept covered for protection.

During passage of the rigid esophagoscope through the cricopharyngeal sphincter, the anesthetist may assist by deflating the cuff on the endotracheal tube and/or pulling forward on the larynx. When insertion of an endoesophageal prosthesis is being considered, a smaller endotracheal tube should be used to ease passage of the prosthesis and its introducer.

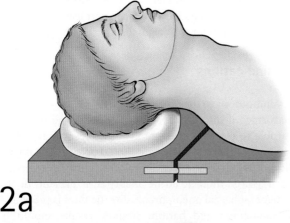

2a

OPERATION

Position of patient

2a, b The patient is positioned supine on an operating table, the head of which can be raised or lowered easily, with the head stabilized on a foam ring. Alternatively, the head and neck may be entirely supported by an assistant. The surgeon stands during insertion of the esophagoscope, then sits during the examination.

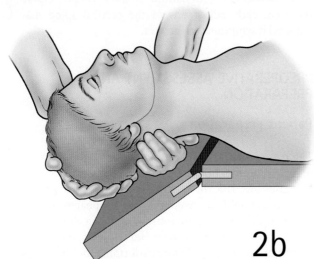

2b

Tooth protection

3 The lubricated esophagoscope is introduced at the base of the tongue with the head in the 'sniffing' position. Throughout the procedure, the upper teeth and gums are protected by a guard, and a gauze swab is positioned over the upper lip. The tongue is gently pushed to the left, and the instrument is held at all times between the operator's thumb and fingers, so that the lips and teeth are protected.

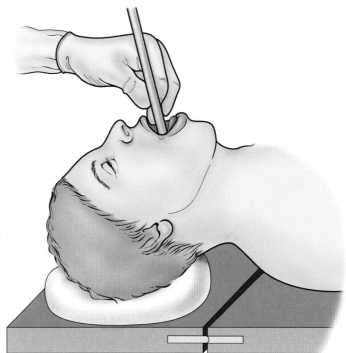

3

Passage of the esophagoscope

4a–c The epiglottis is visualized and pushed out of view by the beak of the endoscope. The endoscope is then advanced to the posterior pharynx, and the neck is extended by approximately 15 degrees. The cricopharyngeal sphincter is identified as a horizontal groove halfway between the posterior larynx and the posterior pharyngeal wall. The esophagus is entered at this point.

No force should be used as this is an area of high risk for perforation. If resistance is met, the balloon on the endotracheal tube should be deflated, and the anesthetist can assist by gently drawing forward on the larynx. If difficulty is still encountered, a small bougie can be threaded through the endoscope into the esophagus to lead the endoscope through.

As the esophagus is gently entered, the head must be lowered to allow a decrease in the angulation of the instrument to bring it into alignment with the long axis of the esophagus.

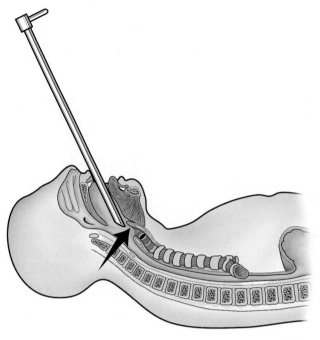

4a

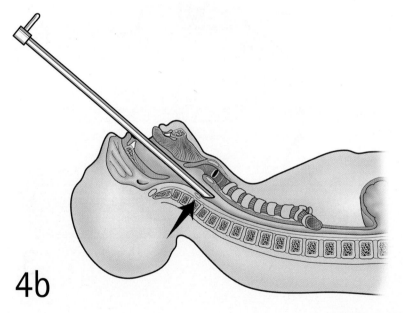

4b

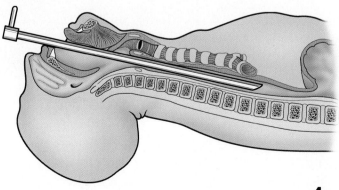

4c

Examination

5a, b The esophagus is examined under direct vision. The areas of natural constriction of the esophagus should be borne in mind, as well as the deviation anteriorly and to the left in the lower third of the esophagus. The position of the gastroesophageal junction is of particular importance and should be noted with reference to its distance from the incisor teeth.

The esophagus should also be examined as the endoscope is being withdrawn, particularly in the area just below the cricopharyngeus, which is poorly seen by other methods. The same care should be taken when withdrawing the esophagoscope as during its introduction, as the esophagus can also be injured during this phase of the examination. Those maneuvers performed on introduction should be replicated in reverse during withdrawal of the instrument.

The opportunity should be taken to palpate the abdomen while the patient is anesthetized and relaxed.

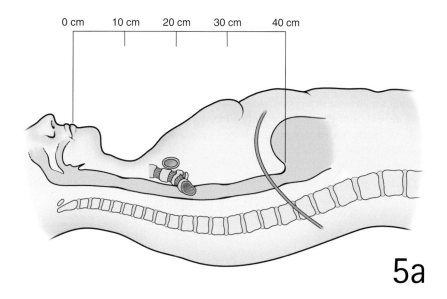

5a

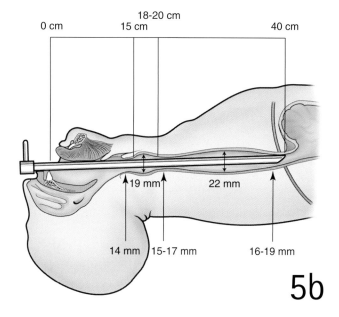

5b

POSTOPERATIVE CARE

Apart from aspiration, perforation is the most common major complication after esophagoscopy, and symptoms and signs of this should be sought in all patients in the early postoperative period. The cardinal features of esophageal perforation are the following:

1 Severe localized pain
2 Subcutaneous emphysema
3 Pneumothorax
4 Pleural effusion
5 Fever

Even in the absence of any of these features, oral intake should be withheld until the patient is fully recovered from the general anesthetic. When an endoesophageal prosthesis has been inserted, a chest radiograph should be obtained to rule out a pneumothorax and verify the position of the prosthesis. If perforation is suspected, an immediate study using water-soluble contrast (meglumine diatrizoate) should be performed.

OUTCOME

Rigid esophagoscopy is mainly a diagnostic procedure but when used for therapeutical dilatation of a stricture is associated with an 80–90% success rate and a less than 5% risk of perforation.

FURTHER READING

Fontana RS, Higgins JA. Endoscopic techniques. In: Payne WS, Olsen AM eds. *The esophagus.* Philadelphia: Lea & Febiger, 1974; 30–8.

Gaer JA, Blauth C, Townsend ER, Fountain SW. Method of endoscopic esophageal intubation using a rigid esophagoscope. *Annals of Thoracic Surgery* 1990; **49:** 152–3.

Orringer MB. Complications of esophageal surgery and trauma. In: Greenfield LJ ed. *The complications in surgery and trauma.* 2nd ed. Philadelphia: JB Lippincott, 1990; 302–25.

Wilson RH, Campbell WJ, Spencer A, Johnston GW. Rigid endoscopy under general anaesthesia is safe for chronic injection sclerotherapy. *British Journal of Surgery* 1989; **76:** 719–21.

33

Sutured anastomoses

JAMIE KELLY BM, BSC, MRCS, FRCS(GEN SURG)
Upper Gastro Intestinal Fellow, University of Adelaide, Department of Surgery, Royal Adelaide Hospital, Adelaide, South Australia, Australia

GLYN G JAMIESON MD, MS, FRACS, FACS, FRCS(GLASGOW)
Dorothy Mortlock Professor and Chairman, Department of Surgery, University of Adelaide, Royal Adelaide Hospital, Adelaide, South Australia, Australia

PRINCIPLES AND JUSTIFICATION

Better staging of esophageal cancer has led to better case selection for esophagectomy, and this has contributed to improved survival figures. As curative resections increase, operative morbidity and mortality becomes even more important. The penalty of an anastomotic leak can be severe, accounting for around 40 per cent of perioperative deaths. Even subsequent survival has considerable morbidity due to a high incidence of anastomotic stricturing, often requiring repeated dilatations

In an effort to reduce complications the surgeon has been left with several decisions to make – the site of the anastomosis, hand sewn Vs stapled anastomosis, and whether or not to combine the anastomosis with an antireflux procedure.

Site – cervical/thoracic

There are two reasons for undertaking a cervical anastomosis. The first is oncological necessity, to provide adequate clearance for an upper third esophageal tumor. The second reason is surgical preference, often dependent on the preferred surgical approach, as with a transhiatal esophagectomy. However, the additional 3–5 cm clearance provided by a cervical over a thoracic anastomosis has shown no survival advantage for middle or lower third tumors.

Traditionally cervical anastomoses have been thought to be associated with a lesser mortality if a leak occurs, since it can be managed by simply opening the cervical wound, for drainage. This has been regarded as less severe than the mediastinal contamination and resultant sepsis from an intrathoracic leak. Nevertheless, cervical anastomoses have higher rates of leakage, stenosis, and recurrent laryngeal nerve injury than thoracic anastomoses. The modified side-to-side stapled techniques described by Collard and Orringer may reduce the morbidity from a cervical anastomosis, and indeed in large centers this has been the case. Nevertheless many surgeons, ourselves included, prefer intrathoracic anastomoses for resectable tumors of the lower two thirds of the esophagus. This preference is influenced by advantages such as avoiding a third incision, better access to nodal disease if node resections are undertaken, lower leakage rates, and the fact that leaks today can often be managed conservatively.

Hand sewn versus stapled

There are a number of variables that make it difficult to compare anastomotic trials. The anastomosis can be located in the thorax or cervical regions; the use of circular or linear stapling devices; and the hand sewn group can be continuous, interrupted, single, or multi layered. These variables, along with the different conduits used, make it difficult to show a significant difference in anastomotic outcomes. Urschel's 2001 meta-analysis confirms that a stapled anastomosis is quicker but suggests it may be associated with a higher mortality. There is no ready explanation for this finding and it is not supported by more recent studies.

OPERATION

Preparation is the key to any gastrointestinal anastomosis and meticulous attention to technical details applies particularly to the easily compromised esophagus and newly formed conduit.

Technique

DOUBLE LAYER – INTRATHORACIC ANASTOMOSIS

1 The anastomosis is undertaken above the level of the azygos vein in the apex of the thoracic cavity.

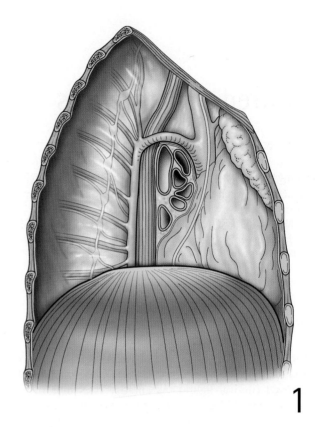

1

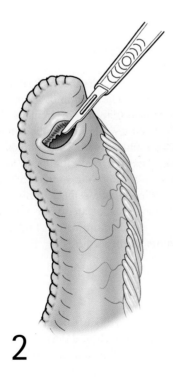

2

2 Following the construction of a gastric conduit, viability in terms of length and vascularity are checked. The oxygen tension of the gastric conduit is lowest at its most proximal point, where an end-to-end esophagogastrostomy would be constructed. To avoid this potential ischemia we favor an anastomosis placed more distally on the gastric conduit. Not only does this give a better vascularized end-to-side anastomosis but it also has the advantage of facilitating the addition of a "fundoplication." The gastrotomy is made on the anterior stomach wall, a minimum of 2 cm away from the newly sutured or stapled margin of the gastric conduit.

3 As the anastomosis is high in the apex of the chest the specimen is first resected and four full thickness stay sutures are placed at the 3, 6, 9, and 12 o'clock positions in the esophagus. The stays help with esophageal manipulation and prevent retraction of the esophageal muscle.

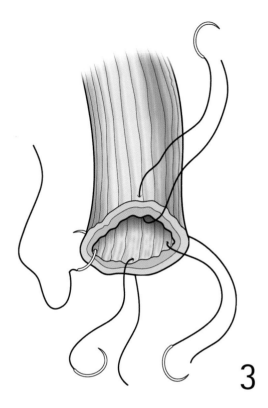

3

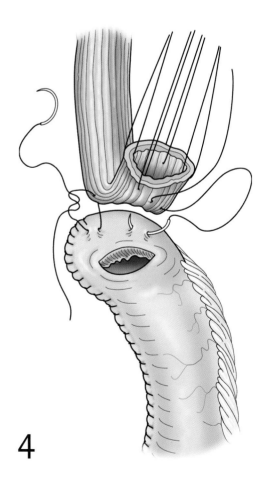

4

4 The esophagus is lifted cranially while the conduit is brought up near to the apex of the thoracic cavity, to lie behind the esophageal remnant. Two nonabsorbable sutures are used to anchor the apex of the conduit to the muscle of the esophagus, as high as is practicable. This allows the esophagus to lie on the anterior stomach wall in preparation for the anastomosis, which begins on the posterior aspect of the esophagus.

5 A row of interrupted horizontal mattress sutures are placed between the esophagus and the conduit. The suture is a 3/0 absorbable monofilament and is placed seromuscularly in the conduit and in the longitudinal and circular muscle layers of the esophagus. These are positioned 3–4 mm apart and taking about 3 mm of the esophagus or stomach wall. The sutures are held in hemostats prior to the conduit being parachuted or snugged into position and the sutures gently tied. The lateral sutures are left long and held in hemostats acting as marker stays.

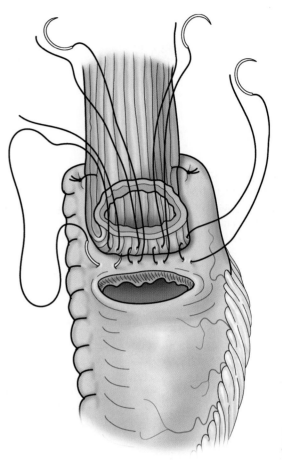

5

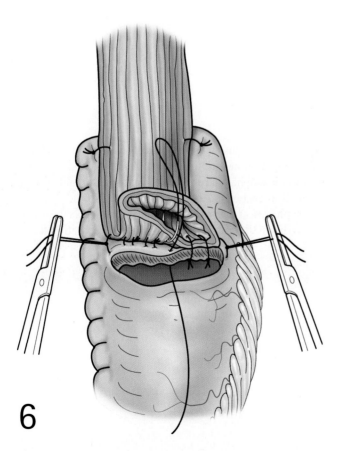

6

6 The back wall of the anastomosis is now completed with full thickness interrupted sutures at approximately 3 mm intervals. These are continued across the anterior wall, knots lying intra- or extraluminally. The initial stays are removed as encountered. The importance of clearly identifying and including the submucosa in each bite is stressed, as this is the strongest layer of the serosal deficient esophagus.

7 The anterior layer of horizontal mattress sutures can be finished using the lateral marker stays to help guide the position of the lateral sutures.

In an attempt to reduce tension on the anastomosis, buttressing sutures from the conduit to the diaphragm or mediastinal pleura are occasionally inserted.

CONTINUOUS SINGLE LAYER – INTRATHORACIC ANASTOMOSIS

The preparation is the same and again stay sutures are placed in the four quadrants of the esophagus. The gastrotomy can be made full thickness initially, but it is our preference to make it through the seromuscular layer only at this stage. This prevents bleeding and spillage of gastric contents.

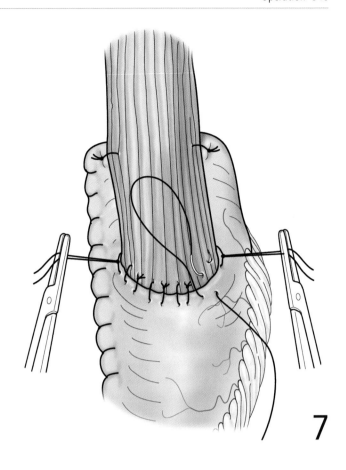

7

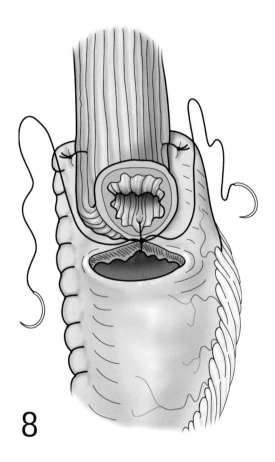

8

8 The back wall of the anastomosis is started in the midline or at the left extremity with a double-ended needled 3/0 monofilament suture. The bite is either full thickness through the stomach wall, or through the seromuscular layer, and full thickness through the esophagus again taking great care to incorporate the submucosa. The knot is thrown intra- or extra-luminally and mid length giving an equal span of suture for each needle.

9 With the gastric seromuscular layer incised, the back and side walls are completed with an over-and-over running stitch from "inside"–out on the stomach and outside–in on the esophagus. Once the posterior aspect of the anastomosis is finished the suture is brought "inside" out of the stomach. If the seromuscular suture on stomach has been used the mucosa is now divided with scissors, taking care to suck away all gastric content. The anterior suture is then inserted, again in an over-and-over fashion passing from outside–in on the stomach and from inside–out on the esophagus. When the posterior suture is reached, the two sutures are tied securely.

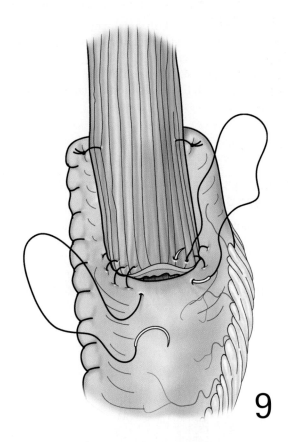

9

An antireflux anastomosis

INTRODUCTION

Rudolf Nissen in 1938 undertook a resection of the gastro-esophageal junction in a young woman, and following an end-to-side esophagogastrostomy he buried the anastomosis to guard against leakage. He found subsequently that the patient developed no reflux and it was this case which led to the anti-reflux operation popularly known as a Nissen fundoplication.

Given that reflux can be a major detrimental factor in quality of life after an esophagectomy, it is perhaps surprising that Nissen's example has not been followed.

The performance of a modified fundoplication requires just two prerequisites. First that approximately 3–4 cm of intrathoracic esophagus is present and second that the gastric conduit can reach up or nearly up to the apex of the thorax.

ANTIREFLUX ANASTOMOSIS WHEN GASTRIC CONDUIT IS MAINLY INTACT

10 The preparation of the esophagus is identical to that described in the hand-sewn technique. It is useful for the surgeon to place his left hand behind the stomach after its apex has been sutured to the esophagus and the anastomosis constructed, by applying upwards pressure on the part of the stomach to be wrapped around the anastomosis. A three-suture fundoplication is now constructed with interrupted nonabsorbable sutures placed 5–10 mm apart on the stomach. The proximinal suture also incorporates the esophageal wall. As with antireflux surgery, the aim is to make a loose wrap. We have not used a bougie but concede it may be helpful.

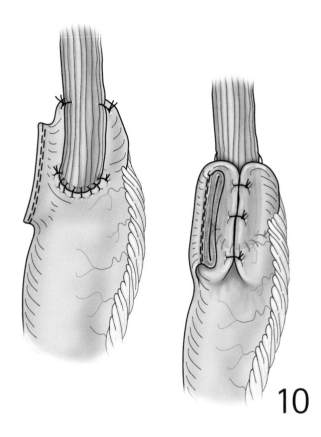

10

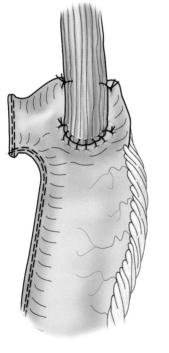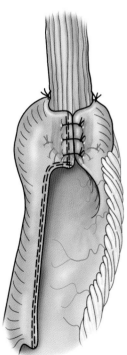

11

ANTIREFLUX ANASTOMOSIS WHEN GASTRIC CONDUIT HAS BEEN MADE MORE TUBULAR

11 The tubed stomach is brought up as an inverted J and the bend in the J is sutured to the esophagus. The limb of the stomach to the right of the esophagus is now brought over the anastomosis and sutured with between two and four interrupted nonabsorbable sutures.

POSTOPERATIVE CARE

It is important to realize that these modified fundoplications can act just as effectively as a one-way valve as fundoplications carried out for reflux disease. Therefore we always use a nasogastric tube to keep the stomach decompressed until day 7 or 8 postoperatively, when a contrast swallow is performed to make sure that the stomach is emptying adequately (and coincidentally to check for an anastomotic leak).

OUTCOME

Clinical anastomotic leak rates of less than 5% are readily achievable using these techniques. Integrating an antireflux anastomosis into our clinical practice has neither affected the anastomotic leak rate nor the anastomotic stricture rate (25%). However, it has significantly reduced symptoms of severe post-operative reflux from 63% to 12%. We stress the basic surgical principles of producing a well vascularized, tension free anastomosis with minimal surgical trauma, but, this must be combined with intensive post-operative care to help maintain tissue oxygenation.

FURTHER READING

Aly A, Jamieson GG, Pyragius M, et al. Antireflux anastomosis following esophagectomy. *Australian and New Zealand Journal of Surgery* 2004;**74:** 434–8.

Chasseray VM, Kiroff GK, Buard JL, et al. Cervical or thoracic anastomosis for esophagectomy for carcinoma. *Surgery, Gynecology and Obstetrics* 1989; **169:** 55–62.

Collard JM, Romagnoli R, Goncette L, et al. Terminalized semimechanical side-to-side suture technique for cervical esophagogastrostomy. *Annals of Thoracic Surgery* 1998; **65:** 814–17.

Dan HL, Bai Y, Meng H, et al. A new three-layer-funnel-shaped esophagogastric anastomosis for surgical treatment of esophageal carcinoma. *World Journal of Gastroenterology* 2003; **9:** 22–5.

Lerut T, Coosemans W, Decker G, et al. Anastomotic complications after esophagectomy. *Digestive Surgery* 2002; **19:** 92–8.

Orringer MB, Iannettoni MD, Marshall B. Eliminating the cervical esophagogastric anastomotic leak with a side-to-side stapled anastomosis. *Journal of Thoracic and Cardiovascular Surgery* 2000; **119:** 277–88.

Patil PK, Patel SG, Mistry RC, et al. Cancer of the esophagus: esophagogastric anastomotic leak – a retrospective study of predisposing factors. *Journal of Surgical Oncology* 1992; **49:** 163–7.

Santos RS, Raftopoulos Y, Singh D, et al., Utility of total mechanical stapled cervical esophagogastric anastomosis after esophagectomy: a comparison to conventional anastomotic techniques. *Surgery* 2004; **134:** 917–25.

Urschel JD. Esophagogastrostomy anastomotic leaks complicating esophagectomy: a review. *American Journal of Surgery* 1995; **169:** 634–40.

Urschel JD, Blewett CJ, Bennett WF, et al. Handsewn or stapled esophagogastric anastomoses after esophagectomy for cancer: meta-analysis of randomized controlled trials. *Diseases of the Esophagus* 2001; **14:** 212–17.

Walther B, Johansson J, Johnsson F, et al. Cervical or thoracic anastomosis after esophageal resection and gastric tube reconstruction: a prospective randomized trial comparing sutured neck anastomosis with stapled intrathoracic anastomosis. *Annals of Surgery* 2003; **238:** 803–12; discussion 812–14.

34

Stapling techniques for anastomoses of the esophagus

GLYN G. JAMIESON MS, MD, FRACS, FRCS, FACS
Dorothy Mortlock Professor of Surgery, University of Adelaide; Professor and Chairman, Department of Surgery, Royal Adelaide Hospital, Adelaide, South Australia, Australia

PRINCIPLES AND JUSTIFICATION

Controlled trials have not established that stapled anastomoses are either better or worse than manually sutured anastomoses. Such trials, however, have usually been performed in units expert in the techniques of esophageal surgery. In the hands of less expert surgeons the stapled anastomosis is quite likely to be safer, because the anastomosis is standardized and probably has a better blood supply than a manually constructed anastomosis.

Attention to detail is still of paramount importance, however, and the overriding principles of lack of tension and provision of the best possible blood supply apply for stapled anastomoses just as for manually constructed anastomoses.

TECHNIQUE

The esophagus receives its blood supply through intramural vascular anastomoses, so that long segments of it can be mobilized without jeopardizing its blood supply. Therefore, 3–5 cm of the esophagus proximal to where it is to be divided should be mobilized.

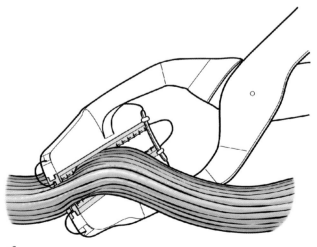

1 If an automatic purse-string device is used, it is applied before dividing the esophagus. If a nasogastric tube lies in the esophagus, it is withdrawn to a point several centimeters above the site of division. The purse-string device is placed in position and closed. A heavy tie is then placed around the esophagus distal to the purse-string device to prevent spillage of esophageal contents.

1

2 The esophagus is now divided flush with the purse-string device, which is opened and removed. The ends of the purse-string suture are retrieved and held in a pair of artery forceps. Esophageal contents in the proximal esophagus are suctioned out. There are two points at which the purse-string may not be held optimally close to the esophagus. These points are at either side where the anterior and posterior rows of staples meet. The author secures the furthest point by placing a single over-and-over suture to incorporate the purse-string. The nearest point is where the purse-string will be tied, and as it lies directly under vision this is not usually a problem. If necessary, an over-and-over suture can be placed here, after the first throw of the knot on the purse-string has been made.

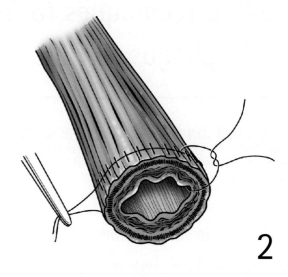

2

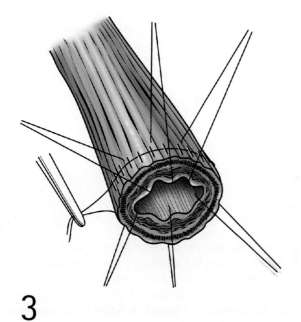

3

3 The esophagus contracts and retracts after being divided, and six stay sutures can be used to give excellent control of the mouth of the esophagus. These stay sutures are placed taking a 5- to 7-mm bite of the full thickness of the esophageal wall, and they usually pass through the esophageal wall incorporating the purse-string suture.

4 Some surgeons prefer to insert the purse-string suture manually. To do this, a 0 polypropylene or monofilament nylon suture on a round-bodied needle is used. The suture begins on the anterior wall of the esophagus, passing from outside to inside, and then is continued around the esophagus with an over-and-over running suture taking bites of 4–5 mm in depth and 4–5 mm apart. When one-third of the circumference of the esophagus has been traversed, the loop of the over-and-over suture can be held by a pair of Allis or Babcock forceps, as this will later be used as a stay suture. Similarly, when two-thirds of the circumference has been dealt with, another pair of Allis or Babcock forceps can be used to hold a second loop. The final suture is brought to the outside of the esophagus, and both ends of the purse-string suture and the two loop stay sutures keep the mouth of the esophagus open.

The esophagus is now dilated with either metal dilators or a large Foley catheter with a 25-mL balloon, which the author has found to be very effective. The catheter is lubricated and then inserted well into the esophagus. The balloon is slowly but firmly inflated, and the catheter is pulled down the esophagus. The bag of the balloon tends to bring a lot of mucus with it, and so a suction device should be held at the mouth of the esophagus as the catheter is withdrawn.

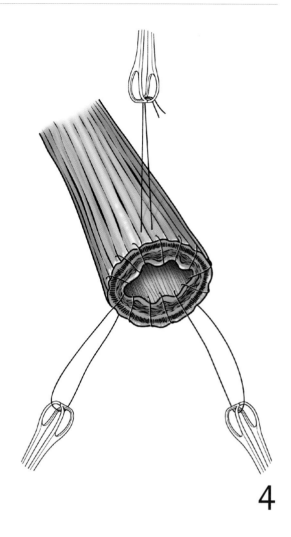

4

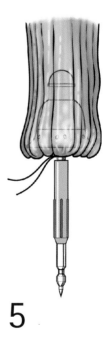

5

5 An appropriately sized staple head is chosen (usually 25 mm or 28 mm). Holding the six stay sutures (or the Allis or Babcock forceps) facilitates the placement of the anvil within the esophagus. Once it is in position, the purse string is tied snugly against the shaft of the anvil. If the surgeon is unhappy with the purse-string suture at this stage, a further purse string can be placed with the anvil in position.

6 The main stapler is introduced into the organ being joined to the esophagus, and the shaft is brought through the wall of the organ.

The anvil is clicked into position on the main shaft of the stapler. The two parts of the stapler are closed, with care taken that no extraneous tissue is caught between the esophagus and the organ to which it is being joined. Closure is completed. A final check is made to see that the tissue is free all the way around the staple head, and the instrument is fired.

The parts of the head are separated by turning the appropriate part of the stapler, and the whole device is removed by using a gently rocking motion while at the same time maintaining a pulling traction on the instrument and supporting the anastomosis with the opposite hand. Once the instrument has been removed, the rings of stapled tissue are inspected to make sure that they are complete. If there is any doubt about the anastomosis, saline can be instilled into the esophagus above the anastomosis to check that the join is watertight.

It is debatable if anything further should be done. If a gastroesophageal anastomosis has been constructed in the chest, the author constructs the anastomosis on the anterior wall of the stomach so that the remaining posterior wall can be brought up above the anastomosis to form a fundoplication. Such a fundoplication may prevent the troublesome complication of reflux.

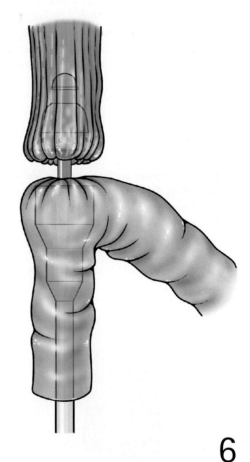

6

35

Use of the stomach as an esophageal substitute

ARNULF H. HÖLSCHER MD, FACS, FRCS
Professor of Surgery and Chairman, Department of Visceral and Vascular Surgery, University of Cologne Medical School; Director, Department of Visceral and Vascular Surgery, Medical Center University of Cologne, Cologne, Germany

J. RÜDIGER SIEWERT MD
Professor, Director, and Chairman, Department of Surgery, Technical University of Munich, Munich, Germany

HISTORY

The use of the stomach as an esophageal substitute was introduced by Kirschner in 1920 as a nonresectional operative bypass. His operation consisted of skeletonization of the greater curvature of the stomach, and the mobilized stomach was then brought subcutaneously up to the divided cervical esophagus. The application of this procedure using either the orthotopic or the retrosternal route after esophagectomy and the standardization of this method was largely due to the work of Ong, Nakayama, and Akiyama.

PRINCIPLES AND JUSTIFICATION

The reconstruction of intestinal transit after esophagectomy is normally made using stomach or colon. The small bowel is used much less frequently for complete substitution of the esophagus. Small bowel interposition does have a place, however, for partial esophageal replacement of both proximal and distal esophagus.

Gastric interposition is the simplest form of esophageal replacement. Furthermore, as it guarantees good long-term functional results, it has become the method of first choice as an esophageal substitute, especially after esophagectomy for cancer. Only when the stomach is not available because of previous operations or in benign esophageal diseases is colonic interposition used.

An important question to be answered in planning an esophageal replacement is where to site the esophagoenteral anastomosis. If intrathoracic anastomoses are performed, they should be carried out near the apex of the pleura. Anastomotic leakage is less likely to occur with intrathoracic anastomosis than with cervical anastomosis, but the consequences of such a leak are much more serious. With regard to

oncologic radicality (remaining esophagus) and long-term results, both types of anastomosis are similar.

Finally, the site for the esophageal substitute must be chosen. Antesternal subcutaneous placement is usually not indicated. This leaves the posterior and anterior mediastinal routes available.

Swallowing, at least in the early postoperative phase, is more normal when the interposition is in the posterior mediastinum. One should also note that the distance through the posterior mediastinum is the shortest. If an intrathoracic anastomoses is performed in the upper thorax, the gastric conduit can only be placed in the posterior mediastinum. In case of cervical anastomoses both routes are possible. The posterior mediastinal route should be avoided for reconstruction if a high-risk for local recurrence exists especially after R1 or R2 resection. If a postoperative radiotherapy of the former tumor site is planned, the anterior mediastinum should be preferred for reconstruction in order to avoid radiation damage of the gastric conduit.

PREOPERATIVE ASSESSMENT AND PREPARATION

The stomach may be used as an esophageal substitute only if it has not previously been operated on. After gastric resections the length will be insufficient and after vagotomy procedures the vascularization is doubtful. If lesser procedures (such as suturing of a bleeding ulcer or closure of a perforation) have been performed, then a transposition of the stomach may be possible, but the vascularity should be checked at the beginning of the operation. A preoperative gastroscopy should be carried out to exclude any mucosal pathology and to confirm the borders of the esophageal tumor. If the cancer is infiltrating the cardia or the subcardial area, the safety margin between the lower edge of the tumor and the resection line of the gastric tube may not be sufficient. Lymph node metastases to the lesser curvature (compartment I according to the classification in gastric cancer) and the celiac trunk (compartment II) should be detected by preoperative endoscopic ultrasonography.

In all cases the colon should be prepared by bowel lavage and colonoscopy so that it may be used if the stomach should prove unusable.

Anatomical points

1a–d A knowledge of the arterial blood supply of the stomach is essential for its use as an esophageal substitute. The arterial supply of the stomach originates from the celiac trunk. This vessel has a short stem that immediately divides into three branches. The left gastric artery runs in a cranial ventral direction, covered by the peritoneum of the posterior wall of the lesser sac. Subcardially it turns to the lesser curvature in an aborad direction, where it supplies the anterior and posterior gastric wall by small branches. The left gastric artery has anastomoses with the right gastric artery, which originates from the common hepatic artery and approaches from the region of the pylorus. By these means, an arterial ring along the lesser curvature is completed, with its strongest inflow being from the left gastric artery.

The second vessel of the celiac trunk is the splenic artery, which runs along the upper border of the pancreas behind the posterior wall of the omental bursa to the hilum of the spleen. At the splenic hilum the short gastric vessels originate; they proceed to the fundus and the cranial third of the greater curvature of the stomach. The left gastroepiploic artery arises from the splenic artery and runs through the gastrocolic ligament parallel to the greater curvature of the stomach in a caudad direction. This artery gives gastric branches to both walls of the stomach and epiploic branches to the greater omentum. It anastomoses with the right gastroepiploic artery, which comes from the region of the pylorus. Thus the greater curvature also has a vascular ring, with its strongest supply being from the right gastroepiploic artery. This artery has a number of anatomical variations, which may be relevant to gastric interposition.

The third vessel of the celiac trunk, the common hepatic artery, turns to the right, in the direction of the hepatoduodenal ligament of the small omentum. There it divides into the hepatic and gastroduodenal arteries. The hepatic artery runs through the hepatoduodenal ligament to the liver and usually gives rise to the right gastric artery, which proceeds to the lesser curvature of the stomach. The right gastric artery may also originate from the gastroduodenal artery. The gastroduodenal artery runs posterior to the superior part of the duodenum distal to the pylorus and comes out caudad to the duodenum, where it divides into the right gastroepiploic and

Anesthesia

The type of anesthesia used depends more on the type of esophagectomy than on the method of reconstruction. If an intrathoracic anastomosis is to be performed, a double-lumen endotracheal tube should be used.

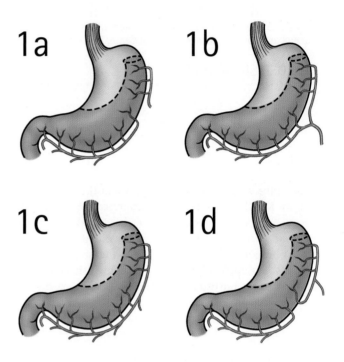

superior pancreaticoduodenal arteries. All gastric arteries anastomose between themselves directly or indirectly by intramural or extramural branches. Therefore, the ligation of two or even three gastric arteries preserves the blood supply of the stomach under normal circumstances.

The veins of the stomach lead the blood to the portal vein. With only minor exceptions they correspond in their courses to the four gastric arteries. From the gastric fundus the short gastric veins run through the gastrosplenic ligament to the splenic vein. The left gastroepiploic vein from the greater curvature also proceeds in this direction to the left side. It reaches the splenic vein through the gastrosplenic ligament. The right gastroepiploic vein accompanies its artery to the area of the pylorus. At this point, the vein turns in a posterior direction and flows into the superior mesenteric vein. At the lesser curvature, a venous arch runs along both arteries (coronary or left gastric vein). This vein flows near the right gastric artery into the portal vein or splenic vein within the hepatoduodenal ligament. At the cardia, the venous arch follows the left gastric artery up to the area of the celiac trunk.

OPERATION (Open technique)

The laparoscopic technique for preparation of the gastric conduit is described in Chapter 48.

Position of patient

2 The patient lies in a supine position with the head turned to the right to provide a free approach to the left side of the neck. A rolled-up towel or a sandbag is placed behind the shoulders to facilitate the approach to the anterior mediastinum, and under the lumbar region to facilitate access to the stomach.

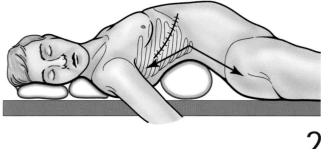

2

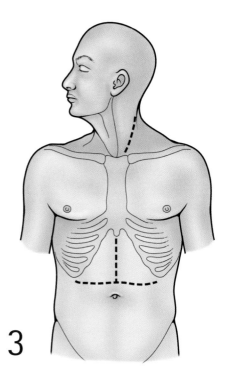

3

Incision

3 The abdomen is opened by a transverse incision extended by an upper midline incision in the direction of the xiphoid process. This ensures a good view of the epigastric area.

Preparation of the stomach

Skeletonization of the stomach begins along the greater curvature outside the gastroepiploic arch. It is performed stepwise in the direction of the fundus. Although the supply to the stomach from the right gastroepiploic artery shows variations (as illustrated in Figure 1), it is sufficient in nearly all cases to guarantee a blood supply to the gastric tube. After division of the left gastroepiploic artery, the preparation of the upper third of the gastric fundus may be performed close to the stomach wall.

4 In an aboral direction the preparation must be done very carefully outside the gastroepiploic arch to the origin of the right gastroepiploic artery from the gastroduodenal artery.

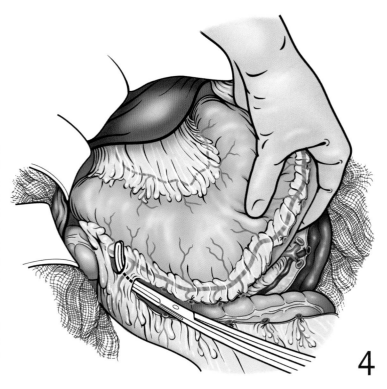

4

5 Maintaining the venous drainage via the right gastro-epiploic vein is also important.

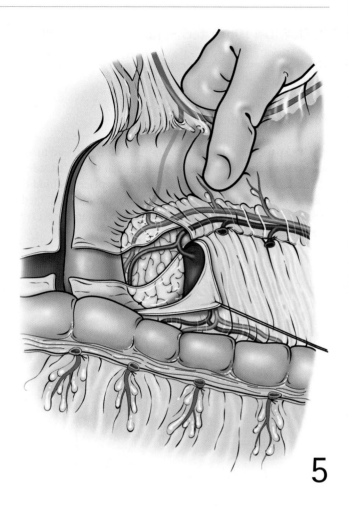

5

Lymph node dissection

The gastroduodenal artery is dissected immediately distal to the pylorus. This allows the common hepatic artery to be easily identified. Dissection proceeds in a medial direction to preserve the origin of the right gastric artery from the common hepatic artery. The right gastric artery may aid the vascularization of the gastric tube, and it should be spared if possible.

6 The lymph nodes are dissected in a manner similar to that used in gastric cancer, which means that all lymph nodes along the common hepatic artery, the celiac trunk, and the medial part of the splenic artery are dissected and taken with the specimen. The ligation of the left gastric artery is performed near its trunk of origin.

After dissection of the lesser omentum, the esophagus, which has previously been dissected by a transthoracic or transmediastinal approach, is pulled out of the esophageal hiatus for the final preparation of the gastric tube.

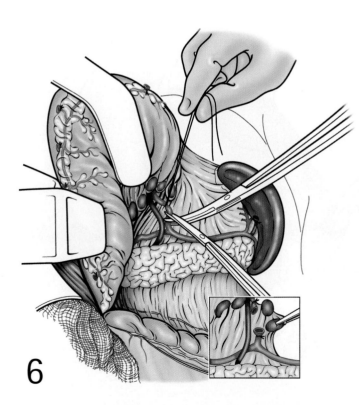

6

Formation of the gastric tube

7 Akiyama recommends that the highest point of the stomach be marked by two stay sutures. This point is located quite a long way to the left of the cardia. The skeletonization of the lesser curvature involves approximately two-thirds of the lesser curvature, which means it starts distal to the third or fourth branch of the left gastric artery, at the region of the 'crow's foot', and continues close to the gastric wall in the direction of the cardia.

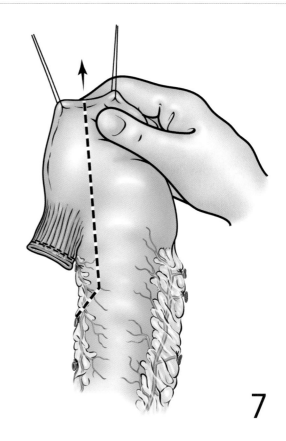

7

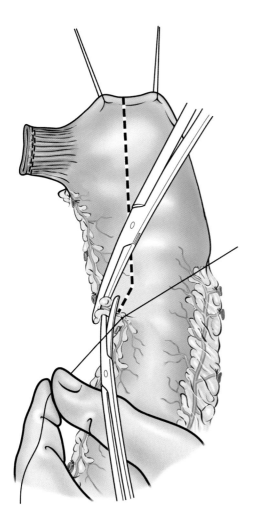

8

8 The lesser omentum should be divided in this area and the vascular arcade suture ligated. The stomach now can be cut in mediastinuman oblique direction between the distal point of skeletonization and the highest point of the gastric fundus (interrupted line in Figures 7 and 8). This means that approximately half of the gastric fundus, including the lymphatic drainage along the left gastric artery (compartment I), is removed. The resulting gastric tube has a width of 3–4 cm.

9a–c Before the stomach is finally cut along this line, the gastric fundus should be opened near the cardia and a pair of long forceps inserted to carry out an intraluminal pyloric dilatation. This helps to avoid early postoperative pylorospasm. The best way to divide the stomach is to use a linear stapler (TA 90). Two applications of this stapler are usually required to close the quite long resection line.

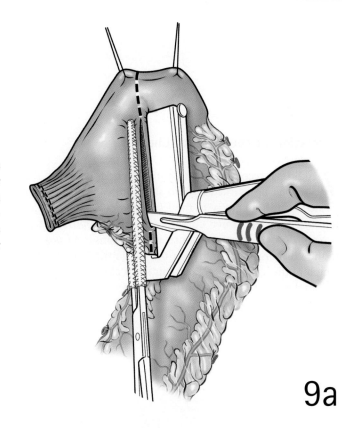

9a

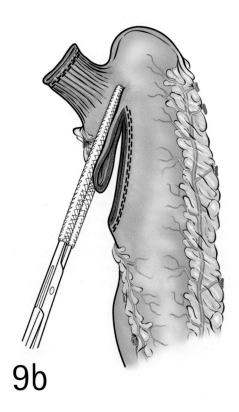

9b

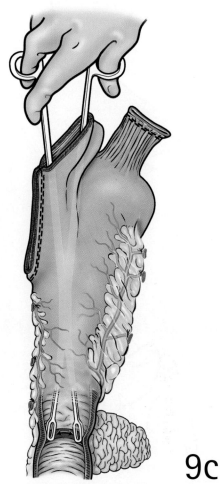

9c

10 If the stomach appears too short for elevation to the neck, cutting the seromuscular layer with a scalpel and then closing the mucosa by stapler results in greater elasticity of the gastric tube.

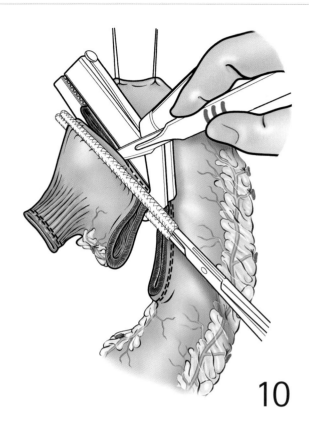

10

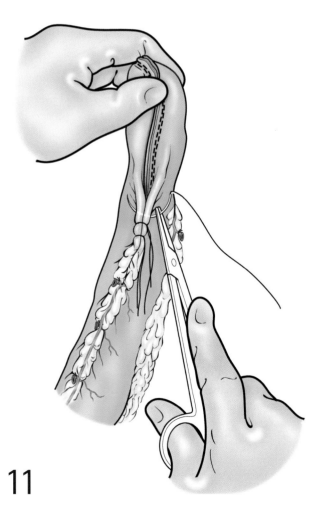

11

11 If additional suturing of the staple line is undertaken, interrupted rather than running sutures are best used to avoid shortening of the tube by a purse-string effect.

Interposition of the whole stomach

The whole stomach, rather than a gastric tube, can be used as the esophageal interposition. This can be done only if the tumor is not infiltrating the gastroesophageal junction. The skeletonization should start at the same point and in the same manner as for the formation of the gastric tube. However, it is continued along the lesser curvature up to the cardia.

12 The staple line (using a TA 55 stapler) is then placed directly below the cardia to preserve the whole gastric fundus.

Pyloric dilatation can be performed through the cardia before stapling.

The advantage of using the whole stomach as the esophageal substitute is that the gastroesophageal anastomosis does not include the tangential staple line at the highest point of the gastric fundus. This may avoid a 'locus minoris resistentiae' of such an anastomosis.

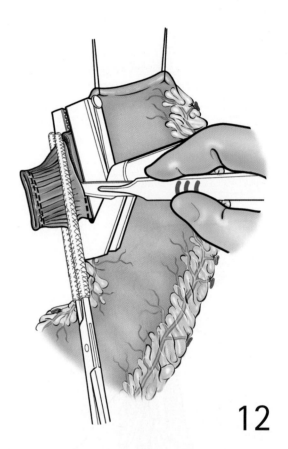

12

Duodenal mobilization

An essential prerequisite for a tension-free stomach interposition is a careful and extensive duodenal mobilization. This Kocher maneuver is performed in the usual way from the right side and should be continued until the vena cava and the aorta up to the superior mesenteric artery are freed. This means that the duodenum and the head of the pancreas are quite mobile.

Another important step is to separate the right colonic flexure from the head of the pancreas and the duodenum. This mobilization should be performed up to the middle colic vein. After this maneuver the pylorus can easily be moved up to the esophageal hiatus or even higher.

Preparation of the tunnel for the interposition

13 If the interposition is to be placed in the posterior mediastinum, some form of tape or Penrose tubing must be drawn down as the esophagus is removed. This is attached to the stomach so that the gastric tube can be pulled upward without further preparation, in the bed of the former esophagus. If the plan is for the interposition to be placed in the anterior mediastinum, a retrosternal tunnel is prepared by blunt dissection.

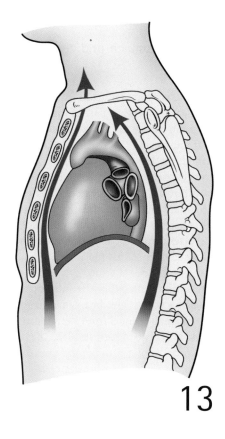

13

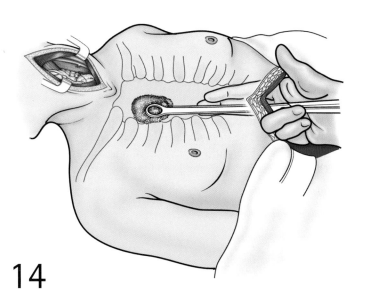

14

14 This blunt dissection can be performed with the help of a swab in sponge-holding forceps. It is essential to limit this preparation strictly to the midline and always with contact to the posterior part of the sternum. Once the sponge-holding forceps has reached the cervical incision, the channel is dilated in a stepwise fashion so that the interposition can be accommodated without compression.

Elevation of the stomach and cervical anastomosis

15 While the abdominal team is operating, another team starts the cervical part of the operation using a left lateral incision along the sternocleidomastoid muscle. The omohyoid muscle and the inferior thyroid artery are ligated and divided, the left thyroid lobe is mobilized, and the recurrent laryngeal nerve is dissected and preserved.

After transthoracic esophagectomy, mobilizing the esophageal remnant and extracting it from the posterior mediastinum is usually easy. The preparation of the esophagus should be extended in the direction of the hypopharynx until it is completely free so that the esophagus passes directly to the anastomosis without kinking.

If the interposition is placed in the anterior mediastinum, the retrosternal space must also be opened from the cervical incision to complete the tunnel from the abdominal and cervical directions. It is a good idea to place the stomach in a plastic bag when drawing it through the tunnel to avoid any trauma to the organ. This part of the operation is facilitated by placing a tube via the cervical incision through the anterior or posterior mediastinum.

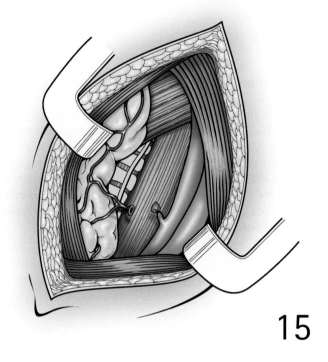

15

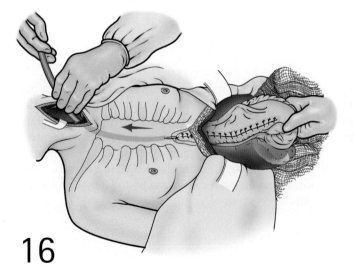

16

16 The stomach is then sutured to the lower tip of the tube. The stomach can be slowly pulled through the mediastinum in an upward direction. It is important to push the stomach upward from the abdomen as well.

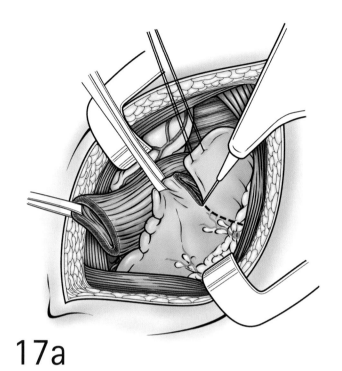

17a–c The gastric interposition usually has sufficient (and sometimes even excessive) length and reaches the neck without tension. Often the cervical esophageal stump overlaps the gastric tube, and an additional resection of the stomach can be performed. The vascularization of the top of the fundus is unreliable and should be resected. The anastomosis with the cervical esophagus is performed in the upper part of the gastric corpus. The anastomosis is usually located just above the clavicle. Before the anastomosis is performed, the back wall of the stomach is fixed to the neck by two or three sutures. The back wall of the anastomosis is constructed using interrupted sutures, which emerge between the mucosa and muscularis; the anterior wall is completed using all-layer interrupted sutures.

17a

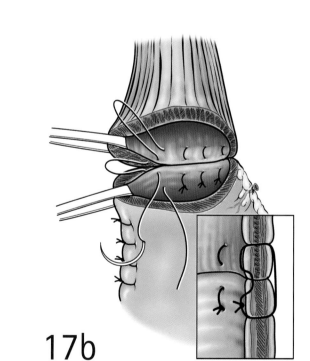

17b

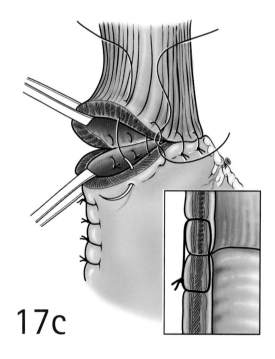

17c

18 The anastomosis is splinted by a transnasal gastric tube to guarantee postoperative decompression of the stomach. The wound is closed by subcutaneous and skin sutures.

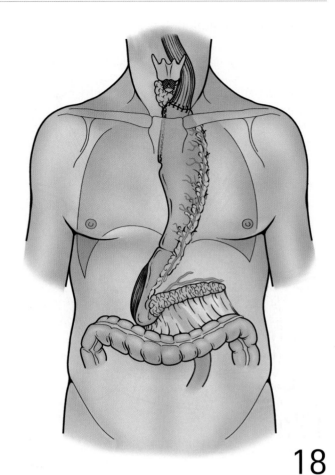

18

As an alternative, the cervical anastomosis can be performed using a stapling technique (see chapter 34). The detachable head of the EEA stapler is introduced into the esophageal stump, which is closed around the mandrel by a purse-string suture. The most appropriate size of stapler is usually size 28; smaller staplers tend to induce postoperative anastomotic stenosis. The recommendation is that the specially designed shorter head of the EEA stapler be used for introduction into the cervical esophagus because it can more easily be placed into the esophageal stump. The stapler is inserted through an incision at the top of the stomach, and the central spike is driven out 5–7 cm aborad through the stomach front wall. After the stapler is turned in the direction of the esophageal remnant, the central pin is connected with the mandrel, and the stapler is closed, fired, and removed. The site of introduction into the stomach is closed using a TA 55 linear stapler.

Elevation of the stomach and intrathoracic anastomosis

If an intrathoracic anastomosis is planned, it should be performed toward the apex of the pleura. It is important for the postoperative long-term results that the stomach be completely transferred into the thorax. This means that the preparation of the stomach is identical to the preparation for an abdominocervical interposition. When the preparation of the stomach has been finished, the gastric tube is pushed through the esophageal hiatus into the posterior mediastinum and the right pleural cavity. The abdominal approach is closed, and the patient is turned for a right thoracic approach to the esophagus. The anastomosis is now performed directly between the esophageal stump and the stomach, either end-to-end or as an implantation of the esophageal remnant on the front wall of the stomach. The suture technique can either be performed by hand or by stapling. If the gastric tube is long enough to preserve a blind oral part of the stomach above the anastomosis, then this can be used to cover the front wall suture line of the esophagogastrostomy. This procedure also has an antireflux effect.

Drainage

The cervical anastomosis is drained by a Penrose or other soft drain. In an intrathoracic anastomosis the pleural cavity is drained by a thoracic tube.

Finishing of the abdominal operation

After the esophagogastric anastomosis in the neck is finished, the abdominal operation should be completed. The operative field is checked for hemostasis. Drainage of the peritoneal cavity is not necessary. When the gastric interposition is positioned well, the pylorus should be located in the area of the diaphragm. The abdomen is closed in layers.

POSTOPERATIVE CARE

Postoperative care should follow the course described for gastroesophagectomy for adenocarcinoma of the cardia in Chapter 46.

Complications

The most common complication of gastric interposition is leakage from the cervical anastomosis. In the authors' experience this complication is unlikely if the gastric tube is elevated as proximally as possible so that the end-to-end anastomosis is performed in a well-vascularized area of the stomach. Other kinds of cervical anastomoses cannot be recommended, as often the gastric part orad to the anastomosis develops necrosis.

If leakage does develop, a salivary fistula results, which usually heals without complications provided sufficient external drainage is present. If drainage is insufficient, a phlegmon may develop in the cervical soft tissue. Therefore, whenever a fever of unknown origin develops postoperatively, the cervical anastomosis should be checked. This can be performed radiologically using contrast medium, but sometimes a safer method is to check the anastomosis directly by opening the cervical incision.

If leakage has occurred, open treatment of the cervical wound is appropriate. Early and adequate external drainage of a cervical leak is necessary to avoid spread of infection into the mediastinum.

More major (or even complete) necrosis of the interposed stomach is extremely rare as the gastric tube usually has a very good blood supply. Very occasionally, postoperative pylorospasm may occur that leads to clinically relevant delay in gastric emptying. Such a situation can easily be treated by a careful endoscopic dilatation of the pylorus. Gastric dilatation as a consequence of postoperative paralysis is extremely rare after gastric tube formation by this technique. A dislocation of the interposed stomach from the mediastinum into one of the pleural cavities is also very rare. If the stomach is shown to be distended with air on postoperative thoracic radiography, temporary placement of a nasogastric tube is suggested. This avoids compression of mediastinal organs and also avoids aspiration.

The most important long-term complication is the development of an anastomotic stricture. This is usually caused by scarring as a result of anastomotic vascular insufficiency, but use of too small a stapler could also cause dysphagia from anastomotic stenosis. In either case the problem can be solved by endoscopic dilatation. If it has no lasting effect, resection of the stenosis and reanastomosis is recommended.

OUTCOME

Functional studies of patients with intrathoracic stomach as esophageal replacement have shown good long-term results. Despite a persistent acid secretion of the vagotomized thoracic stomach, no pathological gastroesophageal reflux or esophagitis was found proximal to the cervical anastomosis. Gastric biopsies mostly reveal mild gastritis of the antral mucosa, and metaplasia is rare. The intrathoracic stomach needs no drainage to facilitate emptying. Postoperative reflux esophagitis is prevented by complete intrathoracic stomach transposition with cervical esophagogastrostomy.

In young patients with benign esophageal diseases requiring an esophagectomy, the authors prefer to use the colon as an esophageal substitute to preserve the gastric reservoir.

FURTHER READING

Aly A, Jamieson GG, Pyragius M, Devitt PG. Antireflux anastomosis following esophagectomy. *Australian and New Zealand Journal of Surgery* 2004; 74: 434–38.

Atkins BZ, Shah AS, Hutcheson KA, et al. Reducing hospital morbidity and mortality following esophagectomy. *Annals of Thoracic Surgery* 2004; 78: 1170–76.

Collard JM, Romagnoli R, Otte JB et al. The denervated stomach as an esophageal substitute is a contractile organ. *Annals of Surgery* 1998; 227: 33–9.

Hölscher AH, Bollschweiler E, Bumm R, Bartels H, Siewert JR. Prognostic factors of resected adenocarcinoma of the esophagus. *Surgery* 1995; 118: 845–55.

Hölscher AH, Schröder W, Bollschweiler E, et al. How safe is high intrathoracic esophagogastrostomy? *Chirurg* 2003; 74: 726–33.

Law S, Fok M, Chu KM, Wong J. Comparison of hand-sewn and stapled esophagogastric anastomosis after esophageal resection for cancer: a prospective randomized controlled trial. *Annals of Surgery* 1997; 226: 169–73.

Siewert JR, Stein HJ, Feith M et al. Histologic tumor type is an independent prognostic parameter in esophageal cancer: lessons from more than 1.000 consecutive resections at a single center in the western world. *Annals of Surgery* 2001; 234(3): 360–69.

Abdominal and right thoracic subtotal esophagectomy

BERNARD LAUNOIS MD, FACS
Professor of Digestive and Transplantation Surgery, Hospital Pontchaillou, Rennes, France

GUY J. MADDERN PhD, MS, FRACS
R. P. Jepson Professor of Surgery, Department of Surgery, University of Adelaide, Adelaide, South Australia, Australia;
Director, Division of Surgery, The Queen Elizabeth Hospital, Woodville, South Australia, Australia

HISTORY

Before 1946, the only widely practiced approach to the thoracic esophagus had been described by Sweet using a left-sided thoracotomy. Although this operation permitted relatively good access to the lower third of the esophagus, cancers of the middle and upper third of the esophagus were dissected with greater difficulty because of the overlying aortic arch. In 1946, Lewis described the abdominal and right thoracic approach for subtotal esophagectomy. This operation was adopted by Tanner in the United Kingdom (Lewis-Tanner operation) and by Santy in France (Lewis-Santy operation), and has remained the favored operation for an abdominal and right thoracic subtotal esophagectomy.

OPERATIONS

Abdominal approach

The operation is usually commenced with the abdominal approach, which enables the assessment of liver metastases, the involvement of draining lymph nodes, and the performance of gastrolysis.

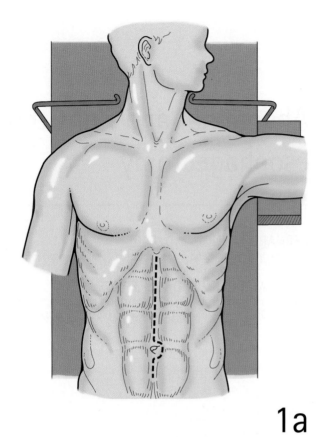

1a

INCISION

1a,b A midline incision is used, with the approach to the hiatus being facilitated by a substernal retractor. This provides improved access to the intra-abdominal esophagus.

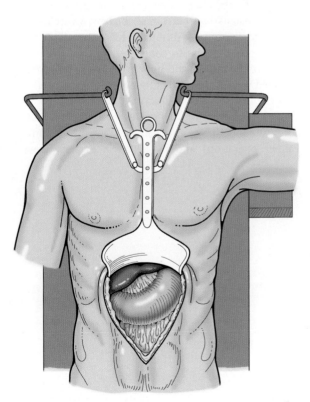

1b

2a,b

The first step is to tie and divide the vessels of the gastrocolic ligament and the short gastric vessels. During the mobilization of the greater curve of the stomach, identification and preservation of the right gastroepiploic vessels is important. The abdominal esophagus is dissected next. The left triangular ligament of the liver is divided, and the left lobe is retracted to the right to reveal the esophageal hiatus. This should be dissected with scissors under direct vision after the peritoneum is divided in front of the esophagus. Opening the tissues to the left and right of the esophagus permits a curved clamp to be introduced and a tape to be passed around the esophagus. The tape can then be used to provide traction on the abdominal esophagus, which aids in the ligation and division of the remaining short gastric vessels.

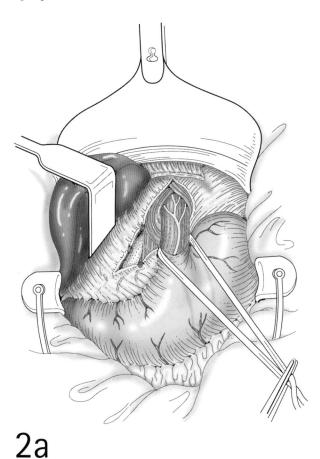

2a

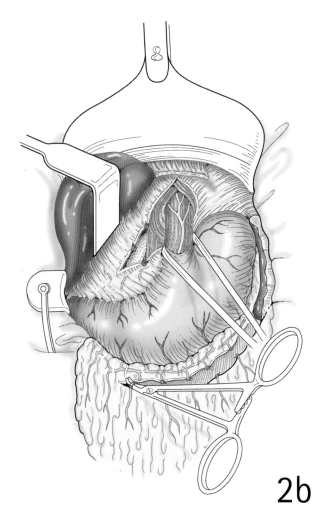

2b

3 From inside the lesser sac, with the mobilized greater curve of the stomach held upward and to the right, the left gastric vascular pedicle and its associated lymph nodes are dissected. The left gastric vein and artery are individually identified, ligated, and divided.

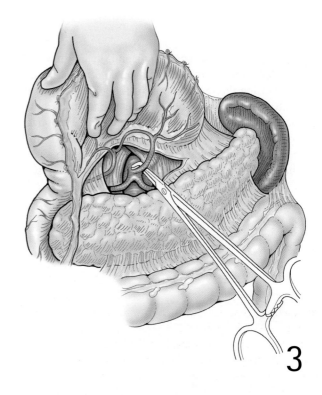

4 The lesser omentum is then ligated and divided from the hiatus down to the pylorus. Mobilization of the duodenum (Kocher maneuver) is not routinely performed for this operation but can be undertaken if increased gastric mobility is required.

A pyloroplasty or a pyloroclasia is performed to help prevent delay in gastric emptying, which sometimes occurs after this procedure. Pyloroclasia is usually performed by using the thumb and middle finger as dilators that pass through the pylorus by invaginating the gastric or duodenal wall to disrupt the sphincteric mechanism.

The right crus is divided and the hiatus opened. The intra-abdominal esophagus is then freed from all its hiatal attachments by a combination of blunt and sharp dissection.

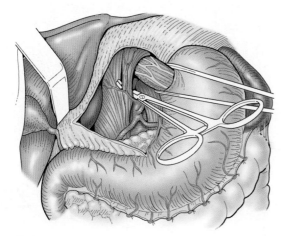

5a,b A gastric tube can be constructed at this stage, although this can be delayed until the thoracic part of the operation. The gastric tube is constructed from below the 'crow's foot' on the antrum of the stomach up to the hiatus. This procedure is most readily performed by using a surgical stapler (e.g. Endo GIA) and leaving the last 5 cm at the cardia unstapled until the esophagus and stomach have been successfully mobilized and delivered into the chest. The danger of completing the gastric tube at this stage is that, should the esophageal cancer prove unresectable, then a complete obstruction has been created unnecessarily. The staple line is oversewn to ensure hemostasis and minimize the possibility of a leak.

A feeding jejunostomy can now be created to facilitate postoperative enteric nutrition.

WOUND CLOSURE

A closed suction drain is placed behind the stomach up to the hiatus, and the abdomen is closed.

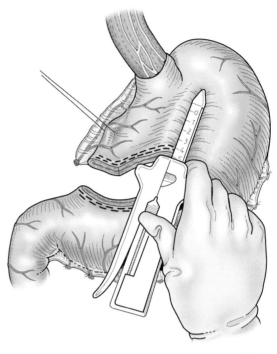

5a

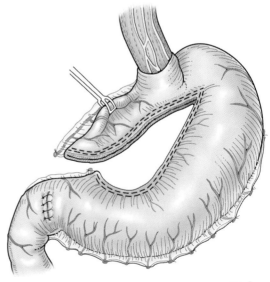

5b

Thoracic approach

POSITION OF PATIENT

6 The patient is placed on the left side with a sandbag under the left ribs. Great care should be taken to ensure not only that the patient is well supported and secured, but that no unsupported pressure points exist. The right arm is most conveniently strapped to a padded overhead rail.

INCISION

Two thoracic incisions are possible, one using a rib resection and the other passing through the intercostal space. The authors have found an unacceptable incidence of paradoxical respiration after rib resection and now recommend an intercostal approach, either through the sixth intercostal space for lower-third cancers or through the fifth intercostal space for cancers of the middle and upper third. Gradual increase in rib retraction at intervals during the procedure can produce adequate retraction without rib fracture, even in elderly patients. The scapula, once freed from its muscular attachments inferiorly, should be retracted upward. At this stage the location of the ribs can be confirmed by counting from the second rib, felt at the apex of the thorax, down to the desired interspace. The periosteum of the rib is lifted with a periosteal elevator, and the intercostal space is opened on the lower border of the rib. The pleura is then opened.

A Finochietto or Lortat-Jacob retractor is positioned and gently opened. Any pleural attachments are freed, and the lung is mobilized to the hilus. The lung is retracted forward and collapsed. It can be held in this position by fixing a broad blade attached to the rib retractor.

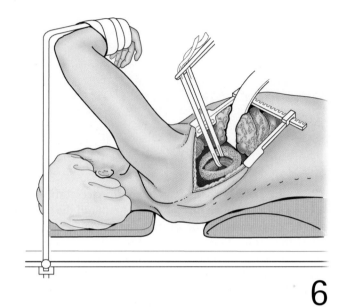

6

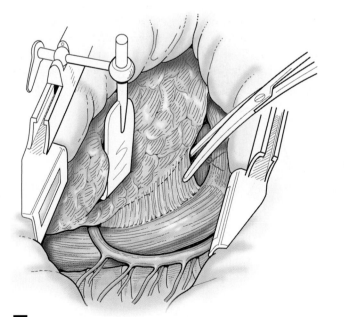

7

7 The right pulmonary triangular ligament is divided close to the posterior edge of the inferior lobe of the right lung, up to the right inferior pulmonary vein.

8 Scissors are introduced vertically between the pericardium and the posterior mediastinum. Opening the scissors reveals a plane close to the pericardium, and one can then dissect upward along this plane.

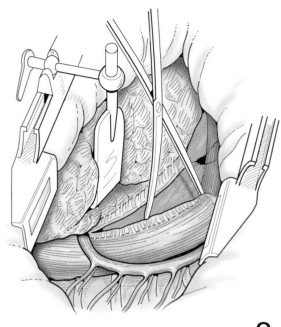

8

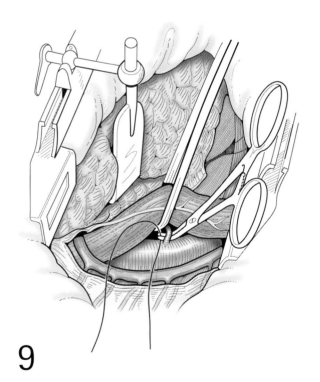

9

9 The fingers of the left hand can palpate the posterior aspect of the esophagus and retract it from the posterior mediastinum. The pleura is then opened along the vertebral column. The scissors are opened horizontally to expose the esophageal arteries, which are tied and divided.

10 The azygos vein is identified and ligated in continuity or transfixed and then divided.

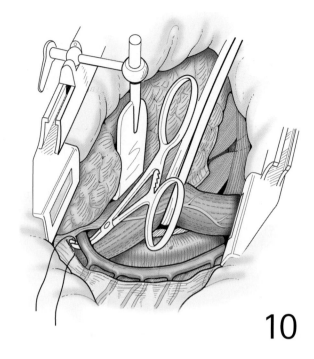

10

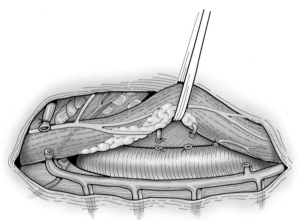

11

11 The esophagus is mobilized above and below the tumor, and tapes are passed around it to aid in retraction during the tumor dissection.

12 The esophagus and tumor are now dissected from the surrounding structures, including the pericardium, the right and left main bronchi, and the aorta. Although avoiding opening into the tumor during the dissection is desirable, this option is preferable to an unexpected aortic or bronchial laceration.

Difficulty in this dissection can occur at the pericardium, the trachea, and/or the aorta. Extension of dissection into the pericardium is not a contraindication to resection, as a portion of pericardium can be excised safely. The pericardium is opened in front of the adhesions and then divided around the margin of the tumor. Dissection is almost never extended into the right inferior pulmonary vein.

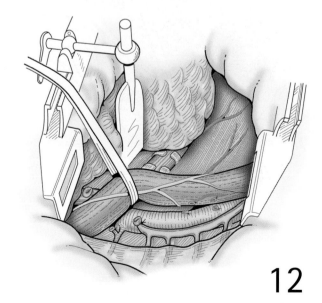

12

13 The aorta is sometimes involved by neoplastic spread. The technique used to free the cancer in these circumstances is to dissect between the intima and the adventitia of the aorta. Returning outside the adventitia once the tumor is freed is important, however. The large esophageal artery that arises from the aortic arch is best ligated and divided. Sometimes the artery is involved in the tumor. Ligation is not then possible, and the artery must be oversewn after the tumor is resected.

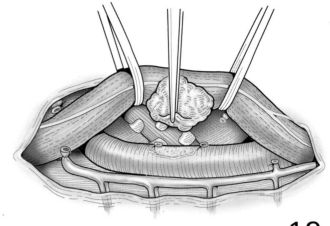

13

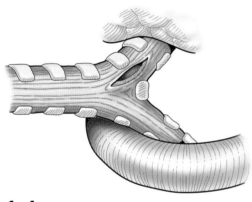

14a

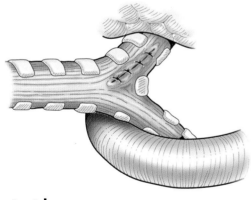

14b

14a,b In some cases the most difficult part of the dissection is to detach the tumor from the trachea and the bronchus. When the neoplastic process involves the cartilaginous rings or the carina, there is little risk of opening the respiratory tree. When the membranous portion is involved, however, dissection is trickier. A plane can usually be found between the trachea and a thin membrane covering it. This dissection should be directed to cutting only the neoplastic adhesions; otherwise, a tracheal tear can occur. If such a tear appears, it can be repaired with interrupted stitches of 5/0 polypropylene (Prolene). This is relatively straightforward and usually successful.

15 The thoracic duct is found in the groove between the esophagus and the vertebral bodies. At least its inferior portion must be ligated if a subsequent chylothorax is to be avoided.

Once the esophagus and cancer are fully mobilized, the stomach is delivered into the chest. Care should be taken to maintain the correct orientation and to avoid possible twists. The nasogastric tube is withdrawn into the cervical esophagus.

A gastric tube can be formed at this stage by using either a GIA stapler or a TA 90, which is easily manipulated in the thorax. The last 5 cm at the cardia is left unstapled.

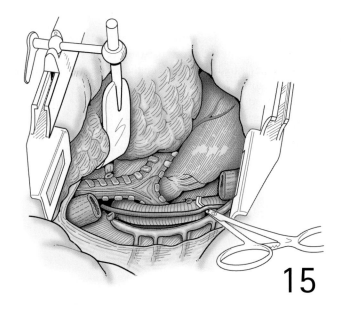

15

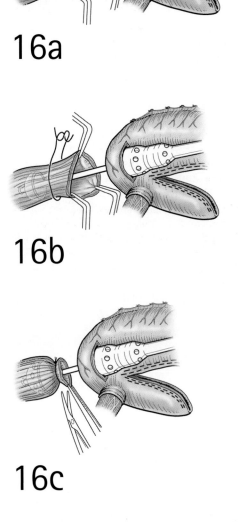

16a

16b

16c

16a–d The proximal portion of esophagus is grasped with a Satinsky clamp and divided below. Two methods can be used to tie a purse string to the anvil of the stapler. The first is to place a tie around the anvil rod after it has been introduced into the esophagus. This is done by placing three clamps on the esophageal wall to hold open the lumen of the esophagus and then introducing the anvil into the lumen and tying a ligature *en masse* around the entire esophageal wall. Excess esophagus distal to the ligature is then trimmed off. The second method is to place an over-and-over purse-string suture in the esophageal stump (see chapter on p. 363).

A gastrotomy is made below the apex of the gastric tube. Often the convenient method is to make the gastrotomy in the portion of the stomach destined to be removed. The stapling device is introduced through the gastrotomy into and through the stomach, the anvil is attached and secured, and the anastomosis is performed by fitting the stapler.

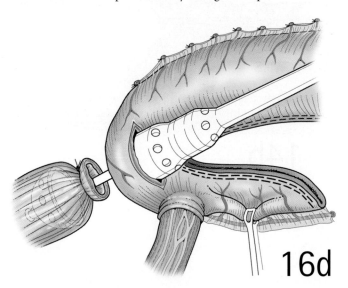

16d

17 The remaining stomach is removed with the gastro-tomy by stapling the remaining section of the tube, and the staple lines are then oversewn. The nasogastric tube is passed down into the stomach and the thoracic drain inserted. The chest is then closed.

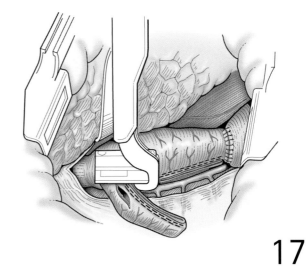

17

POSTOPERATIVE CARE

A nasogastric tube is positioned below the anastomosis under visual control during thoracotomy, and the thoraco-tomy is closed around a thoracic drain placed at the base of the thorax. Another drain is located at the apex in case of air leakage. The patient is then transferred to the intensive care unit and is intubated and ventilated for 24 hours or longer until the blood gas levels are satisfactory. The patient is then moved to the surgical ward. The drain is taken out after 3 or 4 days when less than 150 mL of clear effusion is present. Feeding by the jejunostomy is started as soon as bowel activity commences. The nasogastric tube is usually taken out after 7 days. Oral feeding is then progressively rein-stated.

If anastomotic leakage is established, feeding is continued via the jejunostomy until healing occurs. If leakage is sus-pected (fever), the authors prefer to cease oral feeding and feed the patient by the jejunostomy.

OUTCOMES

This operation has proven overwhelmingly to be the most popular approach in the Western world, for the removal of esophageal cancer.

Overall it is associated with a clinically relevant anasto-motic leakage rate of the order of 10% and an overall morality rate of about 5%.

On a priori grounds one might expect the non thoraco-tomy esophagectomy (see Chapter 38) to have a higher leakage rate and a lower mortality rate. However, randomised studies have never shown significant differences between the two techniques in major outcomes.

FURTHER READING

Campion JP, Grossetti D, Launois B. Circular anastomosis stapler. *Archives of Surgery* 1984; **119:** 232–3.

Lewis I. The surgical treatment of carcinoma of the oesophagus with special reference to a new operation for growths of the middle third. *British Journal of Surgery* 1946; **34:** 18–31.

Santy P, Mouchet A. Traitement chirurgical du cancer de l'oesophage thoracique. *Journal de Chirurgie* 1947; **63:** 505–26.

Sweet RH. Surgical management of carcinoma of the midthoracic esophagus. *New England Journal of Medicine* 1945; **223:** 1–7.

Tanner NC. The present position of carcinoma of the oesophagus. *Postgraduate Medical Journal* 1947; **23:** 109–39.

37

Left thoracic subtotal esophagectomy

JUN-FENG LIU
Professor and Doctor in Chief, Department of Thoracic Surgery, Fourth Hospital, Hebei Medical University, The People's Republic of China

HISTORY

More than 100 years ago, esophagectomy began to be used for obstructive esophageal diseases. Czerny resected the cervical esophagus for a 50-year old woman with esophageal cancer in 1877, and she survived for 15 months. Jejunal interposition was performed in a patient with benign esophageal stricture by Roux and Herzen in 1907. Kelling was the first to use colon as a substitute for the esophagus in 1911. The first successful thoracic esophagectomy was undertaken by Franz Torek in 1913. No attempt was made to perform a reconstruction and the patient fed herself through a gastrostomy until she died from a stroke 13 years later. Ohsawa performed a gastro-esophagostomy through an abdominal approach after resection of a cardiac cancer in 1932. Adams and Phemister performed a left thoracic subtotal esophagectomy for cancer in 1938 and undertook an esophagogastric anastomosis in the thorax. A combined left thoracoabdominal subtotal esophagectomy for cancer was initially reported by Sweet in 1945. Ivor Lewis undertook a three stage esophagectomy first in 1946, and three-field esophagectomy was first used in the treatment for esophageal cancer by Akiyama in 1981.

PRINCIPLES AND JUSTIFICATION

Indications

This operation provides a means for resecting the thoracic esophagus with anastomosis of the esophagus to the fundus of the stomach in the thorax or in the neck from the left side. The principal indication for this approach is resection of tumors of the thoracic esophagus and cardia, but it is also applicable to resection of a benign esophageal stricture. The main advantages of this method of subtotal esophagectomy are that it permits exploration of the tumor, dissection of the esophagus, and mobilization of the stomach through a single thoracotomy incision. This is quicker and simpler than a right-sided three-stage approach, i.e. laparotomy, right thoracotomy, and right neck incision, and it permits dissection of the tumor and its lymphatic or other extensions under direct vision.

In general, indications for surgical therapy of esophageal carcinoma are dictated by cancer stage and fitness of patients for surgery. The stages 0, I, II, and $T_3N_1M_0$ of stage III disease can be radically resected. Palliative resection is usually performed for a T_3 intrathoracic esophageal cancer, but with supraclavicular and/or upper abdominal lymph node metastasis. Although there is a steady increase in surgical mortality with advancing age and a precipitous rise in mortality over the age of 75, left thoracic subtotal esophagectomy can be well tolerated by patients whose age is close to 80 years if they have no obvious cardiopulmonary problems.

Contraindications

The contraindications to this approach are when a tumor is located at or above the aortic arch (judged by barium swallow and not endoscopy) and when the upper part of the stomach is involved by tumor and there is insufficient stomach to reach the anticipated anastomotic site. It is also contraindicated when patients are cachectic, or have significant comorbid disease and are judged unfit to withstand the operation. Clinical factors, which indicate an advanced stage of carcinoma, are recurrent laryngeal nerve paralysis, Horner's syndrome, persistent spinal pain, paralysis of the diaphragm, fistula formation, and malignant pleural effusion, and indicate inoperability. Factors that make surgical cure unlikely are a tumor greater than 8 cm in length, abnormal axis of the esophagus on barium roentgenography, enlarged lymph nodes, invasion of aorta or trachea on CT, and a weight loss greater than 20 per cent.

PREOPERATIVE ASSESSMENT

Routine investigations

Investigations before operation are designed to assess the patient's fitness for operation and to determine whether there is spread of the tumor beyond the limits of surgical resection. Routine investigations include haematological and biochemical tests and measurement of renal and hepatic function. Cardiac status is assessed by chest radiography, electrocardiography, and additional tests if indicated. Respiratory assessment includes routine spirometry, with full tests of respiratory function and blood gases if significant abnormalities are found.

Possible spread of the tumor is investigated by barium swallow, esophagoscopy, and biopsy, computed tomography and/or ultrasonography in all cases, positron emission tomography (PET) scan if available, with bronchoscopy, indirect laryngoscopy, lymph node biopsy, cytology of effusions, and other tests as indicated by symptoms or the findings on physical examination.

Nutritional assessment

Since the predominant symptom of esophageal carcinoma is difficulty in swallowing, most patients are nutritionally depleted. The nutritional status of the patients is important in predicting the outcome. A poor nutritional status decreases host resistance to infection and affects healing of an anastomosis. Physical examination should look for peripheral edema, specifically in the feet and flanks which, if present, gives an initial clue for very poor nutritional status of the patient. Measurement of the serum albumin is a more objective estimate of the status of the patient. A low value of serum albumin (<34 g/L) increases the risk of surgical complications, including anastomotic leakage. A positive nitrogen balance is important for the patient's safe passage through the rigors of this major operation and postoperative stress. Hyperalimentation may be necessary for patients with poor nutritional status before surgery. Albumin or blood plasma can be given to supplement nutrition in patients with hypoproteinemia.

Pulmonary assessment

In addition to the effects of thoracotomy on pulmonary function, the intrathoracic stomach takes up room in the thorax after esophagectomy, and this adversely affects pulmonary function. Thus pulmonary function should be meticulously assessed before resection of the esophagus. Pulmonary complications, including retained secretions, atelectasis, pneumonia, and respiratory failure, are the most severe problems following thoracic surgical procedures. Patients who are heavy smokers have a significantly increased risk of postoperative complications. The ability to cough is important because cough helps avoid postoperative atelectasis. Preoperative pulmonary function testing is undertaken routinely. The tests range from the simplest medical assessment (history taking particularly of past pulmonary disease, physical examination, and stair climbing) to the most sophisticated exercise testing, and even analysis of blood gases.

After deep inspiration, the ability to breath hold for more than 30 seconds suggests normal lung function. A value less than 20 seconds implies a high risk for thoracotomy. After climbing stairs of three stories, a pulse rate of more than 120 beats per minute indicates a high risk for esophagectomy. In our experience, a patient with MVV (maximum volume ventilation) and VC (vital capacity) more than 70 per cent of predicted values will tolerate a transthoracic esophagectomy; however, if the MVV and VC are less than 50 per cent of predicted values, FEV_1/FVC (forced expiratory volume at 1 second/forced vital capacity) less than 60 per cent, and SO_2 less than 90 per cent after exercise, surgery is contraindicated.

Cardiovascular assessment

The risk of both morbidity and mortality from thoracic surgery increases exponentially in patients with respiratory and significant cardiovascular disease. It is important to have an accurate cardiac history and know all cardiovascular medications used. If there is concern, a detailed assessment of the cardiac state should be undertaken in consultation with a cardiologist within a formal risk assessment protocol.

Preparation

Adequate preoperative management will improve the ability of the patient to tolerate the operation. Smoking is stopped for at least 2 weeks before the operation, and all patients are instructed by an experienced respiratory physiotherapist in the breathing and coughing techniques that will be required after operation and in the use of incentive spirometry. Cessation of smoking, aggressive bronchopulmonary toilet, and bronchodilators may improve a marginal FEV_1. Patients with chronic lung disease do better if their operations are scheduled for the afternoon, thus allowing them to ambulate and cough up secretions that have accumulated in the lung overnight.

Most esophageal cancer patients have difficulty swallowing, so preoperative nutritional support is important. Oral intake is usually inadequate in patients with advanced esophageal cancer, and hyperalimentation may be necessary. Enteral alimentation via a nasogastric tube and intravenous hyperalimentation are selected according to the status of the patients.

In resection of the esophagus, the mediastinum is extensively dissected and the bacteriologically contaminated esophagus is opened. Therefore, it is necessary to use prophylactic antibiotics, to reduce the incidence of wound infection and anastomotic breakdown. Adequate doses of a broad spectrum antibiotic with adequate gram-positive and gram-negative coverage is prescribed intravenously. A nasogastric tube is placed before surgery. Washout of esophageal content through the nasogastric tube is necessary for patients who have severe obstruction of the esophagus.

ANESTHESIA

After the administration of general anesthesia and endotracheal intubation with a single- or double-lumen tube (the latter is preferable), the patient is placed in the right lateral decubitus position with the arm flexed at the elbow and shoulder. The table is flexed or a soft pad is placed under the right chest to widen the operative field.

OPERATION

Incisions

1 The site of the incision is decided according to the anatomical level of the tumor and the anticipated site of anastomosis. If the tumor is in the cardia or the lower third of the esophagus and the anastomosis is constructed below the aortic arch, the incision is made through the seventh intercostal space or by resection of the seventh rib. When the tumor is in the middle or upper third of the esophagus and the anastomosis is to be constructed above the aortic arch or in the neck, the incision is made through the sixth intercostal space or by resection of the sixth rib. Usually, the sixth or seventh ribs are identified as the standard left thoracotomy incision, including anterior and posterior extensions when necessary. The basic incision is made from the level of the

costal cartilage in front to the paravertebral region at the angle of the scapula behind. It may be extended upward between the scapula and the vertebral column to the level of the posterior end of the fourth rib. This allows the transection of a higher rib, usually the fifth at the costal end, giving access for a supra-aortic dissection of the esophagus and it also permits an easier high intrathoracic anastomosis.

A left thoracoabdominal incision is usually used for resection of the proximal stomach, or for obese patients. With the patient in the right lateral position, an oblique lateral incision is made starting in the left hypochondrium and continuing over the costal margin and along the line of the seventh rib to the angle of the rib posteriorly. The incision on the abdomen is the oblique extension of the thoracic incision to the edge of the rectus sheath. The peritoneum is opened in the line of the incision, which provides excellent access to upper abdominal organs.

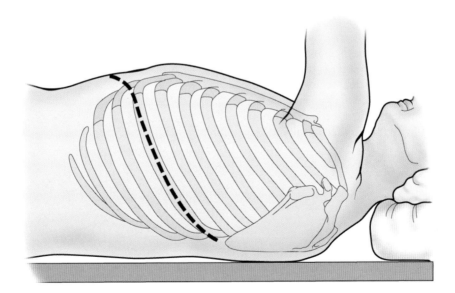

1

Dissection of the esophagus

For resection of the gastric cardia, the dissection of the esophagus needs to be carried out to the level of the inferior pulmonary vein. For cancer arising from the lower third of the esophagus, the dissection of the esophagus should be conducted to the level of the bifurcation of the trachea. The whole of the thoracic esophagus should be dissected for cancers which occur in the middle or upper third of the esophagus and also for cancers involving the cervical esophagus.

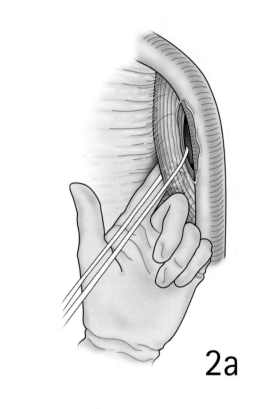

2a

2 After a thorough exploration of the pleural cavity, the mediastinal pleura overlying the esophagus is incised anterior to the aorta and posterior to the pleural reflection at the pericardium, and the tumor is identified and assessed for resectability. If resection of tumor is thought possible, a tape is placed around the esophagus just below the tumor to lift the esophagus for facilitating its dissection. The inferior pulmonary ligament is mobilized to the level of the inferior pulmonary vein, and the lymph nodes within it are removed. The esophagus is dissected from the hiatus below to a level above or at least 5 cm proximal to the tumor. To avoid dissection too close to the tumor, the descending aorta and pericardium are completely bared. The esophageal arterial branches and the bronchial artery on the adventitia of the aorta are divided. Para-esophageal adipose tissue and all mediastinal lymph nodes are completely removed with the esophagus. If invaded by tumor, resection of pulmonary ligament, pericardium, azygos vein, the right mediastinal pleural membrane, and even a wedge of the lung can be undertaken.

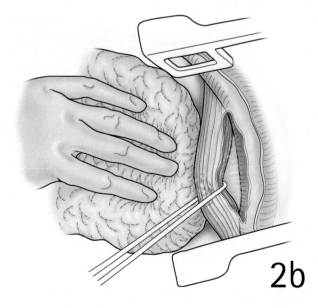

2b

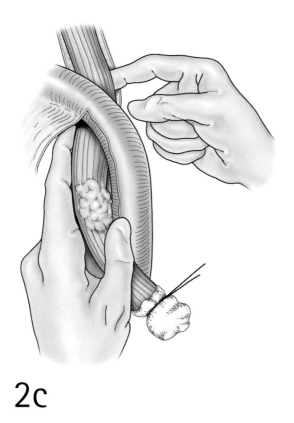

2c

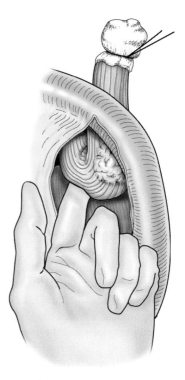

2d

For patients with a middle or upper third esophageal cancer, the whole of the thoracic esophagus is usually mobilized for a curative resection. The technique of esophageal dissection at the aortic arch is critical, particularly for cancers located at this level. The esophagus is freed from behind the aortic arch by blunt dissection in the plane between the esophageal muscle and the adventitia of the aortic arch. A finger is passed behind the aortic arch so that the finger tip appears beneath the mediastinal pleura above the arch. At the level of the upper edge of the aortic arch, the thoracic duct runs from the posterior mediastinum to behind the subclavian artery on the left of the esophagus posteriorly. Therefore, a longitudinal incision of the pleura over the upper mediastinum is made along the front edge of the thoracic spine, in order to prevent damage to the thoracic duct. After the pleura is opened, a tape is passed around the esophagus above the aortic arch. This facilitates mobilization of the upper esophagus into the root of the neck, the level of which is identified by palpation of the inner border of the first rib. If tumor adheres to the arch of the aorta, and blind dissection is not possible,

division of the uppermost intercostal aortic arterial branches may be necessary to help in the mobilization of the arch itself, but care must be taken not to divide more than three branches to prevent the possibility of spinal cord ischemia. The left recurrent laryngeal nerve is carefully preserved to avoid being injured. Because the nerve passes by the side of the aortic arch, loops below it, and ascends behind the aortic arch to the left tracheo-esophageal groove, mobilization of the upper thoracic esophagus should be close to its adventitia. The thoracic duct is usually protected beyond the descending aorta, using the left transthoracic approach, but chylothorax can ensue if the dissection is carried out widely and towards the right pleura. It is always wise to check for possible damage to the duct. If the thoracic duct is injured, it is ligated below the point of injury. In the author's unit, the thoracic duct is routinely ligated at a lower site, usually the level of the ninth or tenth thoracic vertebrae. The azygos arch can also be injured from the left side, and this must be carefully avoided. The left main bronchus is examined to make sure there is no injury to its membranous portion.

Incision of the diaphragm

3 Based on the anatomy, incision of the diaphragm should preserve the branches of the phrenic nerve in the diaphragm. For the transthoracic approach, a radial diaphragmatic incision between the spleen and the liver is commonly used in our unit. The incision is extended from the esophageal hiatus through the aponeurotic portion to the muscular portion of the diaphragm. If the diaphragm is involved by tumor, the affected portion is resected with the tumor. In general, the length of the diaphragm incision is approximately 10 cm, but it can be extended to 15 cm for obese patients, or for large tumors in the gastric cardia. Traction sutures are placed through the cut edges of the diaphragm to aid exposure. The blood vessels in the cut edges are sutured and ligated. For a combined thoraco-abdominal approach, the diaphragm is divided peripherally from its origin on the ribs, around to the hiatus, leaving the phrenic nerve undamaged.

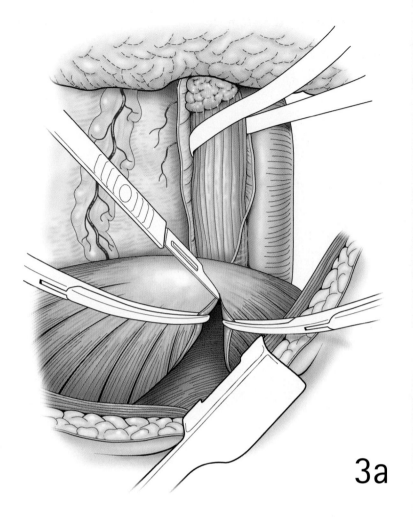

3a

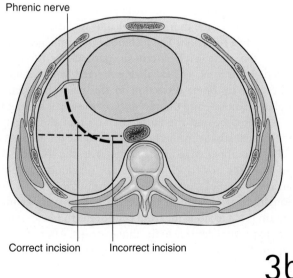

Phrenic nerve

Correct incision   Incorrect incision

3b

Mobilization of the stomach

4 For gastric mobilization, the essential principles are the preservation of a blood supply by preserving the right gastric and right gastro-epiploic vessels and arcades and obtaining maximal length by using the greater curvature for the positioning of the anastomosis.

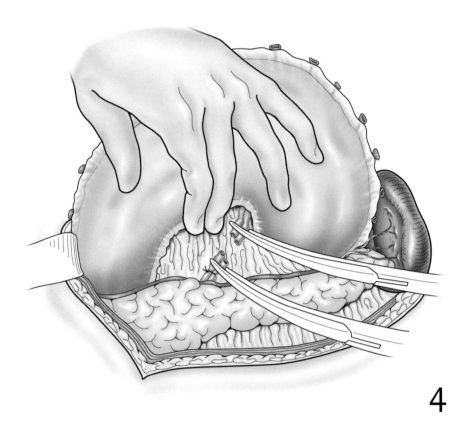

4

Before mobilization of the stomach, the abdominal cavity is thoroughly inspected. The liver, pancreas and lymph nodes of the upper abdominal region are inspected and palpated to determine if potential metastases have occurred to these organs and tissues.

The initial step in detachment of the stomach is division of the phrenoesophageal ligament. Next the greater omentum is divided outside the arch of the gastroepiploic vessels. Care is taken to preserve the gastroepiploic arcade when separating the greater omentum and the spleen from the stomach. The dissection of the greater omentum is carried out to the level of the pylorus, and the rather small omental branches from the epiploic vessels are clamped and divided.

The dissection is then directed toward the spleen, where the left gastroepiploic artery is ligated above its uppermost branch to the stomach wall. The short gastric arteries are divided carefully between hemostatic forceps and are ligated securely. The proximal branches of these vessels may be very short and require the application of suture ligatures. Ligatures on the stomach side must be tied securely because these ties can slip off the stomach if distension of the stomach in the thorax occurs.

Elevation of the stomach to the right by the assistant permits exposure of the left gastric artery and facilitates celiac lymph node dissection from behind the stomach. Much attention should be directed toward exposure of the origin of the left gastric artery at the trifurcation of the celiac axis. It is necessary to divide the filmy, avascular adhesions between the back of the stomach and the retroperitoneum. The left gastric artery is exposed by the surgeon whose thumb and forefinger encircle the lesser curvature attachments. The fat tissue and lymph nodes around the left gastric artery are dissected carefully, starting from the upper edge of the pancreas. Then two hemostatic clamps are applied to the proximal side of the vessel and one to the distal side. The left gastric artery is divided between the second and third clamps. The left gastric artery is doubly ligated at its origin from the celiac axis with a heavy nonabsorbable silk suture. The first ligature is placed and firmly tied proximal to the first clamp, and the clamp is removed. The second tie is then placed on the left gastric artery distal to the first tie. The artery on the gastric side is best managed with a secure suture ligature.

5 Lymph nodes and fat tissue along the left gastric artery and around the gastric cardia are dissected to remain with the resected specimen. For cardia cancer, the transection of the proximal stomach is performed with a linear stapler, and the esophagus is mobilized up to the level of the inferior pulmonary vein. The incision of the stomach is then strengthened with interrupted 4-0 silk sutures placed in the seromuscular layer. For cancer of the esophagus, the stomach itself is transected at, or just below, the esophagogastric junction. The stapler is usually used to close the incision of the stomach, and reinforced with interrupted 4-0 silk sutures in the seromuscular layer. The stump of the esophagus is covered with a sterilized condom to prevent contamination.

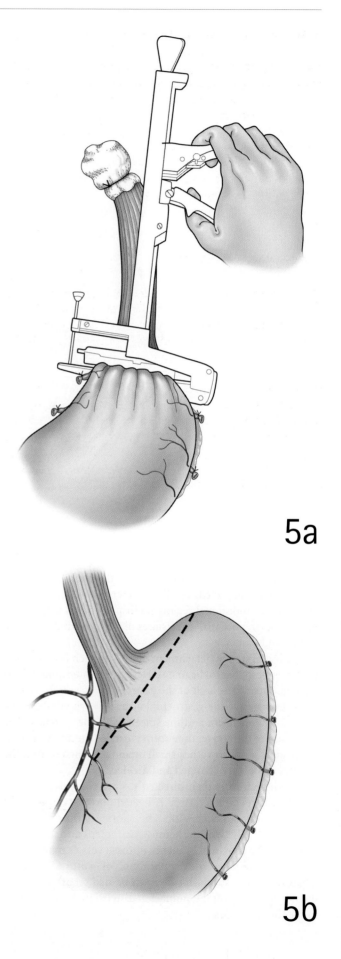

5a

5b

After completion of the detachment of the stomach and its transection, further mobilization of the postesophageal region up to the level of the carina is carried out. Upward lift of the esophagus by an assistant helps resection of subcarinal lymph nodes and freeing of the esophagus from the arch of the azygos vein. Then the total esophagus is pulled to the supra-aortic arch region. The next step is anastomosis in the thorax. However, if an anastomosis in the neck is necessary, the stump of the esophagus is connected to the uppermost region of the stomach with four interrupted stitches, in order to aid pulling the stomach into the neck.

The anastomosis

Although a variety of anastomotic methods have been reported, these can be classified as hand-sewn anastomoses and stapled anastomoses (see Chapters 33 and 34). This chapter describes the anastomotic methods most commonly used in China.

HAND-SEWN ANASTOMOSIS

6 After completion of the mediastinal dissection and gastric mobilization, the stomach can be brought to any level within the thorax by gentle traction on the upper end of the greater curvature. This is where the maximal length of the viscus can be obtained. Traction on the esophageal specimen upward as a sort of handle permits an end (esophagus)-to-side (stomach) esophagogastric anastomosis.

The first row of 4-0 silk sutures is placed in a horizontal mattress fashion between the muscular layer of the esophagus and the seromuscular layer of the uppermost stomach wall. Approximately three or four stitches are placed first. These form the outer posterior row. At 2.5 cm from the first row of sutures, an incision of the gastric wall to fit the diameter of

the esophagus is made, and the intramural plexus of vessels is suture-ligated. Then the sutures forming the first row are tied carefully by the surgeon, who always draws the stomach upward to the esophagus by positioning the tying forefinger above the point of the actual approximation of tissue. The esophagus is a fixed structure that cannot be brought down distally; its serosa-less muscular coat is more fragile and does not hold sutures as well as the stomach. The outer posterior row of sutures covers about a half of the circumference, and the corner ties are left long and marked with hemostats. After completion of the first row of sutures, a soft clamp is applied proximal to the first row of sutures to stop bleeding from the upper stump of the esophagus.

The esophagus is transected 3 cm distal to the first row of sutures and the specimen is removed. Then posterior inner

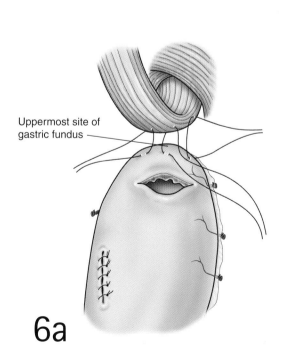

Uppermost site of gastric fundus

6a

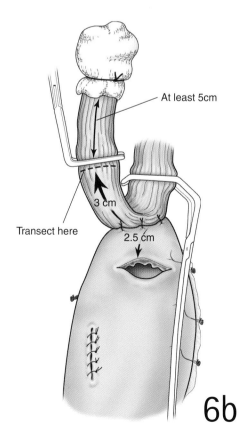

At least 5 cm

3 cm

Transect here

2.5 cm

6b

sutures, also 4-0 silk, are placed and tied with care not to cut the tissue with the suture. Each stitch is placed about 1 cm from the cut margin, and 0.3 cm apart from each other. The needle is pulled through each edge separately, to make sure whole layers of the esophagus and stomach are sutured. The gastric and esophageal mucosa are picked up with a similar bite of tissue. When the suture is tied, it is necessary to press the muscular layer with the tip of a clamp, held by an assistant, to approximate the mucosa of the esophagus and stomach.

The anterior inner row is continued in an interrupted fash-ion; the stitches are placed and tied as the posterior inner row. Whole layers of the esophagus and stomach are sutured. The assistant holds the previous sutures up to facilitate the surgeon placing subsequent stitches. As each suture is tied, the assistant inverts muscular and mucosal layers into the lumen when necessary. This method allows complete inversion of the mucosal layer. This row of sutures is tied from either end toward the middle so that a final suture can be placed anteriorly, which is an easy way to complete the anterior row. After all stitches are tied, sutures are then cut.

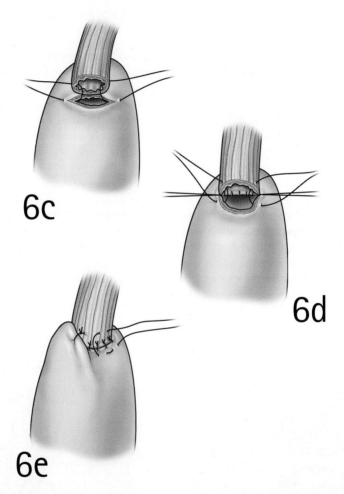

6c

6d

6e

A nasogastric tube is directed downward through the anastomosis to the level of the gastric antrum and is fixed by the anesthetist to the patient's nose to prevent later inadvertent withdrawal.

The anterior outer row is placed in a horizontal mattress fashion over the remaining half of the circumference of the esophagus. Because the anastomosis has been placed 2.5 cm down from the apex of the stomach, this row should bring the anterior wall of the stomach up to the same level as the posterior wall. Three to four horizontal mattress stitches are put between the muscular layer of the esophagus and the seromuscular layer of the stomach which brings it upward circumferentially. This constructs a valve-like luminal orifice which helps to minimize the possibility of gastroesophageal reflux.

The anterior aspect of the anastomosis may further be buttressed by a flap of omentum, which remains at the upper end of the gastroepiploic arcade. The stomach is suspended by a series of nonabsorbable sutures to the fascia that overlies the thoracic spine. This helps to avoid downward traction on the anastomosis.

ANASTOMOSIS WITH A CIRCULAR STAPLER

In order to simplify the anastomotic process, an anastomotic stapler was invented in the former Soviet Union in the 1950s. Since then, the apparatus has been greatly improved. The currently available circular anastomotic stapler has become safe and easy to operate.

7 If an anastomosis using a stapler is planned, the incision in the stomach is left open after transection at the esophagogastric junction for the later placement of a stapler. A purse-string applicator is put on the anticipated site of the anastomosis in the esophagus. After a purse-string suture is applied, the esophagus is transected distal to the clamp. Three Allis forceps are used to grasp the stump of the esophagus at 120 degrees apart after removal of the purse-string applicator, and the anvil is put into the lumen of the esophagus before the purse-string suture is tied. The head of the circular stapler is then put into the cavity of the stomach through the gastric cardia and applied against the gastric wall at the fundus. The turn button at the distal end of the stapler is rotated anticlockwise to allow the tip of the central pole to puncture the gastric wall and connect into the central pole of the anvil. Then the turn button is rotated clockwise to approximate the stomach wall to the esophageal stump to the extent as indicated in the scale plate of the stapler. Examination of the closed stapler is carried out to make sure surrounding structures and tissues (including pleura, the subclavian artery, and foreign bodies such as gauze) have not been caught. Fire the stapler and turn the turn button anticlockwise. The stapler, with anvil, is pulled out through the cardia. Check that two complete circular "doughnuts" from the esophageal and gastric ends are present. If there is any doubt of the integrity of the doughnuts, the anastomosis is reinforced with interrupted nonabsorbable sutures. The incision in the stomach is closed with a linear stapler and strengthened by oversewing the seromuscular layer with interrupted 4-0 silk sutures. A nasogastric tube is placed into the intrathoracic stomach to decrease postoperative gastric distension.

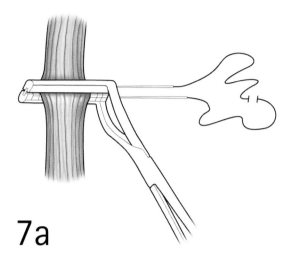

7a

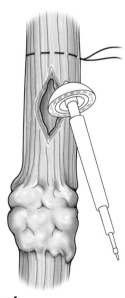

7b

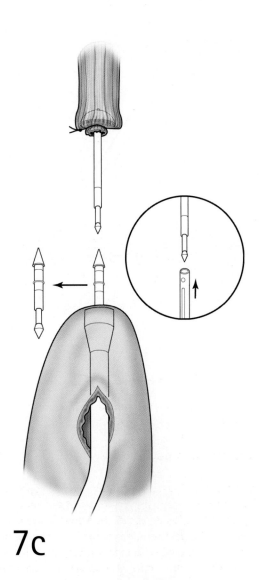

7c

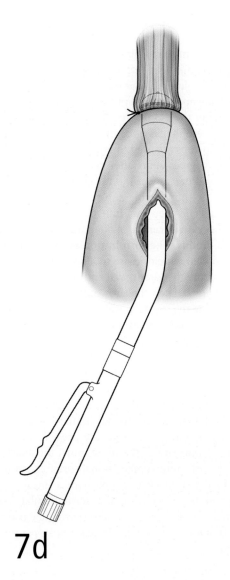

7d

Folding suture of the stomach

8 After completion of the anastomosis, the lesser curvature of the stomach is oversewn. This minimizes the size of the intrathoracic stomach and prevents compression of the stomach on the intrathoracic organs, especially the lung and heart. Interrupted 4-0 silk sutures are put on the anterior and posterior walls which are adjacent to the lesser curvature, at 2 cm apart from each other. After each suture is tied, the stomach is folded in along the lesser curvature.

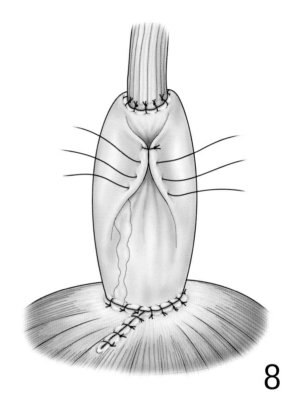

8

Closure of the diaphragm incision and the chest

The incision of the diaphragm is closed with 7-0 interrupted silk sutures and is also sutured to the wall of the stomach with 4-0 thread to prevent prolapse of intra-abdominal contents into the thorax. The space between the edge of the diaphragm incision and the stomach should be snug enough to prevent an index finger passing after completion of the closure of the diaphragm. The pulse in the right gastroepiploic artery is checked. A No. 28 Argyle chest catheter is placed through the eighth intercostal space in the axillary line, for drainage. The chest wall is closed with interrupted heavy nonabsorbable silk sutures and careful approximation of the muscles of the chest wall is undertaken to avoid interference with postoperative shoulder function. Fine interrupted silk sutures are used to suture the skin.

Left cervical approach

The left thoracic or thoracoabdominal cervical approach is an additional procedure for the treatment of carcinoma of the esophagus. The major difference between this method and the classic left thoracic approach is the level of anastomosis. For the cancers located in the upper thoracic esophagus, there is not enough length of normal esophagus to construct an anastomosis in the thoracic cavity according to oncological principles. The left cervical approach is therefore carried out in most of these patients.

LEFT NECK INCISION

9 When the thoracoabdominal incision has been closed the patient is placed in the supine position with a pad under the left shoulder. An oblique incision no more than 8 cm in length is made along the anterior border of the left sternocleidomastoid muscle.

The omohyoid muscle is divided together with the middle thyroid vein and the inferior thyroid artery if these are in the way of the exposure. The carotid artery and jugular vessels are retracted laterally, and the trachea is retracted medially to expose the already mobilized esophagus. The esophagus and fundus of the stomach are delivered through the wound, the stomach being held with a pair of Duval forceps to prevent it slipping back into the chest.

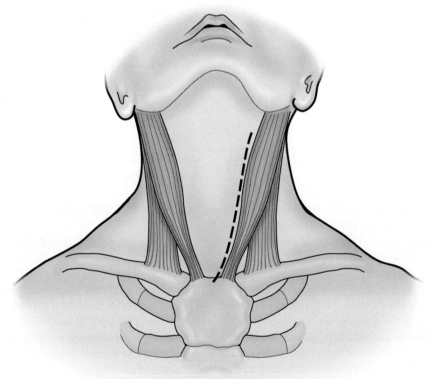

9a

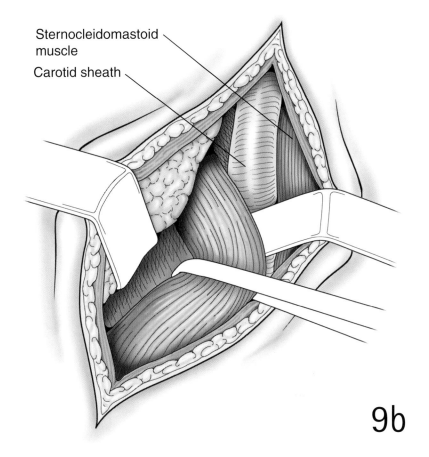

Sternocleidomastoid muscle

Carotid sheath

9b

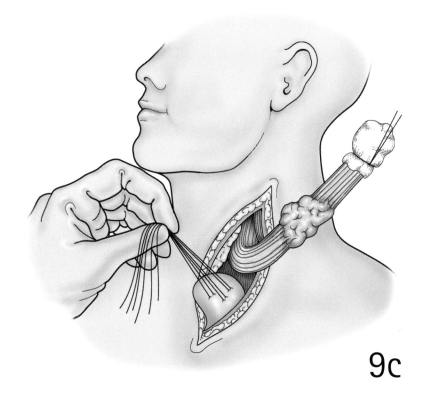

9c

ANASTOMOSIS IN THE NECK

10 A small incision is made in the fundus of the stomach and the esophagus is transected at an adequate level. An end-to-side anastomosis is performed between the two organs, using two layers of interrupted 4-0 silk suture as described above. The fundus of the stomach is then returned to the chest so that the completed anastomosis lies comfortably in the lower part of the incision. The stomach is anchored to surrounding tissue with three stitches at the lowest level of the incision to lessen tension on the anastomosis and to prevent gastric content entering the thorax if leakage should occur. A soft drainage tube is put around the anastomosis before the neck is closed in layers with silk sutures.

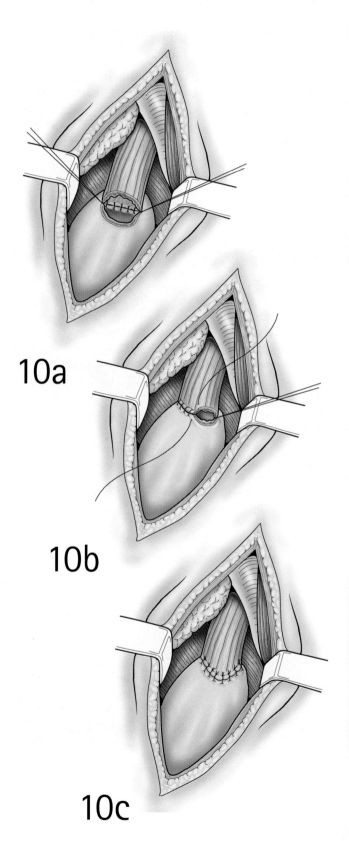

10a

10b

10c

POSTOPERATIVE CARE AND OUTCOME

A nasogastric tube is placed and kept until the fourth or fifth postoperative day when gastrointestinal function usually recovers. Artificial ventilation is not used routinely unless respiratory failure occurs. Intravenous fluids are limited to 3 litres every 24 hours. The chest drain is removed on the third day. Oral fluids are commenced on the fifth or sixth day with 100 ml water every second hour, followed by 200 ml on the eighth day when the intravenous infusion is discontinued. Feeding then progresses gradually to semisolid and solid diets, and a routine barium swallow is obtained before discharge, which is usually on the tenth postoperative day.

Complications related to the reconstruction are uncommon, but include leaks and occasionally complete disruption. Anastomotic leakage is easily demonstrated by swallowing methylene blue which can be seen to drain from the drainage tube. Fasting is not considered necessary for patients with cervical leaks. The area of leakage is dressed, applying mild local pressure to prevent the further leakage of swallowed food and gastric juice. By contrast, intrathoracic leakage usually leads to severe infection, fluid imbalance, and malnutrition. Treatment usually involves adequate control of infection, thorough drainage of the thoracic cavity, maintenance of nutrition, and correction of fluid imbalance. Although parenteral nutrition has been used increasingly in recent years, the preferred current method is feeding jejunostomy.

Another complication related to the operation is chylothorax. The management of chylothorax is still a challenge although it is an uncommon complication. Chylous output of less than 1000 ml/day is managed conservatively by drainage of the thorax and maintenance of nutrition. When daily output of chyle is more than 1000 ml, with no decrease after 4–5 days' observation, reoperation is performed with ligation of the thoracic duct. Supradiaphragmatic ligation of the main thoracic duct is undertaken routinely in Fourth Hospital, Hebei Medical University, as part of esophagectomy for cancer to prevent postoperative chylothorax.

Other common complications occurring before discharge are pulmonary infections, cardiovascular complications, and emphysema. These complications are easily diagnosed and the patients are likely to recover with appropriate treatment.

Late complications are uncommon, but include anastomotic stricture or recurrence, which are treated by dilatation, intubation, or radiotherapy as appropriate.

Using the approach described here, we have undertaken 20 000 esophagectomies in the past 53 years, in which the postoperative mortality rate was 2.0 per cent. In the past 5 years we have undertaken 4337 esophagectomies and the postoperative mortality rate was 0.76 per cent.

FURTHER READING

Adams WE, Phemister DB. Carcinoma of the lower thoracic esophagus: report of a successful resection and esophagogastrostomy. *Journal of Thoracic and Cardiovascular Surgery* 1938; **7**: 621.

Davis EA, Heitmiller RF. Esophagectomy for benign disease: trends in surgical results and management. *Annals of Thoracic Surgery* 1996; **62**: 369–72.

Krasna MJ. Left transthoracic esophagectomy. *Chest Surgery Clinics of North America* 1995; **5**: 543–54.

Liu JF, Wang QZ, Hou J. Surgical treatment for cancer of the esophagus and gastric cardia in Hebei, China. *British Journal of Surgery* 2004; **91**: 90–8.

38

Transhiatal esophagectomy

MARK B. ORRINGER MD, FACS
Professor and Head, Section of Thoracic Surgery, University of Michigan Medical Center, Ann Arbor, Michigan, USA

HISTORY

The feasibility of removing the esophagus from the posterior mediastinum using an instrument similar to a vein stripper was suggested by the German anatomist Denk in 1913. In 1936, the British surgeon Grey-Turner resected the esophagus for carcinoma through abdominal and cervical incisions. Later, restoration of swallowing was achieved with an antethoracic skin tube. This, and subsequent early reports of transhiatal (or blunt) esophagectomy in which the esophagus was resected through abdominal and cervical incisions without the need for a thoracotomy, occurred before the development of endotracheal anesthesia permitted safe transthoracic operations. As endotracheal anesthesia became widely available, however, the technique was all but abandoned. It was still used at times to resect a *normal* thoracic esophagus concomitantly with laryngopharyngectomy for pharyngeal or cervical esophageal carcinoma, with the stomach being used to restore continuity of the alimentary tract. In the 1970s, several authors reported the use of transhiatal esophageal resection for diseases of the intrathoracic esophagus. Orringer and associates repopularized the technique in 1978, and during the ensuing two and a half decades, numerous reports have established that transhiatal esophagectomy is a safe alternative to traditional transthoracic esophageal resection. Based upon a personal experience with more than 2000 transhiatal esophagectomies, the author believes that it is unnecessary to open the thorax in the majority of patients requiring esophageal resection for either benign or malignant disease.

PRINCIPLES AND JUSTIFICATION

The leading causes of morbidity and mortality after standard transthoracic esophagectomy and esophageal reconstruction are pulmonary complications and mediastinitis. Pulmonary complications, typically atelectasis and pneumonia, result from a combined thoracoabdominal operation in a debilitated patient whose nutritional and pulmonary status has been compromised by impaired swallowing.

Mediastinitis follows disruption of an intrathoracic esophageal anastomosis and is associated with an average mortality of 50%. The technique of transhiatal esophagectomy reduces the physiological insult to the patient by avoiding the need for a thoracotomy, and a cervical esophagogastric anastomotic leak is most often managed by simple drainage and establishment of a salivary fistula.

Worldwide experience with thousands of patients undergoing this procedure has demonstrated that with appropriate mobilization, the stomach will reach to the neck in virtually every patient. The advantages of performing a total thoracic esophagectomy and cervical esophagogastric anastomosis in patients requiring esophageal resection are as follows:

1 In patients with cancer, regardless of the level of the esophageal tumor, the maximum vertical surgical margin possible is obtained, thereby minimizing the incidence of suture line tumor recurrence.
2 Postoperative death from mediastinitis and sepsis resulting from anastomotic disruption is virtually eliminated.
3 Clinically significant gastroesophageal reflux is uncommon, in contrast to its frequent occurrence when an intrathoracic esophagogastric anastomosis is performed.

Virtually every patient requiring an esophagectomy for either benign or malignant disease is regarded as a potential candidate for transhiatal esophagectomy. In patients with an upper- or middle-third esophageal carcinoma, bronchoscopy is performed routinely as part of the preoperative assessment. Endoscopic evidence of tracheobronchial invasion by the esophageal tumor is an absolute contraindication to transhiatal esophagectomy. Because of the dismal prognosis of patients with esophageal carcinoma and distant metastases (stage IV) disease, esophagectomy is not undertaken in patients with metastases to the liver, supraclavicular lymph nodes, or other distant sites as proven by biopsy. Computed tomography (CT) is extremely important in evaluating the local extent of the tumor and detecting pulmonary, hepatic, or other distant intra-abdominal nodal metastases, but a tissue confirmation with fine-needle aspiration is generally required before esophageal resection is denied. Although CT scanning may show contiguity of the esophageal tumor and the adjacent aorta, prevertebral fascia, or tracheobronchial tree, it is not a reliable indicator of resectability, as actual invasion of these contiguous structures may not be present. The positron emission tomography (PET) scan has become an important and integral tool in the preoperative staging of esophageal cancer, detecting occult distant metastatic disease which may preclude resection. Esophageal endoscopic ultrasonography (EUS) is now also used routinely to define the depth of tumor invasion and the presence of mediastinal, paraesophageal, and celiac axis nodal metastases.

Transhiatal esophagectomy is feasible even in patients with periesophageal fibrosis from previous esophageal operations, corrosive injuries, or radiation therapy. If, however, significant periesophageal adhesions are discovered on palpation of the esophagus through the diaphragmatic hiatus, the surgeon should be prepared to convert to a transthoracic approach. This is especially so in patients who have undergone previous esophagomyotomy for either achalasia or esophageal spasm in whom adherence between the esophageal submucosa and adjacent aorta may predispose to disastrous intraoperative bleeding during attempted blunt dissection of the esophagus. In every patient undergoing transhiatal esophagectomy, the single most important contraindication to proceeding is the surgeon's assessment that there is excessive fixation of the esophagus to adjacent tissues such as the membranous trachea or the aorta.

Transhiatal esophagectomy has been criticized for ignoring two basic principles of surgery – adequate exposure and hemostasis. As the surgeon gains experience with this technique, however, and particularly when aided by narrow deep retractors within the diaphragmatic hiatus, more and more of the dissection is performed under direct vision (clamping, dividing, and ligating the periesophageal attachments) and less as a blunt or blind procedure. Intraoperative blood loss now averages less than 300 ml, and the need for a blood transfusion is uncommon. An additional controversy surrounds the appropriateness of transhiatal esophagectomy as a "cancer operation," because the procedure precludes a complete mediastinal lymph node dissection as well as accurate staging. From a practical standpoint, however, removal of abdominal lymph nodes and low paraesophageal lymph nodes is readily achieved under direct vision through the retracted esophageal hiatus, and subcarinal lymph nodes are generally accessible for staging as well. Because the overall survival of patients after transhiatal esophagectomy for carci-

noma is similar to that reported after standard transthoracic resections, one has difficulty arguing that the method of esophageal resection determines survival in patients with carcinoma. The additional advantage to the abdominal approach is that it not only provides adequate exposure for the esophagectomy but also permits exposure of all portions of the gastrointestinal tract used for esophageal substitution; if, for any reason, the stomach is found unsuitable, any portion of the colon can be mobilized readily.

PREOPERATIVE ASSESSMENT AND PREPARATION

The initial history taking and physical examination of patients with esophageal carcinoma is extremely important. The presence of supraclavicular lymphadenopathy merits fine-needle aspiration biopsy, which if positive for metastatic cancer precludes esophagectomy. Stigmata of advanced liver disease, particularly cirrhosis, are indicative of markedly increased operative risk that generally precludes esophagectomy. Liver nodularity on physical examination warrants assessment to rule out metastatic disease. The chest radiograph provides important clues as to the degree of associated chronic lung disease or pulmonary metastases. A barium swallow examination is extremely important in assessing the length of the tumor, its proximity to the aorta and carina, and distortion of the axis of the esophagus by the tumor, which suggests local extraesophageal spread. Staging chest and abdominal CT scans, PET scan, and EUS are now a standard part of the preoperative assessment, as only patients with localized tumors or those extending no further than regional lymph nodes are considered as candidates for esophagectomy. As indicated previously, preoperative bronchoscopy to rule out the presence of tracheobronchial invasion is required for cancers of the upper and middle third of the esophagus.

Few, if any, of our patients are admitted to the hospital before the day of planned esophagectomy, and most preoperative preparation is carried out on an outpatient basis. Strict abstinence from cigarette smoking for a minimum of 3 weeks before planned esophagectomy is an absolute requirement in this unit. Vigorous pulmonary physiotherapy, including deep breathing exercises and regular use of an incentive inspirometer, is administered for at least 2 weeks. Patients are instructed to walk 2–3 miles a day when possible. In patients with marked weight loss and dehydration secondary to the esophageal obstruction, a nasogastric feeding tube is inserted, if necessary using fluoroscopic control or dilatation of the malignant obstruction at esophagoscopy. Sufficient tube feedings are then administered at home by the patients and their families to provide between 2000 and 3000 calories per day. In the past, because of the invariable intravascular blood volume depletion in patients with high-grade esophageal obstruction, 1 U of blood was transfused before operation for every 4.5 kg of weight lost. However, in this current era of acquired immunodeficiency syndrome and concern about blood transfusions, rehydration is given primarily through the nasogastric feeding tube, and hetastarch preparations are used as needed for intravascular volume expansion during surgery, so that the need for blood transfusion is generally avoided. Preoperative dental consultation should be undertaken to repair or remove carious teeth, as poor oral hygiene can be a factor in the severity of infection associated with a cervical anastomotic leak. Finally, in patients with gastric scarring and shortening resulting from previous ulceration or ingestion of caustic substances and those with a history of previous antireflux procedures in whom the mobilized stomach may not be suitable as an esophageal substitute, a barium enema should be obtained to assess the suitability of the colon as an esophageal substitute, and the colon should be prepared in the event that a colonic interposition is needed.

Anesthesia

Two large-bore peripheral intravenous catheters are used routinely to permit rapid volume replacement in the event of unexpected intraoperative bleeding. Monitoring of central venous pressure is seldom necessary, but if this is required the right neck should be used and the operative field on the left neck avoided. A radial artery catheter is inserted to detect hypotension, which may occur when the surgeon's hand is inserted into the posterior mediastinum during the transhiatal dissection. This arterial catheter should be sutured into place and protected by padding. The patient's arms are then padded and placed at the sides to provide the surgeon access to the neck, chest, and abdomen. Use of epidural anesthesia for postoperative pain management has become routine and facilitates early extubation and ambulation after the operation.

Endotracheal intubation with a standard unshortened endotracheal tube is used so that in the event of a posterior membranous tracheal tear during the transhiatal dissection, the tube can be guided down the left mainstem bronchus to allow one-lung anesthesia and repair of the injury. Close cooperation between the anesthetist and the surgeon is mandatory to avoid prolonged hypotension during the esophagectomy. As the transhiatal dissection is commenced, administration of the inhalation anesthetic agents is usually discontinued and inspired oxygen concentration increased to minimize the effects of transient hypotension, which is not uncommon. Use of long-acting muscle relaxants during the procedure is kept at a minimum, as patients are typically extubated in the operating room after the esophagectomy, and admission to the intensive care unit is avoided. The bladder is catheterized, and urinary output is monitored during the operation.

OPERATION

The patient is positioned supine with the head turned toward the right and the occiput stabilized on a soft ring. The neck is extended by placing a small folded sheet beneath the scapulae. The operative field extends from the mandibles to the pubis and anterior to both midaxillary lines. The arms are padded and placed at the patient's sides. Two suction lines, one at the patient's head and one at the lower end of the operative field, are routine. If there is unusual concern that a transthoracic exposure may be required for the esophagectomy (e.g. the patient has an upper- or middle-third esophageal tumor or a history of previous esophagomyotomy), the right side may be elevated on a folded blanket, the right arm bent with the hand placed in the small of the back, and the operating table rolled toward the right side to flatten it and provide exposure for a standard upper midline abdominal incision. If necessary, a right anterolateral thoracotomy can be performed, the lung deflated, and more direct access to the esophagus obtained. The author, however, generally uses a standard endotracheal tube with the patient in the supine position as described earlier, preferring to reposition the patient for a posterolateral thoracotomy in the event that a transthoracic approach is required. A posterolateral thorocotomy provides the best exposure of the esophagus in the posterior mediastinum in the rare situation in which a transhiatal mobilization is not possible. A self-retaining table-mounted upper abdominal retractor is used to facilitate exposure of the upper abdomen and hiatus. Transhiatal esophagectomy and cervical esophagogastric anastomosis are performed in four separate phases – the abdominal, the cervical, the mediastinal, and the anastomotic.

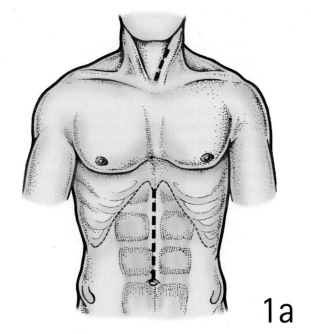

1a,b The abdominal portion of the operation is performed through a midline supraumbilical incision.

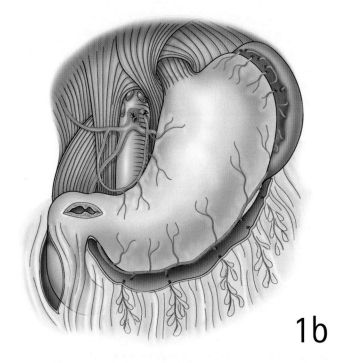

Abdominal phase

After exploring the abdomen to exclude metastases that would preclude resection, the triangular ligament is divided with electrocautery, and the liver is padded and retracted to the right to allow exposure of the diaphragmatic hiatus. The stomach is assessed for its suitability as an esophageal replacement. Extensive gastric scarring and shortening from previous ulcer disease or the sequelae of ingestion of a caustic substance, or involvement by tumor may preclude use of the

entire stomach for esophageal replacement, and in such cases the colon, which has been prepared before surgery, is mobilized. As a general rule, the esophagectomy is not carried out until a viable conduit for replacement has been mobilized.

Gastric mobilization is begun by gently retracting the greater omentum downward and away from the stomach to facilitate identification of the gastroepiploic vessels. The course of the right gastroepiploic artery from the pyloroduodenal area to the middle of the greater curvature, where it generally terminates as it enters the stomach or divides into smaller branches that anastomose with the left gastroepiploic artery, is identified. The lesser sac is entered through an avascular area of the omentum, high along the greater curvature of the stomach. The left gastroepiploic and short gastric vessels are divided between long right angle clamps and ligated along the high greater curvature of the stomach. Injury to the spleen as well as gastric necrosis from ligation of these vessels too near the gastric wall are avoided. As the omentum is then separated from the lower half of the greater curvature of the stomach, clamps are applied as needed at least 2 cm below the right gastroepiploic artery to ensure that this vessel is not injured during gastric mobilization.

Once mobilization of the omentum from the stomach to approximately the level of the pylorus has been completed, attention is directed to the lesser curvature. The filmy gastrohepatic omentum is incised, and the left gastric vein is identified, divided, and ligated. The left gastric artery is divided and ligated at its origin from the celiac trunk, reflecting adjacent lymph nodes with the stomach. The right gastric artery is identified and protected during mobilization of the lesser curvature of the stomach.

The peritoneum overlying the gastroesophageal junction is next incised, and the gastroesophageal junction is encircled with a rubber drain. A narrow Deaver retractor placed into the hiatus anteriorly facilitates exposure of the lower esophagus, which is mobilized under direct vision along with adjacent lymph nodes. The esophagus is retracted from one side to the other in the lower mediastinum to create tension on the tissues on the opposite side and facilitate their elevation with a long right angle clamp and division with a long-tip electrocautery. In this fashion, the distal 5–10 cm of esophagus and paraesophageal soft tissue are progressively mobilized under direct vision. Then, as the drain is retracted downward by one hand, thereby tensing the esophagus, the other hand is inserted through the diaphragmatic hiatus, and further blunt, gentle mobilization of the esophagus to at least the level of the carina is carried out. Mobility of the esophagus within the posterior mediastinum is assessed through the diaphragmatic hiatus by grasping the esophagus (and its contained tumor, if present) and moving it from side to side to determine if fixation to the prevertebral fascia, aorta, or adjacent mediastinal tissues is present. If this assessment indicates that the esophagus is mobile and that a transhiatal resection will therefore be possible, the mediastinal dissection is discontinued for the time being. Throughout the esophageal mobilization, care is taken to minimize direct traction on the stomach, which may injure it.

After gastric mobilization has been completed, a generous Kocher maneuver is carried out to gain maximum upward reach of the mobilized stomach. Sufficient mobilization has been achieved when the pylorus can be grasped and moved from its usual position in the right upper quadrant of the abdomen to a point aligned with the xiphoid process in the midline. Because of the possibility of delayed gastric emptying after the vagotomy that accompanies the esophagectomy, a pyloromyotomy is next performed. The pyloromyotomy extends from 1.5 cm on the stomach through the pylorus and onto the duodenum for 0.5–1.0 cm. The author prefers to use the cutting current of a needle-tipped electrocautery and a fine-tipped vascular mosquito clamp to dissect the gastric and duodenal muscle away from the underlying submucosa when performing the pyloromyotomy. The site of the pyloromyotomy is marked with metal clips for future radiographic localization. If the gastric or duodenal lumen is entered during the pyloromyotomy, the hole is closed with several simple 5/0 polypropylene interrupted sutures, and the pyloromyotomy site is covered with adjacent omentum sutured in place with interrupted fine sutures. A 14-Fr. rubber jejunostomy feeding tube is inserted 15–20 cm distal to the ligament of Treitz and is secured in place with a Weitzel maneuver. The jejunostomy tube emerging from the abdomen is then covered with a towel but is not brought out through the abdominal wall until the transhiatal esophagectomy is completed.

Cervical phase

A 5–8 cm oblique cervical incision parallel to the anterior border of the left sternocleidomastoid muscle is performed (see Figure 1a). This incision is centered on the cricoid cartilage, the origin of the upper esophageal sphincter, and the beginning of the cervical esophagus, and extends inferiorly no further than the suprasternal notch. The platysma and omohyoid fascial layers are incised, and the sternocleidomastoid muscle and carotid sheath and its contents are gently retracted laterally using narrow thyroid retractors. The larynx and trachea are retracted medially using *only* the fingers of the first assistant or surgeon, and no metal retractor is placed against the tracheoesophageal groove so that the chance of recurrent laryngeal nerve injury is minimized. The middle thyroid vein and inferior thyroid artery are typically divided and ligated. The dissection is carried directly posterior to the prevertebral fascia, which is followed bluntly with the index finger into the superior mediastinum. With the first assistant's index finger elevating the esophagus out of the superior mediastinum by traction superiorly on the cricoid cartilage in the tracheoesophageal groove, the plane between the trachea and esophagus is developed by sharp dissection; the dissection is kept as posterior to the tracheoesophageal groove as possible to avoid injury to the recurrent laryngeal nerve. The cervical esophagus is bluntly mobilized from adjacent tissues circumferentially, with particular care taken not to injure the posterior membranous trachea, and is encircled with a rubber drain. At no time should metal come in contact with the recurrent laryngeal nerve. With upward traction on this drain, blunt mobilization of the upper esophagus from the superior mediastinum is carried out, the dissection proceeding in the midline and the fingers kept against the esophagus at all times. The upper thoracic esophagus is generally mobilized circumferentially almost to the level of the carina through this approach.

Mediastinal (transhiatal) dissection

2 Attention is now redirected to the abdomen, and transhiatal dissection of the esophagus is initiated. This dissection is carried out in an orderly, sequential fashion, with the posterior aspect of the esophagus mobilized first, then the anterior surface, and finally the lateral attachments. With the left hand retracting the esophagus downward using the rubber drain encircling the gastroesophageal junction, the right hand is inserted behind the esophagus through the diaphragmatic hiatus, which is progressively dilated one finger at a time until the entire hand and forearm can be inserted into the posterior mediastinum.

A surgeon whose glove size is larger than a size 7 may have difficulty negotiating the hiatus without incising the muscle of the hiatus anteriorly to enlarge it, but this is not routine. Transhiatal esophagectomy should be performed as a midline dissection, with the volar aspect of the fingers closely applied to the esophagus to minimize the chance of entry into the pleural cavities or of injury to the tracheobronchial tree, particularly in the region of the carina.

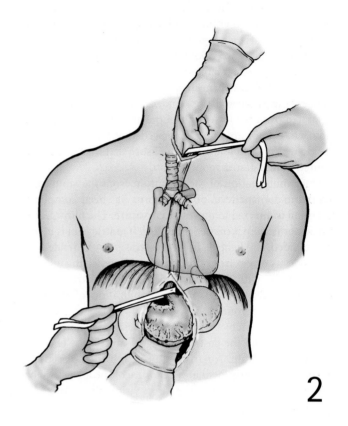

2

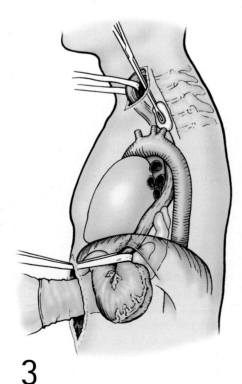

3

3 With the hand inserted through the diaphragmatic hiatus behind the esophagus, blunt dissection of the esophagus from the posterior mediastinum may be facilitated by holding a small gauze square in sponge forceps and introducing it through the cervical incision into the superior mediastinum posterior to the esophagus. This sponge stick is guided along the prevertebral fascia and into the inferior mediastinum, gently sweeping away periesophageal attachments as it is advanced. When this sponge stick can be felt by the hand inserted in the abdomen, the final filmy attachments separating the sponge from the fingertips are gently avulsed, and mobilization of the posterior esophagus from the prevertebral fascia is completed.

During this and subsequent portions of the transhiatal esophagectomy, careful continual monitoring of intra-arterial blood pressure is necessary to avoid prolonged hypotension which can result from cardiac displacement. After the sponge stick and hand are removed from the posterior mediastinum, a 28-Fr. Argyle Saratoga sump catheter is inserted through the neck wound into the posterior mediastinum, and blood is evacuated with suction.

4 The anterior esophageal dissection is next begun by retracting the rubber drain encircling the gastroesophageal junction downward with one hand and inserting the other hand palm down against the esophagus and advancing it into the mediastinum. As the fingers are advanced into the mediastinum, attachments between the esophagus and the posterior aspect of the pericardium and carina are gently avulsed.

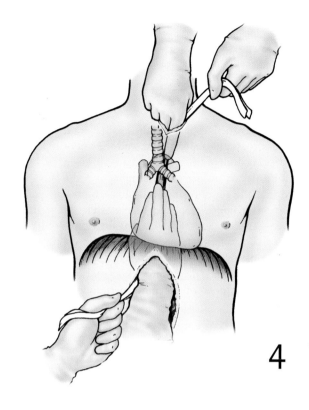

4

5 During the anterior esophageal mobilization, the hand should be kept as far posterior as possible to minimize cardiac displacement and hypotension. The characteristically filmy fibroareolar attachments posterior to the trachea are bluntly divided by simultaneous dissection through the abdominal and cervical incisions along the anterior surface of the esophagus.

With the anterior and posterior esophageal mobilization now completed, the lateral upper esophageal attachments still remain to be divided. Upward traction on the rubber drain encircling the cervical esophagus is once again delivered, and as the esophagus is elevated into the neck wound from the superior mediastinum, the lateral attachments are swept away by the index finger applied closely to the esophagus. In this fashion, 5–8 cm of upper thoracic esophagus is circumferentially mobilized. The upper esophagus is then permitted to retract back into the mediastinum.

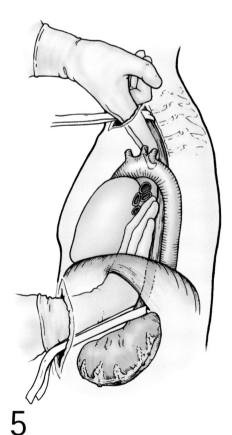

5

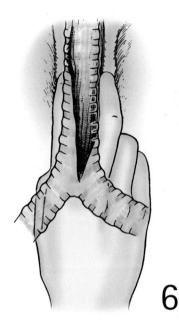

6 Traction is then applied on the rubber drain encircling the gastroesophageal junction, and the opposite hand is inserted palm downward through the diaphragmatic hiatus along the anterior surface of the esophagus and is advanced upward into the superior mediastinum behind the trachea. The portion of upper esophagus that was circumferentially mobilized can be identified with the fingertips. Once the intact lateral attachments are palpated, the esophagus is trapped against the prevertebral fascia by the index and middle fingers, and a gentle downward raking motion of the hand avulses the remainder of the filmy periesophageal attachments.

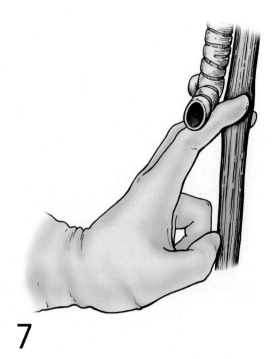

7 Sizable vagal branches may be palpated along the middle and distal esophagus at this point, and by placement of narrow deep retractors into the diaphragmatic hiatus, they can be identified, divided, and ligated using long right-angled clamps. At times, finger fracture between the index finger and thumb of subcarinal or subaortic periesophageal adhesions may be required.

8a–c In elderly patients with cervical arthritis which prevents extension of the neck, or obese patients with a "bullneck" habitus, access to the cervical and upper thoracic esophagus may be facilitated by a partial upper sternal split, which provides exposure almost to the level of the carina.

Once the entire intrathoracic esophagus is mobile, an 8- to 10-cm length is delivered into the cervical wound, where an Endo GIA surgical stapler is applied and fired obliquely in an anterior to posterior direction, leaving the anterior tip of the divided esophagus slightly longer than the posterior corner. The stomach is then drawn out of the abdominal wound with the attached esophagus.

Once the esophagus has been delivered from the posterior mediastinum, narrow deep retractors are inserted into the diaphragmatic hiatus so that the posterior mediastinum can be inspected for bleeding and the mediastinal pleura for lateral rents that indicate the need for a chest tube. Blood is again evacuated from the posterior mediastinum using the Argyle Saratoga sump catheter inserted through the cervical wound. A 28-Fr. chest tube is inserted into the appropriate pleural cavity if entry has occurred during the esophagectomy. A large abdominal pack is then placed in the low posterior mediastinum through the diaphragmatic hiatus and a narrow "thoracic" pack in the superior mediastinum through the cervical incision to tamponade any vascular oozing. Attention is then turned toward preparing the stomach for its transposition into the chest. The stomach and attached esophagus are placed on the anterior abdominal wall, and the point along the high greater curvature that will reach most cephalad to the neck is identified and held by the assistant with a moist pack. The lesser curvature of the stomach is then cleared of fat by dividing the vessels and fat between clamps at the level of the second vascular arcade from the cardia.

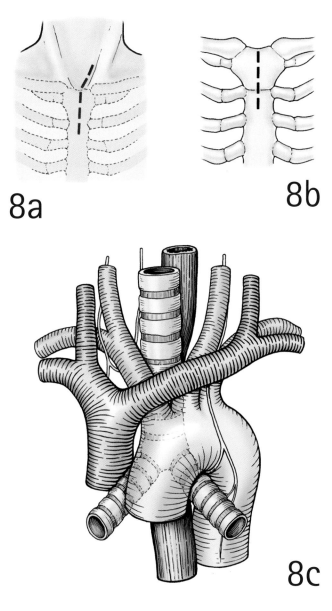

8a

8b

8c

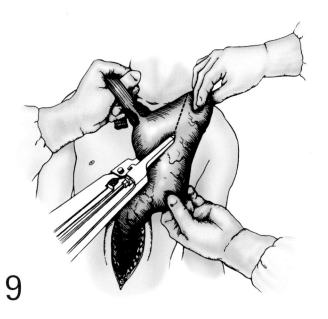

9

9 A GIA stapler with a 6-cm cartridge is then applied beginning at this point on the lesser curvature and proceeding toward the gastric tip. Each time the stapler is removed, traction is applied to the gastric fundus to allow the stomach to be straightened progressively so that its cephalad reach is maximized. The GIA stapler is applied on average three times. As wide as possible a gastric tube is created to maximize submucosal collateral circulation and vascularity of the conduit; a narrow gastric tube is avoided.

10 Once the partial proximal gastrectomy has been completed, the esophagus and attached proximal stomach are removed from the field, and the gastric staple suture line is oversewn with two running 4/0 polypropylene Lembert stitches. This same technique is used when resecting carcinomas localized to the cardia and proximal stomach. Rather than carry out a traditional proximal hemigastrectomy, which wastes valuable stomach (stippled area of Figure 10) that can be used for esophageal replacement and commits the surgeon to an intrathoracic esophageal anastomosis, the surgeon divides the stomach as described earlier 4–6 cm distal to the palpable tumor, thereby preserving the greater curvature and the point along the gastric fundus that reaches to the neck (asterisk in Figure 10).

Attention is now redirected to the diaphragmatic hiatus. The previously placed mediastinal packs are removed, and with the narrow deep retractors placed into the hiatus, a last inspection is made for any bleeding, which can be controlled under direct vision through the diaphragmatic hiatus. Again, the 28-Fr. Argyle Saratoga sump inserted through the neck wound provides a dry field as the posterior mediastinum is inspected through the hiatus. To ensure an adequate posterior mediastinal tunnel for the stomach, the surgeon inserts the entire hand and forearm through the diaphragmatic esophageal hiatus and advances them through the posterior mediastinum until three or four fingers are visible in the cervical incision. During this procedure, the blood pressure must be watched carefully.

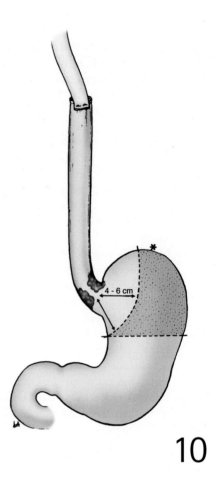

10

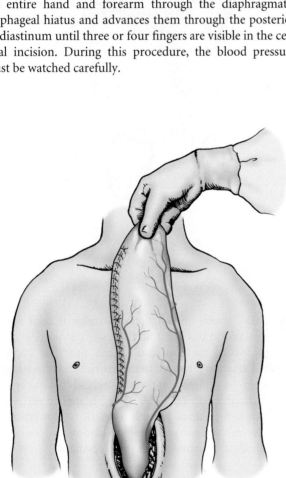

11

11 The stomach is then again delivered onto the anterior chest wall, and the point along the gastric fundus that will extend most cephalad is identified.

12 The diaphragmatic hiatus is elevated with a narrow Deaver retractor, and the stomach is gently grasped and manipulated progressively upward through the diaphragmatic hiatus into the posterior mediastinum. No drain is sutured to the stomach, and no suction device to pull the stomach through the mediastinum is used to minimize trauma to the stomach. Once the gastric fundus can be palpated with the index finger inserted through the cervical incision, a Babcock clamp is inserted downward into the superior mediastinum through the cervical incision, and the tip of the gastric fundus is manipulated into the clamp by the hand within the posterior mediastinum. The gastric tip is grasped with clamp, which is not ratcheted closed, and is drawn into the cervical wound more by pushing the stomach upward beneath the aortic arch by the hand in the posterior mediastinum than by pulling the Babcock clamp. As soon as there is sufficient stomach visible within the cervical incision, the clamp is removed from the field in order to minimize gastric trauma, and the tip of the stomach is grasped with the fingertips and guided into the neck wound. (inset) The hand in the posterior mediastinum is withdrawn.

The anterior surface of the intrathoracic stomach is greatly palpated through the diaphragmatic hiatus and the cervical incision to insure that the stomach has not been twisted during its positioning in the chest. When the stomach has been brought through the posterior mediastinum without torsion, the oversewn staple suture line should be oriented toward the patient's right side. The stomach is not sutured to the prevertebral fascia in order to avoid traumatizing an already relatively ischemic gastric tip. The position of the stomach in the cervical wound is maintained by inserting a small moistened thoracic gauze pack alongside the stomach in the thoracic inlet to prevent it from slipping back downward into the mediastinum.

To avoid contamination of the abdomen by intraoral contents, the cervical gastroesophageal anastomosis is not begun until the abdominal incision is closed completely and excluded from the field. Before the abdomen is closed, however, a final inspection for bleeding, particularly in the area of the spleen, is made. The diaphragmatic hiatus is narrowed with one to three #1 silk sutures so as to admit three fingers along the side of the stomach easily. The edge of the diaphragmatic hiatus is tacked to the adjacent anterior gastric wall with one or two 3/0 silk sutures to prevent intrathoracic herniation of bowel. The pyloromyotomy is covered by adjacent omentum, and the previously retracted left hepatic lobe is returned to its normal position. The feeding jejunostomy tube is then brought out through a left upper quadrant stab wound, and the jejunum is fixed to the anterior abdominal wall with several interrupted sutures. The abdominal incision is then closed and isolated from the field by covering it with a sterile towel and sheet. Attention is now redirected to the neck, where the cervical gastroesophageal anastomosis is performed.

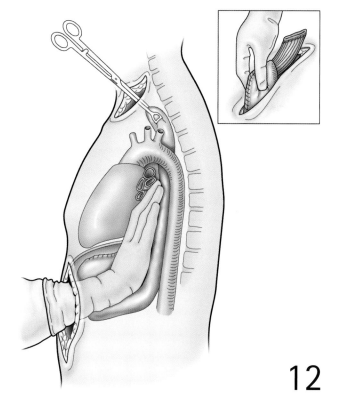

12

Cervical gastroesophageal anastomosis

13a When the stomach has been properly mobilized, 4–5 cm of the gastric tip rest in the neck above the level of the clavicles against the prevertebral fascia and well behind the divided cervical esophagus.

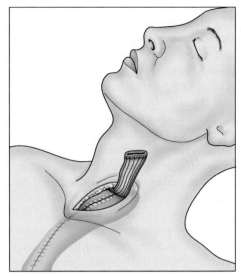

13a

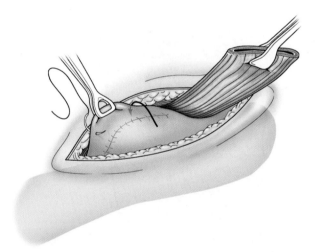

13b

13b The end of the divided esophagus is grasped and elevated to the right with an Allis clamp. The anterior surface of the stomach as near to the sternum as possible is grasped with a Babcock clamp, elevated further into the cervical wound, and rotated medially in order to displace the gastric staple suture line away from the site of the subsequent anastomosis. A 3-0 silk seromuscular gastric traction suture is placed as far inferiorly near the sternum as possible.

14 The traction suture is used to elevate the anterior surface of the stomach to the level of the skin and is secured to the drapes with a hemostat. The site of the anastomosis (dotted line) is determined by lowering the divided end of the esophagus against the gastric wall, and a 1.5- to 2-cm vertical gastrotomy is made with the cutting electrocautery current. This gastrotomy must be placed low enough on the stomach so that a 3-cm staple cartridge can be accommodated in the tip of the stomach superior to this point.

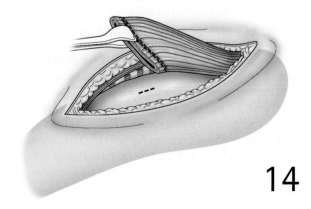

14

15 The esophageal staple suture line is retracted inferiorly with two Allis clamps, the esophagus grasped obliquely with a DeBakey forceps, and the staple line amputated sharply using the forceps as a guide against the knife. This end is submitted to pathology as the "proximal esophageal margin." It is important to remember that once the anastomosis is completed and the gastric traction suture cut, the stomach will partially retract downward toward the mediastinum. Therefore overaggressive shortening of the remaining esophagus should be avoided in order to minimize tension on the anastomosis. Alternatively, if the residual esophagus proximal to the anastomosis is too redundant, the ultimate functional outcome may not be good.

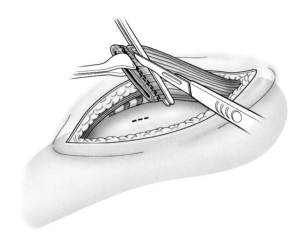

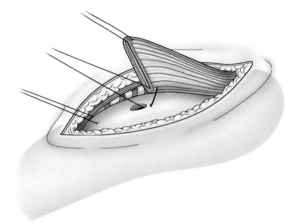

16

16 Placement of two stay sutures is extremely important in insuring alignment of the posterior esophageal wall and the anterior wall of the stomach. One suture passes through the anterior tip of the divided esophagus. The other suture passes in and out of the upper corner of the gastrotomy and then from outside in on the posterior end of the esophagus.

17a,b While applying continual downward traction on the above two sutures, the thinner blade (anvil) of an Endo GIA 30-3.5 staple cartridge (United States Surgical Corp, Norwalk, CT, USA) is inserted into the stomach, and the thicker staple-bearing portion into the esophagus. The jaws of the stapler are partially approximated as the stapler is gradually rotated so that the cartridge points toward the patient's right ear, carefully aligning the posterior esophageal and anterior gastric walls.

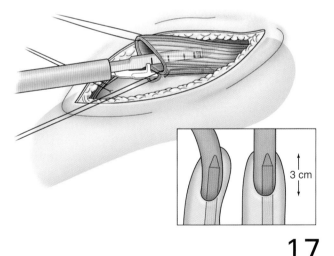

17

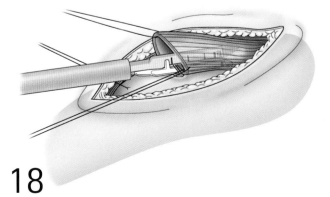

18

18 After closing the stapler, but before firing it, two "suspension" absorbable 4-0 sutures are placed on either side between the gastric wall and adjacent esophagus.

19 The knife assembly of the stapler is advanced, thereby joining the anterior wall of the stomach and the posterior wall of the esophagus and creating a 3 cm long side-to-side anastomosis. The stapler is removed from the field, and a nasogastric tube is inserted by the anesthesiologist and guided into the intrathoracic stomach by the surgeon.

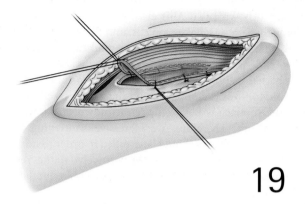

19

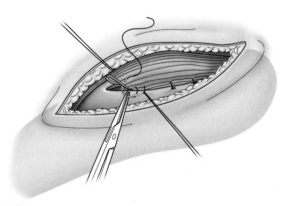

20

20 An absorbable 4-0 "corner stitch" is placed on either side of the opened stomach and esophagus. The opened esophagus and stomach are approximated in two layers of 4-0 monofilament absorbable suture, the first, a running full-thickness inverting suture.

21 The second layer consists of interrupted full thickness inverting sutures. Overaggressive inversion of this closure will not compromise the anastomosis, which is more posterior under the "hood" of the esophagus. A silver metallic hemostatic clip is placed on both of the corner sutures, which are then cut. The clips serve as markers of the anastomosis for future radiographic studies. The cervical wound is then irrigated, and a ¼-inch rubber drain placed to its depth. Muscle fascia is approximated loosely with three to five absorbable 3-0 interrupted sutures, and the skin with a running 4-0 nylon suture. After placement of dressings on the abdominal and cervical incisions and the chest tube(s) and jejunostomy tube sites, a portable chest radiograph is obtained in the operating room to document full expansion of the lungs and exclude an unrecognized hemo- or pneumothorax.

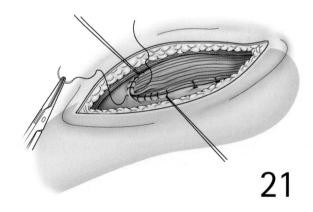

21

COMPLICATIONS

Intraoperative complications associated with transhiatal esophagectomy include entry into one or both pleural cavities during the transhiatal dissection, disruption of the tracheobronchial tree, and hemorrhage. As indicated earlier, the mediastinal pleurae are inspected after removal of the esophagus from the posterior mediastinum, and if pleural entry has occurred, a chest tube is inserted and connected to suction before the stomach is positioned in the posterior mediastinum. Tracheal tears during transhiatal esophagectomy are rare, generally small and linear, and involve the posterior membranous trachea. They are heralded by a rush of air from the ventilator felt either through the diaphragmatic hiatus or the neck wound during the transhiatal dissection. If the air leak is sizable, the endotracheal tube balloon should be deflated and the tip of the endotracheal tube guided into the left mainstem bronchus by the hand inserted through the diaphragmatic hiatus. One-lung ventilation may then be achieved in a more controlled fashion. Addition of a partial upper sternal split may provide sufficient exposure of the membranous trachea for direct repair. Before tracheal repair is begun, however, the transhiatal esophagectomy should be completed, if possible, to improve exposure of the posterior membranous trachea. Larger tears may necessitate a right thoracotomy and direct suture closure. Major intraoperative hemorrhage should not occur during transhiatal esophagectomy if proper patient selection is used, and attempts to resect an esophagus that is fixed to adjacent structures by tumor or fibrosis are abandoned. Should untoward bleeding occur during the transhiatal dissection, the 28-Fr. Argyle Saratoga sump catheter inserted through the neck incision is used to evacuate the posterior mediastinum as the anterior surface of the aorta is inspected and direct control of the bleeding is obtained. If hemostasis is not possible using this technique, the posterior mediastinum should be packed with large laparotomy pads, and several minutes should be allowed to elapse and intravascular volume replaced before the mediastinum is again inspected. If bleeding resumes, the pack should be reinserted, the abdomen quickly closed, and the patient repositioned and turned to the appropriate side for a thoracotomy – left if the intraoperative bleeding occurred during dissection of the lower third of the esophagus – and right if the bleeding occurred during dissection of the middle or upper thoracic esophagus.

Intraoperative recurrent laryngeal nerve injury should not occur if care is taken to avoid direct injury to the recurrent laryngeal nerve in the tracheoesophageal groove. No metal retractors should be placed against the trachea during the cervical portions of the operation to prevent this complication.

If the patient develops fever of 101°F or more 48 hours after transhiatal esophagectomy, this is presumptive evidence of an anastomotic leak until proven otherwise and is an indication for a contrast study of the esophagus regardless of how uninflamed the cervical wound may be. A water-soluble contrast material such as Gastrografin may result in severe chemical pneumonitis if aspirated and should be avoided. It is best to use dilute barium for this study, as this better defines the mucosal detail. If, on the other hand, the patient begins to drain swallowed liquids from the cervical wound drain site, obviously a leak has occurred, and the neck wound should be opened at the bedside in its entirety by removing the five or six sutures used to close it. Good mechanical cleansing of the open neck wound can be obtained by having the patient swallow water while at the same time aspirating with a suction catheter any liquid that issues from the cervical wound. The neck wound is packed loosely with saline-moistened sponges several times a day. Most cervical esophagogastric anastomotic leaks will close within 1 week. Closure is often facilitated by passage of 36-, 40-, and 46-Fr. tapered Maloney dilators at the bedside. This dilation ensures that no associated distal obstruction (edema or spasm) is present.

Postoperative chylothorax may occur after transhiatal esophagectomy and manifests as prolonged and excessive chest tube drainage (typically greater than 200–400 ml per 8-hour shift). If chylothorax is suspected, cream can be administered through the feeding jejunostomy tube, which will result in a change of the character of the chest tube drainage from serosanguineous to milky white fluid. An aggressive approach is adopted toward treatment of postoperative chylothorax in the patient who has undergone transhiatal esophagectomy. A transthoracic approach to the thoracic duct with direct identification and suturing of the leak facilitated by administration of cream through the jejunostomy tube is preferred to prolonged chest tube drainage and intravenous hyperalimentation.

POSTOPERATIVE CARE

Patient's are typically extubated in the operating room, as epidural anesthesia provides sufficient pain management so that postoperative mechanical ventilation is unnecessary. After several hours in the recovery room, patients are transferred to a monitored hospital bed, but admission to an intensive care unit is seldom indicated. Because of the routine preoperative emphasis on use of an incentive inspirometer to facilitate postoperative pulmonary hygiene, resumption of use of the inspirometer is begun the afternoon of the operation. Ambulation is begun on the first postoperative day. Because transhiatal esophagectomy is basically an upper abdominal procedure requiring little manipulation of the intestines or the root of the mesentery, postoperative ileus beyond 48–72 hours is unusual, and administration of 5% dextrose and water through the jejunostomy feeding tube may begin at a rate of 30 ml/hour on the second or third postoperative day. If this rate is tolerated for 12 hours, the volume is increased to 60 mL/hour, jejunostomy tube feedings are begun the next day and advanced as tolerated. The arterial catheter is removed in the recovery room the day of operation once the endotracheal tube has been removed. The intravenous catheters are removed once jejunostomy feedings are tolerated, the cervical wound drain on the third postoperative day, and the nasogastric tube on the third postoperative day when jejunostomy feedings are started. Once the patient has tolerated having no nasogastric tube for 24 hours, oral intake is progressively advanced from a liquid to a soft diet during the first postoperative week. A barium swallow examination is obtained on the seventh postoperative day. The barium swallow assesses: (1) anastomotic integrity; (2) emptying of the intrathoracic stomach; and (3) passage of contrast past the jejunostomy tube site. Oral intake should not be withheld until the barium swallow study is obtained, because the patient is swallowing saliva from the moment he or she emerges from general anesthesia, and it is unrealistic to think that nothing is going across the anastomosis because of the presence of a nasogastric tube. As oral intake is advanced, the rate of jejunostomy tube feedings may be progressively decreased, and eventually tube feedings delivered only at night so as to not interfere with the patient's appetite during the day. Complaints of postvagotomy dumping (varying degrees of cramping and diarrhea) typically respond to an appropriate antidumping diet, avoiding overdistension of the intrathoracic stomach by minimizing the amount of liquid consumed with meals, and antispasmodics such as tincture of opium or diphenoxylate hydrochloride (Lomotil).

The patient is commonly discharged from the hospital after a satisfactory postoperative barium swallow examination on the seventh postoperative day. Supplementation of oral caloric intake at night with two or three cans of tube feedings through the jejunostomy tube may be helpful early after discharge from the hospital, but this is not mandatory if the patient is eating relatively well in the hospital. When the patient returns for the initial postoperative assessment 2–4 weeks after discharge, if the feeding jejunostomy tube is not being used, it is removed.

Early mild postoperative cervical dysphagia may result from anastomotic edema, but this is far less common with the 3-cm stapled side-to-side esophagogastric anastomosis. This complaint generally requires no specific therapy and gradually subsides with time. However, any complaint of cervical dysphagia occurring 2–4 weeks after discharge is managed by passage of 36-, 40-, and 46-Fr. Maloney dilators through the anastomosis on an outpatient basis.

OUTCOME

In the past two and a half decades, Orringer and associates have performed transhiatal esophagectomy without thoracotomy in more than 2000 patients. In their 1999 report of their initial 1085 transhiatal esophagectomies, 285 (26%) had benign disease and 800 (74%) carcinoma (4.5% upper, 28% middle, and 73.5% lower third and/or cardia). Benign esophageal disease included neuromotor dysfunction (33%); strictures (26%); Barrett's mucosa with high grade dysplasia (19%); recurrent gastroesophageal reflux (7%); acute perforation (5%); acute caustic injury (5%); and others (5%). Of the patients with benign disease, 52% had undergone at least one previous esophageal operation. Transhiatal esophagectomy was possible in 98.6% of the patients in whom it was attempted, the remainder requiring conversion to a transthoracic approach. The stomach was used as the esophageal substitute in 96% of these patients, firmly establishing the principle that the properly mobilized stomach will virtually always reach to the neck for construction of a cervical esophagogastric anastomosis. In 98% of these patients, the esophageal substitute was positioned in the posterior mediastinum.

The hospital mortality rate for these 1085 patients was 4% (44 deaths), and in most cases death was unrelated to the technique of operation. There were three intraoperative deaths due to uncontrollable hemorrhage. Complications included intraoperative entry into one or both pleural cavities requiring placement of one or more chest tubes (77%), anastomotic leak (13%), clinically significant pneumonia or atelectasis (<2%), recurrent laryngeal nerve paralysis (<1%), and chylothorax and tracheal laceration (less than 1% each). Reoperation for mediastinal bleeding was required within 24 hours of operation in five patients (<1%). The average intraoperative blood loss was 689 ml (795 ml for benign disease and 652 ml for carcinoma). The Kaplan–Meier actuarial survival of our patients undergoing transhiatal esophagectomy for carcinoma was similar to that reported after more traditional transthoracic esophagectomy; the overall 2-year survival was 47% and the 5-year survival, 23%. Among the patients with benign disease, long-term follow-up has indicated good or excellent functional results after a cervical gastroesophageal anastomosis in nearly 80%. It is the author's practice to pass a Maloney esophageal dilator on an outpatient basis for any complaint of cervical dysphagia after transhiatal esophagectomy, no matter how mild. With this liberal use of dilatation, nearly 75% require an esophageal dilatation at some time, but at last follow-up 81% were swallowing well without the need for dilatations. With the side-to-side stapled cervical esophagogastric anastomosis we have used for nearly 6 years, the anastomotic leak rate has been reduced to less than 3%, and predictably, the need for postoperative anastomotic dilatations concomitantly decreased. Clinically troublesome gastroesophageal reflux is unusual after a cervical esophagogastric anastomosis and has occurred in less than 8% of these patients. Our results support our contention that a thoracic incision is seldom required to resect the esophagus for either benign or malignant disease. Transhiatal esophagectomy is safe and well tolerated if performed with care and for proper indications.

FURTHER READING

Hulscher JB, Tijssen JG, Obertop H, et al. Transthoracic versus transhiatal resection for carcinoma of the esophagus: a metaanalysis. *Annals of Thoracic Surgery* 2001; **72**: 306–13.

Orringer MB. Partial median sternotomy: anterior approach to the upper thoracic esophagus. *Journal of Thoracic and Cardiovascular Surgery* 1984; **87**: 124–9.

Orringer MB, Bluett M, Deeb GM. Aggressive treatment of chylothorax complicating transhiatal esophagectomy without thoracotomy. *Surgery* 1988; **104**: 720–6.

Orringer MB, Marshall B, Iannettoni MD. Transhiatal esophagectomy: clinical experience and refinements. *Annals of Surgery* 1999; **230**: 392–400.

Orringer MB, Marshall B, Iannettoni MD. Eliminating the cervical esophagogastric anastomotic leak with a side-to-side stapled anastomosis. *Journal of Thoracic and Cardiovascular Surgery* 2000; **119**: 277–88.

Orringer MB, Sloan H. Esophagectomy without thoracotomy. *Journal of Thoracic and Cardiovascular Surgery* 1978; **76**: 643–54.

39

Long esophageal myotomy and excision of diverticula

ANDRÉ DURANCEAU MD

Professor, Department of Surgery, Université de Montreal; Chair, Department of Surgery, Division of Thoracic Surgery, Centre Hospitalier Universitaire de Montreal, Montreal, Quebec, Canada

PRINCIPLES AND JUSTIFICATION

Pulsion diverticula of the distal esophagus are considered to be complications of abnormal intraesophageal pressures. The work of Cross and colleagues supported the concept that spasm of the inferior sphincter accompanied by increased contraction pressures in the esophageal body is responsible for both the symptoms and the appearance of the diverticulum. Allen and Claggett and Benacci *et al.* have reported significantly fewer leaks with secondary sepsis when a myotomy is combined with diverticulectomy than when a diverticulectomy alone is performed. When surgical treatment is indicated for a distal esophageal diverticulum, the diverticulum should be excised if it is large enough and the underlying motor abnormality corrected. After myotomy, a significant weakening of the gastroesophageal junction results, and an antireflux repair is added to the myotomy to prevent reflux damage to the esophageal mucosa. A partial fundoplication is preferred, as a more complete wrap causes functional obstruction to an esophagus made powerless by the myotomy.

Indications

Significant symptoms related to swallowing and to the presence of the diverticulum constitute the main indication for surgical treatment. Asymptomatic diverticula do not require operative treatment.

PREOPERATIVE ASSESSMENT AND PREPARATION

Assessment

Radiological assessment is important to identify the size and location of the diverticulum. Videoscopic radiography usually allows visualization of the accompanying motor dysfunction. Although optional, radionuclide transit studies using liquid and solid markers quantify esophageal retention.

Esophageal motility studies are essential to characterize the motor disorder accompanying the diverticulum and to determine the extent of dysfunction.

Endoscopy and 24-hour pH monitoring are important to rule out reflux disease and mucosal damage or other mucosal abnormality.

Patient preparation

The patient is put on a liquid diet for 24 hours before the operation. If there is any possibility of significant esophageal retention, lavage of the esophageal cavity is performed with the patient awake on the morning of the operation.

A cephalosporin and antibiotics active against anaerobes (such as metronidazole [Flagyl], 500 mg, or clindamycin, 600 mg) are administered before induction of anesthesia. Subcutaneous heparin sodium, 5000 U, is administered routinely 2 hours before the operation and every 12 hours thereafter until the patient is fully ambulatory and ready to leave the hospital.

OPERATION

Incision

1 The esophagus is approached through a left thoracic incision. The pleura is opened at the superior border of the eighth rib, and a small posterior segment of the rib is removed. Anesthesia via a double-lumen endotracheal tube allows exclusion and retraction of the left lung during the operation.

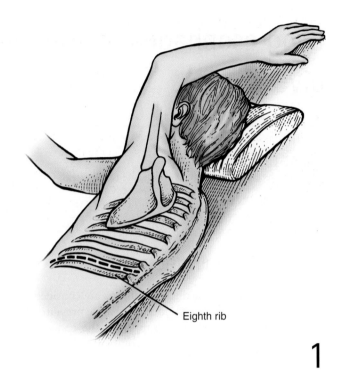

Eighth rib

1

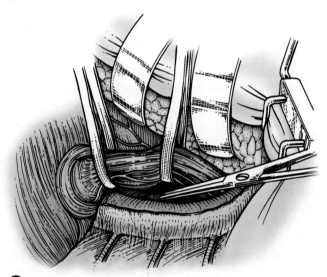

2

2 The mediastinum is opened 1 cm anterior to the aorta, from the aortic arch to the diaphragm. At the distal extent the pleura is incised as an inverted T to provide free access to the hiatus. The inferior pulmonary ligament is divided up to the inferior pulmonary vein.

The esophagus is mobilized proximally and at the level of the hiatus, below the diverticulum. Penrose drains are passed around it to facilitate traction and dissection.

3 The esophageal body is freed completely from its fascial and vascular attachments up to the inferior border of the aortic arch.

Progressive dissection of the diverticulum is then undertaken, with care given to ensure that the right pleura is protected.

If the hiatus is small and without a hernia, free access to the peritoneal cavity is obtained through a peripheral diaphragmatic incision 2–3 cm from its insertion at the chest wall. This allows complete and easy dissection of the fundus, gastrosplenic vessels, and hiatal structures. The phrenoesophageal ligament and the peritoneum are opened, and the whole gastroesophageal junction is delivered into the chest through the hiatus. The gastroesophageal fat pad is removed.

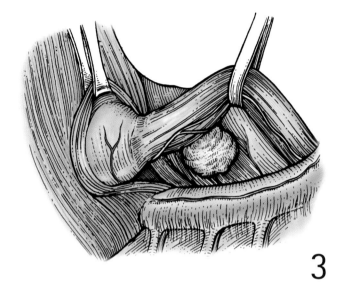

3

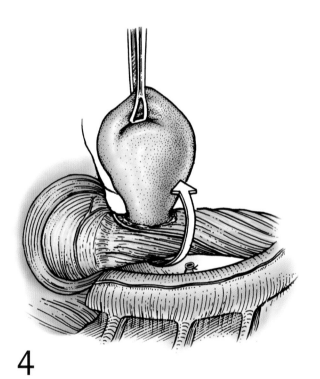

4

4 When the esophagus and proximal stomach have been fully mobilized, the diverticulum and the distal esophagus are rotated toward the left chest. Usually a layer of fibromuscular tissue invests the diverticulum. The mucosa of the diverticulum is freed progressively toward its neck, and the muscular defect surrounding the neck is thus clearly identified.

If the diverticulum is not directed toward the right chest, it may have to be included in the planned myotomy and then suspended rather than removed.

5a–c On completion of the dissection, a large mercury bougie (No. 50) is placed into the esophagus and stomach. This stent serves to distend the esophageal lumen and prevent undue narrowing at the point of excision of the diverticulum.

With the bougie safely in place, resection of the diverticulum is now undertaken, using one of two methods.

6 The first technique is a manual one for resection of the diverticulum. Traction sutures are placed on the proximal and distal borders of the neck, and the diverticulum is resected by opening a straight line of mucosa.

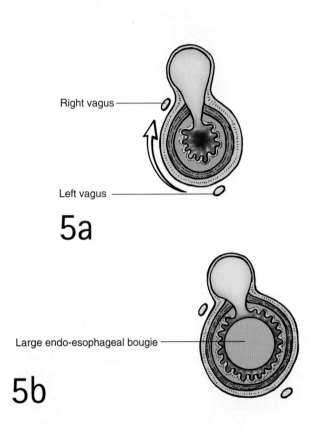

Right vagus

Left vagus

5a

Large endo-esophageal bougie

5b

5c

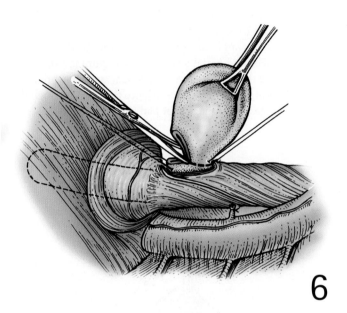

6

7 The esophagotomy is closed longitudinally, as for any esophageal anastomosis, with an interrupted single layer of inverting sutures. Both ends are closed with internal knots. The last three or four sutures are tied externally.

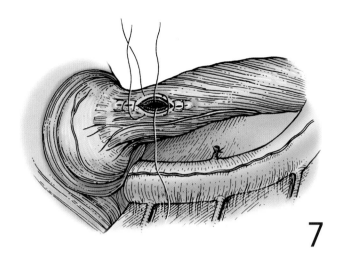

7

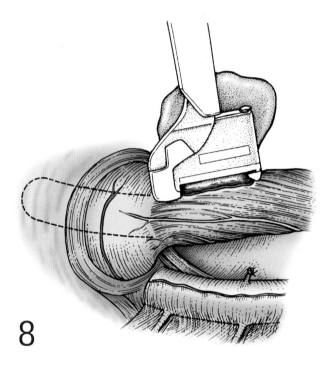

8

8 The second technique is to use a 5- to 6-cm stapler to close the neck of the diverticulum. This is again accomplished with a large bougie protecting the esophageal lumen. A small cuff of mucosa is left distal to the stapling line, and a second row of sutures reapproximates the muscle over the staple line, anchoring it to the cut rim of the mucosa.

9 When the rotation traction is eased, the site of the diverticulectomy resumes its normal position facing the right chest. A long myotomy is performed on the left posterolateral esophagus. The mercury bougie remains in place and serves as support for the mucosa. The use of magnifying spectacles helps in identifying the esophageal structures and encourages stringent hemostasis. A No. 15 scalpel blade is used, and the longitudinal muscle is opened along the whole length of the planned myotomy. The myotomy is then completed through the circular muscle layer, with care taken to avoid perforating the mucosa. The lower esophageal sphincter area may be recognized as the muscle is usually thinner here.

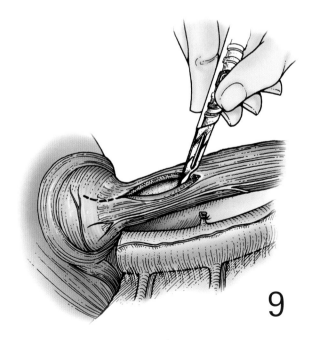

9

10 The myotomy is extended for 1 cm onto the gastric wall muscle, and the gastric submucosa can then be seen as a richly vascularized layer.

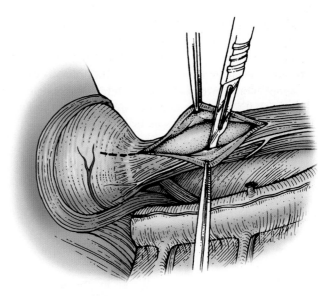

10

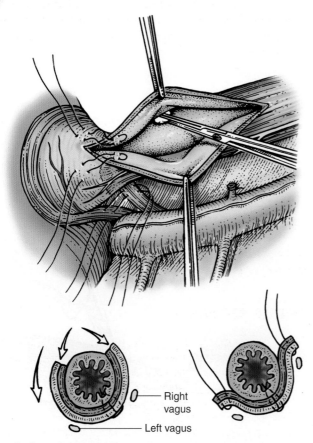

11

Right vagus

Left vagus

11 Lateral dissection of the muscle from the mucosa is carried out with scissors. The assistant pulls the muscle outward while the surgeon holds the mucosa against the bougie with a dissector swab. This exposes a cellular tissue plane between the layers that affords easy dissection. Approximately 50% of the esophageal circumference is freed from the muscle. Once the myotomy is completed, hemostasis is obtained and the mucosa of the myotomized zone is checked to make sure that it has not been breached. The transverse sections show the points of dissection between layers, the placement of sutures to evert the dissected muscle, and the position of the sutures in relation to the right and left vagi.

The bougie is removed, a nasogastric tube is placed in the esophageal cavity, and 50–100 mL of air is introduced into the esophagus while it is kept under saline. Any leak will be shown by bubbles of escaping air.

12 A two-thirds fundic wrap of the Belsey type is next carried out. Two 2/0 silk sutures anchor the fundoplication on each side of the myotomized zone and at two levels. The two layers of the muscle are transfixed from outside to inside to evert the muscle while anchoring the seromuscular layer of the fundus to the esophageal wall. This is accomplished to prevent any closure of the myotomy at the gastroesophageal junction.

The first two sutures are completed at the level of the former insertion of the phrenoesophageal ligament. The two sutures of the second layer are placed in a similar fashion, 2–3 cm more proximal, from the esophagus to the fundus and then through the diaphragm to tie both sutures on the thoracic side of the hiatus.

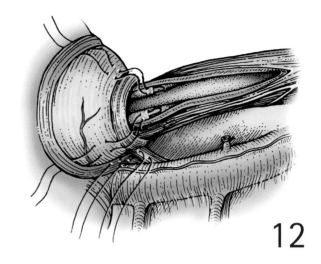

12

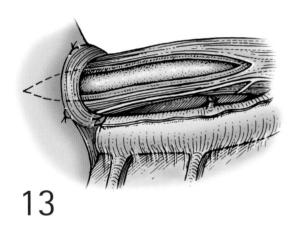

13

13 With this partial fundoplication, the distal 4–5 cm of the myotomized esophagus is reduced without any tension under the diaphragm. It affords good antireflux protection while allowing proper food transit at the gastroesophageal junction.

POSTOPERATIVE CARE

The nasogastric tube is left in place until normal bowel activity has resumed. Once gastric drainage is discontinued, an esophagogram is obtained using water-soluble contrast medium. If the mucosal configuration is considered adequate, liquid barium is added to complete the immediate postoperative evaluation.

The chest tube is removed when normal pulmonary reexpansion is obtained with less than 100 mL of drainage over a 24-hour period.

A liquid diet is resumed once the myotomy and diverticulectomy sites have been shown to be intact. The patient progresses to a semiliquid diet for the following 10 days. Normal alimentation is then resumed.

Complete functional reassessment is obtained 2 years after the operation and at regular intervals thereafter. Documentation of emptying capacity and reflux damage over time in these patients is particularly important.

FURTHER READING

Allen TH, Claggett OT. Changing concepts in the surgical treatment of pulsion diverticula of the lower esophagus. *Journal of Thoracic and Cardiovascular Surgery* 1965; **50:** 455–62.

Benacci JC, Deschamps C, Trastek V, Allen MS, Daly RC, Pairolero PC. Epiphrenic diverticulum: results of surgical treatment. *Annals of Thoracic Surgery* 1993; **55**(5): 1109–13.

Cross FS. Esophageal diverticula related neuromuscular problems. *Annals of Otology, Rhinology and Laryngology* 1968; **77:** 914–26.

Cross FS, Johnson GF, Gerein AN. Esophageal diverticula. *Archives of Surgery* 1961; **83:** 525–33.

Thoracoscopic management of esophageal diverticulum

GLYN G. JAMIESON MS, MD, FRACS, FRCS, FACS
Dorothy Mortlock Professor and Chairman, Department of Surgery, University of Adelaide, Royal Adelaide Hospital, Adelaide, South Australia, Australia

ROBERT LUDEMANN MD, PHD
Research Fellow, University of Adelaide, Department of Surgery, Royal Adelaide Hospital, Adelaide, South Australia, Australia

JOHN HUNTER MD
Professor and Chairman, Department of Surgery, Oregon Health Sciences University, Portland, Oregon, USA

INTRODUCTION

The principles and justification for surgery in patients with diverticula of the esophagus are detailed in Chapter 40, and will not be repeated here.

When planning for a minimal access approach to a diverticulum, there are two possible approaches. First, in mid esophageal or lower esophageal diverticula, the approach can be through either a right or left thoracoscopy. If the diverticulum is in the mid esophagus or proximal lower esophagus, our preference is for a right-sided thoracoscopy. If the diverticulum is epiphrenic, our preference is either a left-sided thoracoscopy or latterly, via laparoscopy. The second approach via laparoscopy can be used for most lower third diverticula, as it is usually feasible to mobilize the lower third of the esophagus via a laparoscopic approach through the esophageal hiatus.

OPERATION

Mid to lower third diverticulum of the esophagus via right thoracoscopy

POSITION OF PATIENT

The patient is intubated with a double-lumen endotracheal tube. If the diverticulum is large (the usual situation requiring operation) the aspiration risk in these patients is substantial, and care should be taken during induction. The patient is then placed either in the full left lateral decubitus position, or our preference is for the patient to be placed in the fully prone position. The advantage of the fully prone position is that the lung falls forward, so with minimal insufflation gas pressure there is usually no need to deflate the right lung.

TROCHAR PLACEMENT

1 A small amount of gas at 5 mmHg pressure is then introduced into the right hemithorax. This can be done using
a Veress needle, or our preference is to introduce a 10 mm
round-ended rod blindly through a 1 cm cut, and then introduce a 10–11 mm trochar over the rod. Two other trochars
(10–11 mm) are placed under direct vision in the sites shown,
with site A being for the camera. As stated above, it is not usually necessary to deflate the right lung, although if it obscures
the view it can be collapsed.

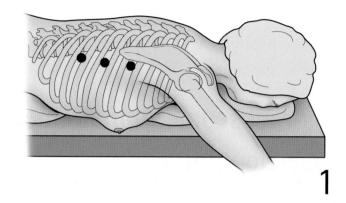

1

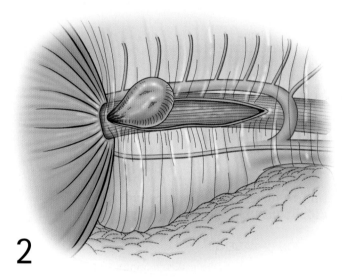

2

ESOPHAGEAL EXPOSURE

2 Identification of the esophagus is facilitated by introducing a flexible endoscope, with the endoscope
transilluminating the esophageal body. The pleura over the
esophagus is picked up and longitudinally incised for the
whole length of the esophagus up to the azygos vein, using
endoscissors. Sharp and blunt dissection is then used to
mobilize the distal esophagus. Particular care needs to be
exercised in the region of the diverticulum, since it can be
associated with peridiverticular inflammation in this area.
Certainly this is not always the case, but if present, it makes
dissection of the diverticulum more difficult.

3 The esophagus itself is not usually difficult to dissect
from its bed, although the most difficult maneuver is get-
ting around the esophagus with a curved instrument in order
to place a tape around the esophagus. The tape is brought out
through one of the ports, the blunt-ended rod reinserted, the
port removed, and the tape picked up outside the patient, and
then the port is reinserted over the rod, leaving the tape outside the port. Next, the diverticulum is dissected out in its
entirety. It may be necessary to rotate the esophagus so that
the neck of the diverticulum can be clearly displayed.

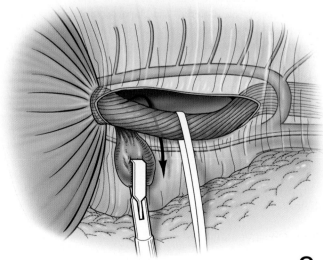

3

DIVERTICULECTOMY

4 Both intraluminal (through the endoscope) and extraluminal views (through the thoracoscope) help to provide a complete demonstration of the anatomy of the diverticulum. Sometimes it can prove helpful to use an additional port if those already in place do not give optimal entry, particularly for the stapling instrument. An Endo GIA stapler with a roticulating head is then introduced. The endoscope is removed and a 52 French bougie is passed down the esophagus. The neck of the diverticulum is then stapled across, the diverticulum is removed, and the longitudinal muscle of the esophagus is approximated across the staple line using either a 5-0 monofilament or braided suture.

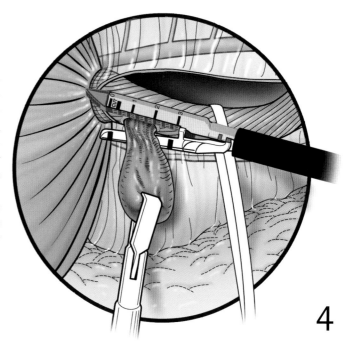

4

5

MYOTOMY

5 A myotomy is performed at a different site from the staple line in the esophagus, preferably at a site 90–180 degrees from the site. The myotomy is undertaken using a combination of endoshears and the hook diathermy. It is helpful to use a curved instrument such as a Mixter clamp, which helps to separate the mucosa from the muscle, and by spreading the jaws of the instrument the muscle is put under tension for division with the diathermy hook. The proximal extent of the myotomy should be at least equal to the proximal extent of the neck of the diverticulum. The distal extent is directed by manometric findings, but in any case is taken well below the diverticulum. The diverticulectomy and myotomy sites are then checked for leaks, sites are submerged in saline, and the esophagus is gently filled with air via the endoscope, the bougie having been removed. If a leak is found, it is usually a very small perforation, and is closed using a 5/0 prolene suture with intracorporeal suturing. We believe it is important to loosely close the myotomy using several interrupted sutures in the longitudinal muscle layer of the esophagus. This is done to prevent future herniation of the mucosa.

CLOSURE

The skin wounds are closed in standard fashion and a chest drainage tube is brought out through one of the trochar sites.

POSTOPERATIVE CARE

Most patients are immediately extubated and the chest tube is placed on underwater seal drainage. A barium swallow is obtained on the first postoperative day and if satisfactory, the patient is allowed a liquid diet. The chest tube is usually removed on the first postoperative day and the patient may be discharged on the second or third postoperative day with instructions to slowly introduce soft foods until reviewed 14 days later.

Alternative approach for lower third (epiphrenic) diverticula

6 A laparoscopic approach is being used increasingly for diverticula in the lower third of the esophagus (see "Discussion" below). The mobilization of the esophagus is a standard approach, as used for antireflux surgery. The only difference is that the mobilization is taken more proximally in the mediastinum, and the diverticulum is dissected free in its entirety. Once again, intraoperative endoscopy is very helpful. A 52 French bougie is then passed and the diverticulectomy is carried out using an Endo GIA. It is usual to require more than one application of the stapler in order to encompass the whole of the neck of the sac of the diverticulum. As with the thoracoscopic approach, several tacking sutures of a fine suture of either prolene or a braided suture are then inserted to close the muscle defect where the neck of the diverticulum has been stapled. A myotomy is then carried out in a different plane from the diverticulectomy, using the same principles as with the thoracoscopic myotomy. This means that if the myotomy is taken down through the gastroesophageal junction, a Dor patch is added to the procedure, but again we believe that it is important to close the longitudinal muscle layer of the esophagus above the Dor patch.

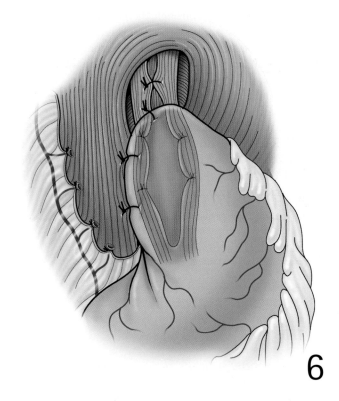

6

DISCUSSION

Esophageal diverticulum is not a common problem, so experience with the minimal approach to its management has been slow to accumulate. Nevertheless, from reports at recent international meetings, several points have emerged. First, is that the procedure seems to be associated with a relatively high leak rate, and the reason why this leakage rate should be higher than with open surgery is not clear. Thus, in the largest experience reported to date in 20 cases there were three staple line leaks, and at 15% this is a much higher rate than reported in open series. Other smaller and therefore virtually anecdotal series have reported even higher leak rates than this. For instance, our own combined experience of three cases was associated with two leaks (but no deaths).

Second, there seems to be a move away from the thoracoscopic approach to the laparoscopic approach for distal third diverticula (which are by far the majority). Dr Peracchia's group performed their first ten cases thoracoscopically with two leaks, and their last ten laparoscopically with one leak.

When a diverticulum is removed at open surgery, the stapler used is a transverse one which has an extra row of staples compared to the Endo GIA. Perhaps this is one reason why the leak rate is lower in the open setting.

For the present, it is clear that the minimal access approach should only be used with great caution, and with patients fully informed that the possibility of leakage is probably higher than with the open approach. Nevertheless, the gains of minimal access surgery for this condition are so undeniably greater when the patient's course is uncomplicated that there seems little doubt the procedure will establish a place in the treatment of this condition.

FURTHER READING

Fumagalli U, Bona S, Zago M, Bisagni P, Rosati R, Peracchia A. Laparoscopic approach to epiphrenic esophageal diverticula. V061 ISDE Meeting Sao Paulo, 2001.

41

Perforation of the esophagus

BAIYA KRISHNADASAN MD
Assistant Professor, Department of Surgery, Division of Cardiothoracic Surgery, University of Washington School of Medicine, Seattle, Washington, USA

OLIVIER HUBER MD
Associate Professor, Department of Surgery, University of Geneva; Head, Foregut Surgery, University Hospital of Geneva, Geneva, Switzerland

CARLOS PELLEGRINI MD
The Henry N. Harkins Professor and Chairman, Department of Surgery, University of Washington School of Medicine, Seattle, Washington, USA

HISTORY

The first reported spontaneous rupture of the esophagus was described by Herman Boerhaave, a 'leading physician of the age,' in early mid 18th century Germany. His patient, the Baron de Wassenaer, consumed a large meal and subsequently 'strove to excite vomiting by tickling his fauces,' resulting in a post emetic esophageal perforation. Not unexpectedly, the Baron died within 24 hrs, and his post mortem revealed a linear esophageal perforation that had ruptured into both pleural spaces. A number of similar reports followed Boerhaave's seminal description. Attempted suture repair was only contemplated in the mid 20th century, and initial attempts in the United States (1944) and England (1946) were unsuccessful. Successful suture repair was performed by Norman Barrett in 1947, the year following his insightful and comprehensive review of the subject. Although post emetic perforation is no longer the principal etiology for esophageal perforation, it is notable that successful surgical repair followed two centuries later.

PRINCIPLES AND JUSTIFICATION

Despite improvements in supportive therapies, including ventilator management, antibiotics and nutrition, perforation of the esophagus can be fatal unless diagnosed promptly and treated effectively. The most common cause of perforation is passage of instruments down the esophagus, especially during forced dilatation of an esophageal stricture. Injury to the cervical esophagus is particularly common following endoscopy and endotracheal intubation, and these iatrogenic events account for 60% of cervical perforations. External trauma due to stab or gunshot wounds is also common in both the cervical and thoracic esophagus. Other etiologies include the 'spontaneous' or emetogenic disruption of the esophagus (Boerhaave's syndrome), perforation of an esophageal cancer, sloughing of the esophageal wall after injection sclerotherapy or caustic injury, foreign body impaction, surgical injury and infectious processes.

A number of recent studies have reported mortality rates of less than 10% in contrast to the 10–30% historical mortality from esophageal perforation. These contemporary reviews, which typically investigate a small group of patients, are predominantly concerned with patients who have had instrumental injury to the esophagus. This cohort of patients typically have their diagnosis made more expeditiously and represent a healthier group of patients compared to individuals who have post-emetic esophageal perforation. The current overall mortality rate for all patients who develop esophageal perforation is 18%.

The risk of dying from an esophageal perforation varies markedly with location and extent of the perforation, time elapsed prior to treatment, the age and general condition of the patient, and the presence of intrinsic esophageal disease. A key to understanding the pathophysiology of esophageal perforation is the recognition that it causes a rapidly evolving infection of the mediastinum, with substantial spread and necrosis of poorly vascularized mediastinal fat tissue. In addition, and particularly pertinent to treatment options, there is prompt deterioration of the esophageal wall at the site of the rupture. Thus, ideally an esophageal perforation should be treated within 12 hours of its occurrence – attempts at primary repair after the first 36–48 hours are more challenging.

Contrast radiography should be used liberally after pneumatic dilatation and whenever the circumstances related to esophageal instrumentation cause any concern about the possibility of a perforation.

PREOPERATIVE ASSESSMENT AND PREPARATION

Clinical diagnosis

The most common symptom is pain, which is first felt during, or immediately after, the completion of the instrumentation. Pain is constant, most often radiates to the back, and may be felt in the upper abdomen and chest, particularly in the case of thoracic esophageal injury. Perforations in the neck often present with pain on neck flexion or manipulation of the thyroid cartilage. Subcutaneous emphysema and crepitation are often evident following cervical perforation and are present in approximately twenty percent of thoracic esophageal perforations. Most patients also complain of dysphagia, odynophagia, occasionally aphagia, and profuse salivation. Fever and leukocytosis are common within the first 4–6 hours after perforation and some patients develop hypotension, sweating, and all the features of shock. Airway compromise is uncommon following injury to the esophagus, but may be of concern in the case of a cervical perforation.

The commonly quoted triad of symptoms described by Mackler, including thoracic pain, following vomiting, associated with cervical emphysema, is only present in approximately 40% of patients. These findings are only relevant to post emetic esophageal perforation.

Radiological diagnosis

1, 2 Chest and abdominal radiography are invaluable in the diagnosis of esophageal perforation. The perforation may be suspected from plain films of the neck, chest, or upper abdomen, as free air may dissect adjacent tissues, creating subcutaneous emphysema, pneumomediastinum, pneumoperitoneum, or even pneumothorax. Cervical perforation may present with subtle findings such as air in fascial planes, widening of the retroesophageal space and loss of normal cervical lordosis. Thoracic perforations often demonstrate widened mediastinal shadow and air fluid levels within the mediastinal space. A left pleural effusion is also an indirect sign of esophageal perforation. In the experience of the authors and of others, however, these signs are present only in approximately 30% of cases.

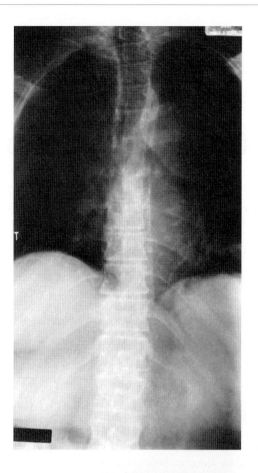

1

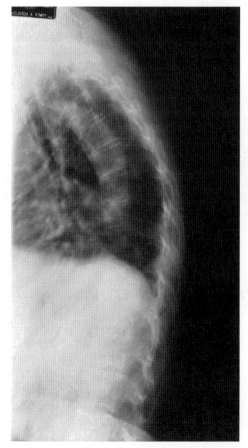

2

3 The essential radiological investigation in these patients is a contrast study of the esophagus, which will reliably indicate an esophageal perforation. More importantly, however, contrast studies will define the site and extent of the perforation, the amount of extravasation, the communication with the pleural or peritoneal cavity, and the presence of distal obstruction. Thus, a contrast study is not only important to diagnose esophageal perforation but is essential to correct planning of surgery.

The authors prefer to use meglumine diatrizoate 66%, sodium diatrizoate 10% (Gastrografin), as the contrast medium in the initial investigation. This water-soluble material is rapidly absorbed from the gastrointestinal tract and from the pleural or peritoneal cavity if extravasated. It allows even small amounts of extravasation to be detected by a follow-up computed tomographic (CT) scan. Gastrografin may be more caustic to the airway if aspirated and generates a false negative study in approximately 20% of cervical esophageal perforations. In cases where aspiration is a concern or a false negative is suspected, a thin barium swallow may be more informative.

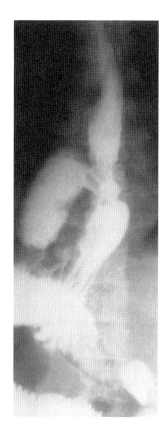
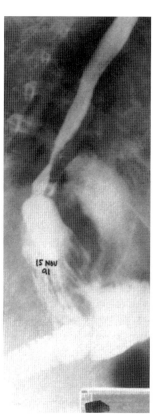

3

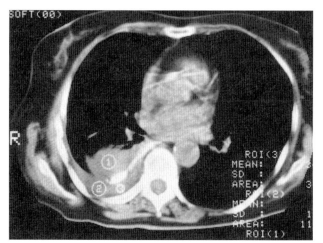

4

4 CT scanning may detect a small perforation that did not appear on the esophagogram and is indicated in patients in whom the swallow examination was negative but who are suspected of having esophageal perforation. Often the CT scan is the first study that is performed, and may reveal subtle signs of a perforation, including mediastinal air or fluid, or small pleural effusion. In these cases the CT scan should be followed by an appropriate contrast study of the esophagus.

5 A CT scan provides invaluable information on patients who present with delayed perforations. These are patients who survived the initial insult and who have developed an abscess that effectively contains the perforation and prevents further mediastinal or pleural soiling.

To plan adequate drainage, one must define the site, the extent, and the relation of the abscess to adjacent structures, and CT scanning is the test of choice.

Endoscopic diagnosis

Endoscopic examination adds little information to that gleaned from high-quality contrast radiography. In some patients, however, particularly those suffering from foreign body perforation or penetrating trauma, endoscopy may help to identify and characterize the injury. For example, a patient who has stab or gunshot wounds may also have a perforated esophagus. These patients are too unstable to undergo contrast esophagography, and the risk of esophageal perforation is low. Notably, the sensitivity of esophagoscopy in detecting subtle injuries is inferior to contrast study and not unexpectedly, it is operator dependent. Another example is a patient who is undergoing dilatation of an esophageal stricture and who is suspected of having had a perforation. Insertion of the endoscope at the end of a difficult procedure may provide invaluable information at an early stage. It has been recommended that the endoscope be passed through a perforated esophagus to assess the damage inflicted to adjacent structures, but the authors believe the risks of this maneuver outweigh its potential benefit.

Endoscopic examination may be helpful in those patients that have intrinsic esophageal disease and esophageal perforation. In these cases, discovery of a cancer, stricture or other esophageal pathology, will effect planning of the operation. For this reason, the authors routinely perform endoscopy on all patients who are undergoing an operation for esophageal perforation immediately following induction of anesthesia.

Initial management

The initial management of an esophageal perforation involves several steps.

AGGRESSIVE RESUSCITATION

These patients suffer rapid dehydration and overwhelming contamination if the perforation is large and in the chest. Large bore intravenous access or central access is warranted, particularly if the patient is being transferred to another institution. A secure airway is also paramount in elderly patients requiring large volume resuscitations and who have compromised ventilation. Occasionally, a chest drain may be required to drain a pneumothorax or large pleural fluid collection.

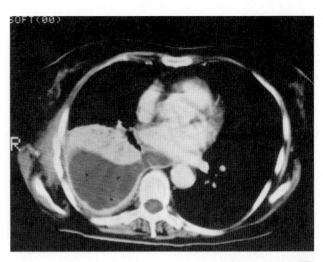

5

ANTIBIOTIC ADMINISTRATION

As soon as a perforation is suspected, the patient should be started on broad-spectrum antibiotics directed against oral flora to adequately cover aerobic Gram-positive and Gram-negative bacteria, as well as anaerobic micro-organisms. Antifungal coverage is also routinely administered at our institution because of the high incidence of pathologic oral fungal flora.

ASSESSMENT OF THE INJURY

The surgeon should determine the following before deciding on the kind of treatment:

1 The type of perforation: 'contained' (i.e. limited to the tissue immediately adjacent to the esophagus) or 'free' (the most common type of perforation, with free extravasation of contents into the neck, the pleural cavity, or the peritoneal cavity)
2 The etiology of the perforation – post instrumentation, spontaneous, traumatic etc. (The gastroenterologist who performed the endoscopic procedure that led to the perforation may have important information related to the esophagus itself and to the injury)
3 The time elapsed since the perforation occurred
4 The location and extent of the perforation
5 The presence of pre-existing esophageal disease, most commonly an obstruction, usually distal to the perforated area
6 The age and general health of the patient.

Indications for surgical intervention

The strategy for intervention should be chosen by following the steps described earlier.

CONTAINED PERFORATIONS

Contained perforations, which affect a small area of tissue adjacent to the esophagus, may be treated without surgery, provided that: (1) the perforation is small; (2) the contrast material flows immediately back into the esophagus and distally into the stomach; (3) no underlying esophageal disease is present distal to the perforation (i.e. stricture); and (4) the clinical manifestations are minimal (i.e. low-grade fever, minimal pain, etc.). Some have argued that patients that have had symptoms for greater than 24 hrs or that have eaten following the onset of symptoms should be excluded from this non-operative approach. It should be noted that this 'conservative' management is the exception, not the rule, when treating esophageal perforation. In fact, in some instances the surgeon ought to look 'beyond the horizon' in making the decision. Such may be the case of a patient who has achalasia and has a 'minimal' perforation. It is unlikely that anyone will attempt subsequent dilatation of this achalasia; thus, operating early, closing the perforation and performing a myotomy will deal with both aspects of the problem: the underlying disease and the complication of treatment.

One perforation that may be treated successfully with conservative (non-operative) management is that which occurs a few weeks after injection sclerotherapy. The inflammatory reaction caused by the sclerosing agent adheres the periesophageal tissues to the wall of the esophagus, effectively blocking the perforation and decreasing the chance of mediastinal spread of infection. However, the underlying general state of the patient (cirrhosis) and the esophagus (varices) would make any attempt at surgical intervention very difficult. When this strategy is followed, the patient should be given enteral or parenteral nutrition, a nasogastric tube should be placed with fluoroscopic guidance, broad-spectrum antibiotics should be administered for at least 7 days or until no sign of infection is present. Most importantly, the esophagus must be evaluated periodically with contrast radiography and CT scanning to monitor the progress. Any evidence of spread of infection or lack of adequate response to this treatment should elicit an immediate change of treatment, most probably prompting surgical intervention.

FREE PERFORATIONS

Free perforations, which are much more common than contained perforations, should almost always be treated operatively, regardless of location or size. The principles of surgical repair include (1) control/drainage of the esophageal leak, (2) eradication of mediastinal and pleural sepsis, (3) reexpansion of the lung.

TIME ELAPSED SINCE INJURY

The time elapsed since the perforation determines to some extent the intervention to be used. Patients who suffered their perforation 24–36 hours previously should undergo an exploration of the area, and if possible, the perforation should be closed with buttressing. The mediastinal and pleural spaces should be debrided and drained and the lung decorticated. Patients who present several days after perforation are likely to have a periesophageal abscess. In these cases closure of the perforation may no longer be possible; if mediastinal and pleural sepsis is controlled and the lung is reexpanded, interventional radiological techniques may be utilized to drain the infected areas.

LOCATION AND EXTENT OF PERFORATION

Injuries to the esophagus above the thoracic inlet should be treated by neck incision on the side of the extravasation, or on the left side (the esophagus is easier to access from the left). Occasionally, cervical esophageal perforations will extend into the mediastinum or right chest and require open mediastinal and pleural debridement through a right fifth intercostal space posterolateral thoracotomy. Nonoperative treatment of perforations in the neck has been advocated, on the basis that most heal by apposition of adjacent tissue (no 'real' space is present around the esophagus in the neck). The authors believe that early closure or drainage of these injuries accelerates recovery and allows for treatment of associated injuries, which are common when external trauma is the cause of the perforation. If the perforation has occurred in a Zenker's diverticulum, resection of the diverticulum and a concomitant cricopharyngeal myotomy are recommended. Most other esophageal perforations should be approached through a thoracotomy. High and mid esophageal injuries are best approached by thoracotomy in the right posterolateral fifth intercostal space. Most low lesions should be approached through the left posterolateral seventh intercostal space, even if the extravasation is in the abdomen. Occasionally bilateral thoracotomies will be required to decorticate both pleural spaces.

PRESENCE OF UNDERLYING ESOPHAGEAL DISEASE

Underlying esophageal disease plays a critical role in determining the kind of procedure to be performed. Because perforation occurs most commonly during dilatation of strictures, and because the mechanism of injury is such that the wall of the esophagus is injured at or just above the stricture, therapy should be planned accordingly. If the stricture is fixed and fibrotic, the best treatment is to resect the stricture and perforated area, and immediately reconstruct the gastrointestinal tract. If the perforation is caused by dilatation for achalasia, closure of the perforation and a Heller myotomy on the other side of the esophagus are recommended. Whatever the choice, the important principle is to *never* close primarily a perforation above an esophageal stricture.

GENERAL HEALTH OF THE PATIENT

Unfortunately, early discovery of a free perforation mandates an operation, regardless of the fitness of the patient. A poor general state of health of the patient, however, may lead to a decision for nonoperative treatment of a perforation of the neck or a small mediastinal perforation.

Preoperative preparation

The preoperative preparation involves adequate resuscitation including tube thoracostomy, antibiotic administration, and a thorough evaluation of the injury as described earlier.

Anesthesia

During induction of anesthesia, care must be taken to avoid causing tension pneumothorax, which is possible if vigorous mask ventilation is performed before intubation (because of the hole in the esophagus). The anesthetist must prevent aspiration of blood, secretions, and any residual contrast medium from the esophagography that may have accumulated in the esophagus. Inserting a nasogastric tube blindly in these patients is unwise, as the tube is likely to exit through the perforation and cause further damage. A single lumen endotracheal tube is placed initially to facilitate endoscopy. Finally, a double-lumen endotracheal tube should be used, as independent ventilation of the lungs is required to be able to collapse the lung on the side of the operation. Appropriate monitoring and IV access should be ensured prior to induction; liberal use of pulmonary artery catheters and central venous monitoring is reasonable in elderly or critically ill patients.

OPERATIONS

Unobstructed esophagus

6 Most spontaneous and instrumental perforations occur in the distal esophagus. The best way to approach these lesions is by thoracotomy through the left posterolateral seventh intercostal space. We routinely harvest an intercostal muscle flap prior to entering the chest. This pedicle can be harvested by stripping the periosteum of the seventh and eighth rib or it can be taken with cautery, with care not to disrupt the underlying neurovascular pedicle. The pedicle is then wrapped in a warm saline sponge and left in the chest till it is required during closure of the perforation. Once the chest has been entered and the lung adequately collapsed, the inferior pulmonary ligament is incised and the lung is packed into the upper chest. The parietal pleura overlying the esophagus should be opened at a site near the perforation and extended both cephalad and caudad to permit adequate exposure. Occasionally the esophageal lesion has lacerated the pleura, and the site of perforation is obvious from the beginning. With care taken not to injure the contralateral mediastinal pleura, the esophagus is dissected off its bed and surrounded with a one inch Penrose drain above and below the perforation. The plane of dissection on the esophagus is on the longitudinal muscular coat and not in the periesophageal tissue.

Adequate mobilization of the esophagus may require extensive dissection, particularly if the perforation has occurred in the right side of the esophagus. The area of injury must be clearly identified, as well as the normal esophagus above and below. If the perforation is not evident, the chest should be filled with saline while the anesthetist blows air through the esophageal lumen. Bubbles of air will appear at the site of perforation. Alternatively an endoscope can be passed transorally and an examination performed while the patient is anesthetized and the chest is open. The air insufflated will in most instances be enough to identify the site of injury but further insight can be gained by directly inspecting the mucosa. Most often the perforation is easily identified by surrounding inflammation as well as the presence of Gastrografin or thin barium in the esophageal lumen. At this stage a nasogastric tube should be carefully passed transorally and advanced into the stomach under direct vision to help during closure of the perforation.

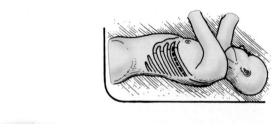

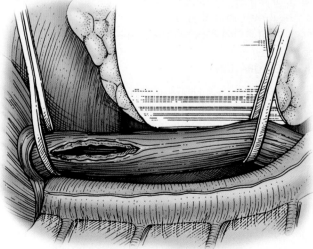

6

7 The edges of the perforation are trimmed with scissors to obtain clean edges and to expose the mucosal rent entirely. Routinely the muscular layer requires additional debridement and dissection to clearly define the ends of the mucosal injury. Failure to demonstrate the entire extent of the mucosal injury will lead to incomplete closure of the esophageal perforation. If the mucosa is healthy it should be approximated using an interrupted suture of 3/0 or 4/0 polyglyconate, and the muscular coat closed with interrupted sutures of nonabsorbable material (3/0 silk or similar). If the perforation is several hours old and the tissues are edematous, all the layers may have to be closed together. In this case, interrupted sutures of nonabsorbable material of adequate size (2/0 or similar) are preferred, as thinner and monofilament material tends to cut the inflamed tissues.

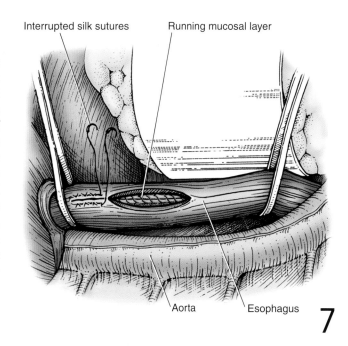

Interrupted silk sutures   Running mucosal layer

Aorta   Esophagus

7

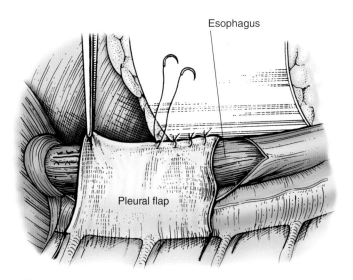

Esophagus

Pleural flap

8

8 Whenever possible, the esophageal closure should be buttressed with the previously harvested intercostals flap or by stripping a flap of pleura from the posterolateral chest wall. The buttress should be securely sutured to the esophagus to provide an additional layer of tissue to secure the closure. The intercostals flap should be placed parallel and on top of the repair and sutured to healthy muscular layer with interrupted 3/0 silk sutures. The pleura may be too edematous to dissect because of the inflammatory reaction. If this is the case, and if the stomach is accessible, the area may be buttressed using the stomach or omentum.

Finally, any fibrinous membrane and necrotic tissue is debrided and the lung decorticated. The control of mediastinal and pleural sepsis is a critical aspect of the care of esophageal perforation, and this aspect of the patient's operative management cannot be overlooked. The chest is drained with a large (No. 36) straight tube placed with its tip in the apex of the pleural cavity and a similar (No. 36) right-angled tube left on the surface of the diaphragm with its tip near, but not touching, the area that has been repaired. The proximity of this chest drain to the repair allows adequate drainage of the esophagus if the repair is not successful. The chest is then irrigated and closed. In critically ill patients both gastrostomy and feeding jejunostomy are performed.

Obstructed esophagus

The two most common conditions are perforation occurring during pneumatic balloon dilatation of a patient with achalasia and perforation occurring during instrumentation of a benign or malignant stricture.

PERFORATION FROM PNEUMATIC DILATATION FOR ACHALASIA

The approach and the initial procedure are similar to that described for the treatment of the unobstructed esophagus. This perforation always affects the lower esophagus and is approached from the left side.

9 Simply closing the perforation may result in early dehiscence (because of the concomitant obstruction) and leaves the patient with untreated achalasia. Thus, after closing the perforation in a manner similar to that described earlier, the opposite side of the esophagus is exposed, exactly 180 degrees from the perforated area, and a longitudinal myotomy approximately 6-8 cm along the esophagus is performed. After the phrenoesophageal ligament is divided, the fundus of the stomach is brought up and the myotomy is extended one to two centimeters onto the stomach. A partial fundoplication (Dor, Thal, Belsey) over the area of the perforation is made. The wrap is secured with interrupted sutures to each side of the myotomy. This not only buttresses the repair well but also acts as an antireflux procedure and helps to keep the edges of the myotomy far apart, which prevents it from healing. The 360 degree plication, as described by Nissen, should not be used as it is contrary to the principle of diminishing the lower esophageal sphincter pressure.

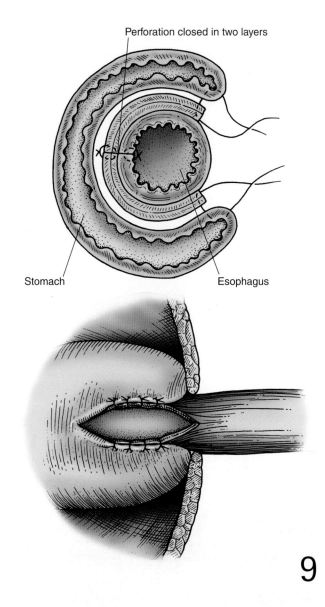

Perforation closed in two layers

Stomach

Esophagus

9

PERFORATION ABOVE A FIBROTIC, BENIGN, OR MALIGNANT STRICTURE

Whenever possible, resection of the esophagus by the transhiatal approach and esophagogastrostomy at the neck are recommended. This treats the perforation and underlying disease, and brings a graft of well-vascularized tissue into the posterior mediastinum that fills the space and helps treat the mediastinal infection. The patient is placed in the supine position, anesthesia is induced, a single lumen tube is used and both lungs are ventilated. A midline laparotomy is performed and, after a Kocher maneuver, the omentum is divided outside the gastroepiploic arcade, with care taken to preserve this arcade.

10 The gastrohepatic ligament is divided, with the right gastric vessels preserved. The gastroesophageal junction is then isolated, a tape is passed around the distal esophagus, and the short gastric vessels and the left gastric artery are divided. The left diaphragmatic vessels are ligated and the diaphragm is opened anteriorly as far as needed to perform the mediastinal dissection.

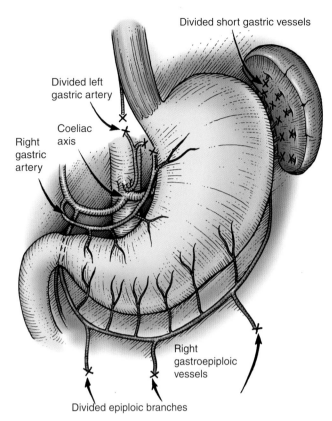

Divided short gastric vessels

Divided left gastric artery

Coeliac axis

Right gastric artery

Right gastroepiploic vessels

Divided epiploic branches

10

11 The lower esophagus can usually be dissected under direct vision to the inferior pulmonary vessels and then bluntly to the thoracic inlet. At this stage a pyloroplasty is performed.

A seven centimeter incision is made in the left side of the neck following the anterior aspect of the sternocleidomastoid muscle. The platysma and omohyoid muscle layers are incised. The sternocleidomastoid and carotid sheath are retracted laterally and the airway is reflected medially. The middle thyroid vein is ligated between ties and dissection proceeds just posterior to the prevertebral fascia. Care is taken to identify and preserve the recurrent laryngeal nerve and to avoid devascularization of the trachea. Retractors are used sparingly to preserve the function of the recurrent laryngeal nerve. Dissection of the esophagus is performed bluntly into the superior mediastinum after it has been encircled with a Penrose drain. Using the Penrose drain for gentle countertraction, the esophagus can be bluntly dissected into the superior mediastinum to the level of the carina.

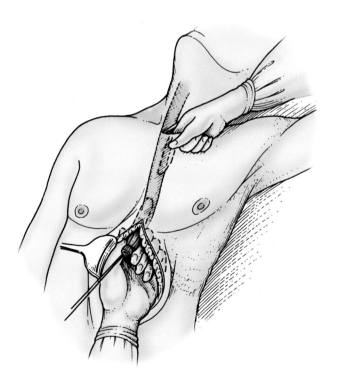

11

12a,b The stomach is then divided using an Endo GIA instrument, starting 2–3 cm lateral to the gastroesophageal junction in the greater curvature and continuing to the midportion of the lesser curvature. This suture line is oversewn with interrupted 3/0 silk suture.

A wide Penrose drain is sutured to the lower end of the divided esophagus, and the esophagus and top of the stomach are removed by pulling from the neck to leave the Penrose drain in the posterior mediastinum. The inferior end of the drain is then attached to the fundus of the stomach to serve as a guide to direct the stomach to the neck, where a two-layer anastomosis is performed to the cervical esophagus just above the thoracic inlet.

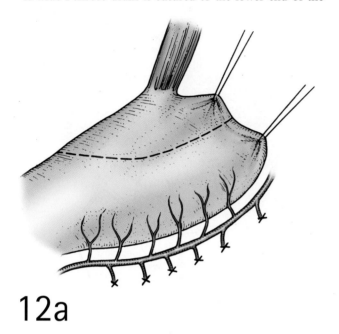

12a

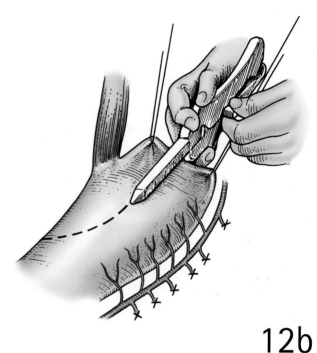

12b

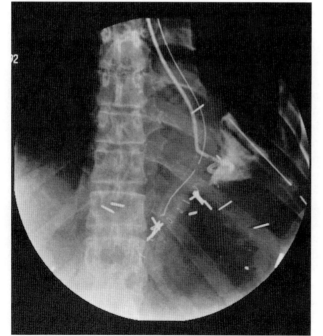

13

Perforation diagnosed several days after occurrence

Patients in whom the perforation is diagnosed several days after occurrence are treated primarily by interventional radiological techniques, although some authors have used operative techniques. The strategy is to drain the cavity adjacent to the perforation and the abscesses as adequately as possible.

13 This involves placing a transoral-transesophageal tube through the perforation to aspirate the cavity. In addition, a percutaneous gastrostomy is performed, and through it another tube is advanced in a retrograde direction into the esophagus. This tube may also be used to decompress the cavity. Finally, a thoracostomy tube may be placed to drain the abscess directly, but this may lead to a temporary esophagocutaneous fistula.

Because the patient will not be able to eat for some time, a feeding jejunostomy catheter should be placed. This can be done laparoscopically to obviate the need for laparotomy.

Alternative approach

In some patients it may not be possible to close the perforation because of a delay in diagnosis, because the patient is too sick for the thoracotomy, or because sepsis persists after interventional radiological management or dehiscence of a previous closure.

14 The treatment of choice in these cases is to divide the esophagus at the neck, bringing out an end-esophagostomy and closing the thoracic esophagus as low as possible in the neck. A long length of cervical esophagus is critical in this situation, as it makes subsequent reconstruction easier. The stoma can be tunneled onto the anterior chest wall and matured at an appropriate location. The cardioesophageal junction is closed with a stapling device via laparotomy or laparoscopy. This effectively isolates the perforated segment and stops mediastinal and pleural soiling.

Unfortunately, this procedure requires a second operation to re-establish continuity of the gastrointestinal tract. This is best accomplished 2–3 months later via a total esophagectomy by the transhiatal approach and a gastroesophageal anastomosis at the neck. Not unexpectedly, this therapy is associated with a high mortality and significant morbidity.

A similar therapy for esophageal perforation that is not amenable to primary repair is the insertion of a T-tube. The T-tube is inserted into the esophagus and an appropriate sized cut chest drain, to ensure that the distal holes have been removed, is inserted into the T-tube. A nasogastric tube is passed through the T-tube into the stomach, securing it into place. In this manner, the esophagus is drained and a controlled esophocutaneous fistula is created. Although this therapy has been used successfully by a number of surgeons, it is not recommended as a routine measure and should only be utilized when the esophagus cannot be reconstructed or closed in a poor risk patient.

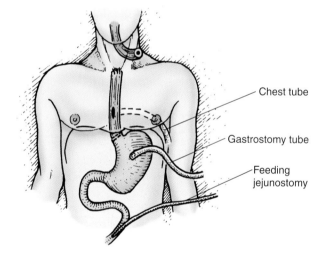

Chest tube

Gastrostomy tube

Feeding jejunostomy

14

Cervical esophageal perforation

Surgical access to the cervical esophagus has been described in a previous section. A similar approach to thoracic esophageal injury is undertaken, including debridement of muscular tissue to identify the mucosal rent and closure in two layers. The repair may be buttressed with strap muscle, but this aspect is less critical in the neck. In fact, many authors advocate simple drainage of cervical esophageal perforations because of the tendency of these injuries to heal without direct suture repair. Adequate drainage can be provided with either closed suction drains or Penrose drains. Debridement of the mediastinal space through a right thoracotomy should be considered if there is significant undrained abscess on CT scan.

POSTOPERATIVE CARE

The patient is intubated for the first 12–24 hours. Good ventilation and full lung expansion are essential to prevent atelectasis, pneumonia and to allow the decorticated lung to expand. Also, if the endotracheal tube is removed at the end of the operation, not uncommonly emergency reintubation is necessary. Forceful mask ventilation before emergency re-intubation increases esophageal pressure and may lead to dehiscence of the suture lines. These patients need intensive care during the first few days. The nasogastric tube must be carefully cared for and routinely flushed, as draining the stomach and esophagus is imperative. To decrease gastric acid secretion H_2-receptor antagonists are administered. The apical chest tube is removed as soon as good lung expansion is achieved and no evidence of air leaks is seen (usually 2 days after surgery).

Antibiotics and antifungals are continued for 7–10 days, depending on the degree of contamination: in patients with positive results on preoperative blood cultures, antibiotics should be continued for 14 days. Enteral feeds using the feeding jejunostomy are started 48 hrs after surgery. If no feeding tube is inserted total parenteral nutrition is administered for the first 8–10 days.

Eight or nine days after surgery, a barium swallow examination should be performed (water-soluble material should be used if there is any suspicion of dehiscence). If this study demonstrates no extravasation, the angled chest tube is removed, and the patient is started immediately on a mechanically soft diet. Patients are discharged home as soon as they can eat and have no evidence of residual infection. If dehiscence is noted and it is contained and asymptomatic, they are kept on enteral or parenteral nutrition for an additional 10 days and the study is then repeated. If symptoms of abscess are present, treatment should be the same as if a delayed perforation is discovered.

Late-diagnosed perforation

Management of the tubes is very important to the success of the procedure to treat late-diagnosed perforation. The tube placement should be inspected periodically (every 2–3 days or more frequently if there is evidence of infection) and cavity size measured by fistulography. The tubes are advanced back into the esophageal lumen as soon as the cavity becomes smaller to allow for more rapid closure of the perforation.

FURTHER READING

Attar S, Hankins JR, Suter CM, Coughlin TR, Sequeira A, McLaughlin JS. Esophageal perforation: a therapeutic challenge. *Annals of Thoracic Surgery* 1990; **50:** 45–51.

Backer CL, LoCicero J 3rd, Hartz RS, Donaldson JS, Shields T. Computed tomography in patients with esophageal perforation. *Chest* 1990; **98:** 1078–80.

Brinster CJ, Singhal S, Lee L, Marshall MB, Kaiser LR, Kucharczuk JC. Evolving options in the management of Esophageal Perforation. *Annals of Thoracic Surgery* 2004; **77:** 1475–83.

Dolgin SR, Wykoff TW, Kumar NR, Maniglia AJ. Conservative medical management of traumatic pharyngoesophageal perforations. *Annals of Otology, Rhinology and Laryngology* 1992; **101:** 209–15.

Engum SA, Grosfeld JL, West KW, Rescorla FJ, Scherer LR, Vaughan WG. Improved survival in children with esophageal perforation. *Archives of Surgery.* 1996; **131:** 604–10

Flynn AE, Verrier ED, Way LW, Thomas AN, Pellegrini CA. Esophageal perforation. *Archives of Surgery* 1989; **124:** 1211–15.

Gayet B, Breil P, Fekete F. Mechanical sutures in perforation of the thoracic esophagus as a safe procedure in patients seen late. *Surgery, Gynecology & Obstetrics* 1991; **172:** 125–8.

Jones WG 2nd, Ginsberg RJ. Esophageal perforation: a continuing challenge. *Annals of Thoracic Surgery* 1992; **53:** 534–43.

Maroney TP, Ring EJ, Gordon RL, Pellegrini CA. Role of interventional radiology in the management of major esophageal leaks. *Radiology* 1989; **170:** 1055–7.

Port JL, Kent MS, Korst RJ, Bacchetta M, Altorki NK. Thoracic esophageal perforations: a decade of experience. *Annals of Thoracic Surgery.* 2000; **75:** 1071–4

Sauer L, Pellegrini CA, Way LW. The treatment of achalasia. A current perspective. *Archives of Surgery* 1989; **124:** 929–32.

Skinner DB. *Instrumental perforation and mediastinitis.* Philadelphia: WB Saunders, 1988; 783–98.

Tilanus HW, Bossuyt P, Schattenkerk ME, Obertop H. Treatment of oesophageal perforation: a multivariate analysis. *British Journal of Surgery* 1991; **78:** 582–5.

Tomaselli F, Maier A, Pinter H, Smolle-Juttner F. Management of iatrogenous esophagus perforation.*Thoracic and Cardiovascular Surgery.* 2002; **50:** 168–73.

White RK, Morris DM. Diagnosis and management of esophageal perforations. *American Surgeon* 1992; **58:** 112–19.

42

Open antireflux operations through a left thoracic approach

ANDRÉ DURANCEAU MD
Professor of Surgery, Chair, Division of Thoracic Surgery, Centre hospitalier de l'Université de Montréal, Montréal, Québec, Canada

HISTORY

Hiatal hernia and its symptoms became recognized during the initial half of the twentieth century. The deranged anatomy of the hiatus with protrusion of the stomach into the chest influenced surgeons to treat this condition and its associated reflux by restoration of the normal anatomy of the gastro-esophageal junction by operative techniques as proposed by Harrington, Sweet, Lertat, Jacob and Allison. Allison, however, documented that in a 20-year assessment of the patients he had treated, 49% showed an anatomical recurrence. Allison recognized that the reflux of gastric contents into the esophagus was responsible for the symptoms and he proposed the term reflux esophagitis. Woodward and Pope documented that approximately 50% of patients with an anatomical repair had pH documentation reflux after their operation.

Development of more effective antireflux operations were reported mainly during the 1960s and 1970s, and associated with the parallel development of more objective methods to document reflux disease and its complications. The Belsey technique, the Nissen total fundoplication, and the Hill operation were assessed with their respective approach, their respective morbidity and recovery. Collis proposed an esophageal lengthening operation for reflux associated with a shortened esophagus consequent to mucosal damage and peri-esophagitis. This elongation procedure was subsequently coupled to a partial or a total fundoplication with excellent long-term results.

Standard antireflux repairs and modified repairs lengthening the esophagus with an added partial or total fundoplication have now been described using minimally invasive techniques. The long-term results and the durability of these procedures in relation to the level of reflux and the inflammatory change encountered are awaited.

The aim of this chapter is to describe the detailed techniques of selected antireflux repairs when they are performed through the chest.

PRINCIPLES AND JUSTIFICATION

The basic principles of surgical reconstruction of the esophagogastric junction to insure competency of the cardia against gastroesophageal reflux have been well described and apply to all types of antireflux repairs:

1 The operation should restore the deficient lower esophageal sphincter to physiological levels (gradient of 15–20 mmHg above resting intragastric pressure).
2 Adequate length of the distal esophagus, including the lower esophageal sphincter pressure zone, should be reduced to an intra-abdominal position, to be exposed to positive intra-abdominal pressure.
3 The reconstructed cardia should not create a resistance that will exceed the propulsive force of the esophagus.
4 The operation should be made without tension, and ensure that the repair will not migrate into the mediastinum.
5 If the esophagus is shortened, either by inflammation within its wall from long-term reflux or by peri-esophagitis encountered at surgery, an elongation gastroplasty with an added partial or total fundoplication should be constructed. A repair which has placed the oesophagogastric junction without tension to the infra-diaphragmatic position, associated with a partial or total fundoplication, is offered as the ideal treatment.

PREOPERATIVE ASSESSMENT

Symptoms usually bring the patient for investigation. These symptoms are not reliable indicators of the presence of reflux disease, the degree of esophageal damage, or provide an indication for surgery.

Radiological assessment aims to document the anatomy of the esophagus and stomach and to classify a hiatus hernia when present. Visual demonstration of reflux on radiology is a poor indicator of endoscopically proven esophagitis.

Objectivity in documenting reflux disease in the esophagus requires the use of investigative methods whereby reflux can be quantified.

1 Endoscopy using the Los Angeles classification or the MUSE classification gives credit to mucosal damage when mucosal breaks are documented.

2 Esophageal biopsies will document unequivocal evidence of reflux damage when acute epithelial or subepithelial inflammation and/or ulceration are present. Fibrosis in the submucosa, in the muscle or the presence of a columnar lined esophagus are signs of more advanced disease.

3 Manometry documents the physiological abnormalities and is the scientific basis of gastroesophageal reflux disease. An absent lower esophageal sphincter with esophageal contractions showing poor strength and deficient or incoordated propulsion is highly suggestive of the diagnosis.

4 Long-term recording of an acid refluxate (24-hour pH) or of a biliary-pancreatic refluxate (Bilitec) are used to document abnormal levels of reflux exposure.

5 Radionuclide scintigrams are used mostly to assess the emptying capacity of the esophagus before and after treating esophageal diseases.

OPERATION

1 A double-lumen tube is positioned in the trachea, and the patient is placed in a right lateral decubitus position. The left arm is supported by an arm rest, and the incision follows the upper border of the eighth rib. The posterior arc of the rib is divided, and 1 cm of the rib is removed to avoid postoperative end-to-end rib contact.

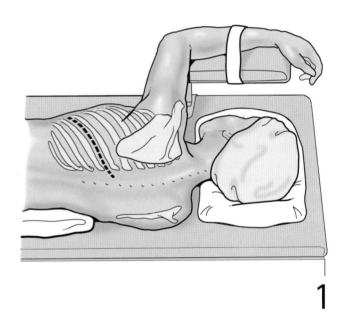

1

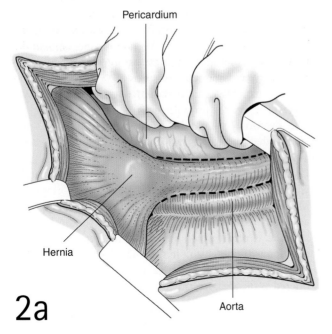

Pericardium

Hernia

Aorta

2a

2a Adhesions between the lung and the chest wall are freed if necessary. The inferior pulmonary ligament is divided using electrocautery. The collapsed left inferior lobe is retracted anteriorly and kept in place by large intrathoracic pads. The mediastinum is opened as an inverted T, and the vertical incision is made 1 cm anterior to the descending aorta and along the pericardium. Both incisions meet behind the inferior pulmonary vein.

2b The horizontal part of the T is made along the left crus of the diaphragm and extended anteriorly, where the pericardium is freed from the fibrous portion of the diaphragm. The mediastinum is opened widely, and vessels from the aorta to the esophagus are clamped and divided.

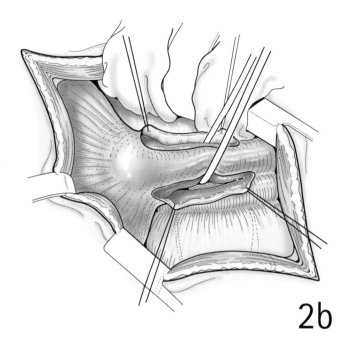

2b

Pericardium

Penrose drain

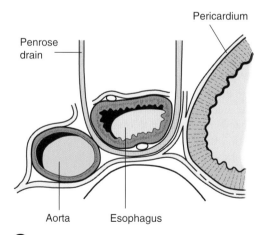

Aorta   Esophagus

2c

2c After being freed from the aorta and pericardium, the esophagus is encircled by blunt dissection, protecting both the anterior and posterior vagi. Doing so exposes the contralateral pleura. The esophagus is dissected completely free between the hiatus and the area above the inferior pulmonary vein just under the aortic arch.

3a Complete dissection of the hiatus is made easier when the peritoneal cavity is opened. The diaphragmatic hiatus is freed with easy identification of the left crus. Anterior to the herniated stomach or the esophagus, the incision follows the circular limits of the hiatus.

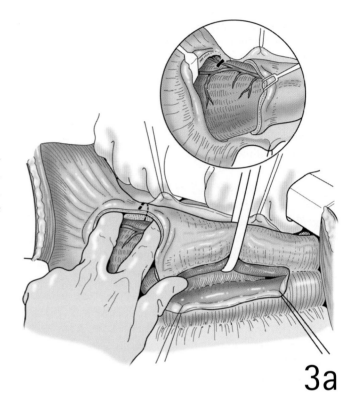

3a

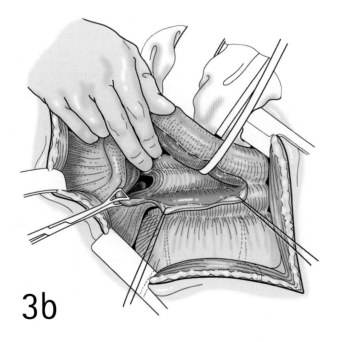

3b

3b The right crus is exposed posterior to the esophagus. With the hiatus widely opened to the abdominal cavity, the index finger is passed behind the esophagus and across the hiatus. The proximal gastrohepatic ligament is opened, exposing the caudate lobe of the liver. With the index finger behind the right crus, all posterior cardial attachments to the diaphragm are divided. Circumferential clearing of the hiatus is completed. The pleura to the right chest is then opened and divided so that the pleura over the right crus is left intact. The entire esophageal diaphragmatic hiatus is well identified with normal peritoneum covering the abdominal surface and normal pleura over the thoracic side. Left and right crura are ready to be reapproximated by wide, tension free 1-0 silk sutures.

4a If a massive hernia is present (types II, III, or IV), the hiatus is usually very wide, and the peritoneum is easily opened anteriorly. In this situation, the fundus and greater curvature are easily identified, and the short gastric vessels are dissected free and ligated. More than 50% of patients with severe complications of idiopathic reflux disease (i.e. esophageal stricture or Barrett's esophagus) actually reveal no evidence of a hiatal hernia. In such a situation, two techniques allow access to dissection of the greater curvature. The first technique opens the retrogastric cavity behind the esophagogastric junction and left crus. Progressive freeing of the stomach is then accomplished by ligation of the short gastric vessels. The second approach creates a lateral opening in the diaphragm, approximately 2–3 cm from the muscular insertion on the chest wall. A GIA stapler is used to create a 6- to 8-cm-long diaphragmatic division. Thus exposed, the short gastric vessels are ligated under direct vision, and the entire greater curvature is freed. With two or three fingers positioned through the abdominal hiatus, the phrenoesophageal ligament is put under tension and divided around the limits of the hiatus. The anterior and posterior aspects of the lesser curvature are easily identified and dissected using this approach. When completely free, the esophagus and proximal stomach are delivered into the chest through the hiatus.

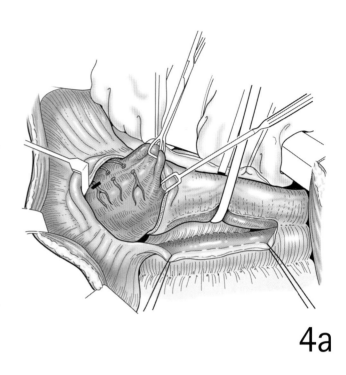

4a

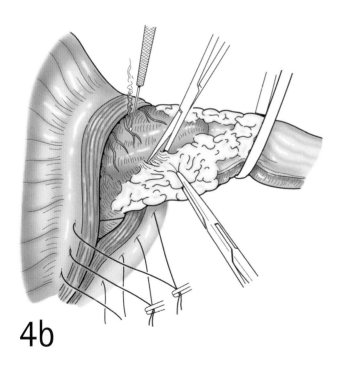

4b

4b When a lengthening operation needs to be added, the anterior and posterior portions of the proximal lesser curvature are dissected as for a highly selective vagotomy. The fat pad of the esophagogastric junction is resected, the anterior and posterior vagi are dissected free from the stomach wall and pushed away to allow the creation of the gastroplasty, and 6 to 7 cm of lesser curvature is denuded from the surrounding tissue. Closure of the hiatus behind the esophagus is accomplished at this point. These sutures cannot be easily placed once the esophagogastric junction repair is completed. The right crus is grasped with a small Duval clamp, holding the crus with the peritoneum under and the pleura above. This maneuver creates an eversion of the right crus toward the chest, allowing an excellent visualization of the inferior vena cava. The left crus is seized in the same way with a second clamp. 1-0 silk sutures are initially passed posteriorly with bites taking all the tissue layers, including the transversalis fascia and the fibrous portion of the crus. A distance of 0.5–1 cm is left between each suture, and when the last suture is installed, easy passage should remain for the index finger between the esophageal wall containing the number 50 bougie and the last suture reapproximating the crura.

The Belsey mark IV repair

5 With the esophagus and gastric fundus completely mobilized and the phrenoesophageal ligament divided at 2 cm from its esophageal insertions, the esophagogastric junction is brought into the chest through the hiatus. The fat pad covering the anterior portion of the junction is then removed, creating a raw surface that will favor healing of the plication against the esophageal wall.

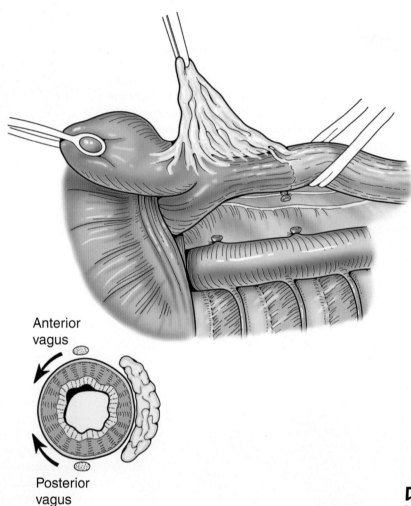

Anterior vagus

Posterior vagus

5

6a,b The goal of the Belsey repair is the creation of a partial fundoplication covering two thirds (240 degrees) of the circumference of the distal esophagus. This is accomplished using two rows of sutures. The first row of 2-0 silk material is passed through the muscularis of the distal esophagus and then through the seromuscular layers of the proximal gastric fundus. Three stitches are placed to appose the raw surfaces between the anterior vagus and the posterior vagus.

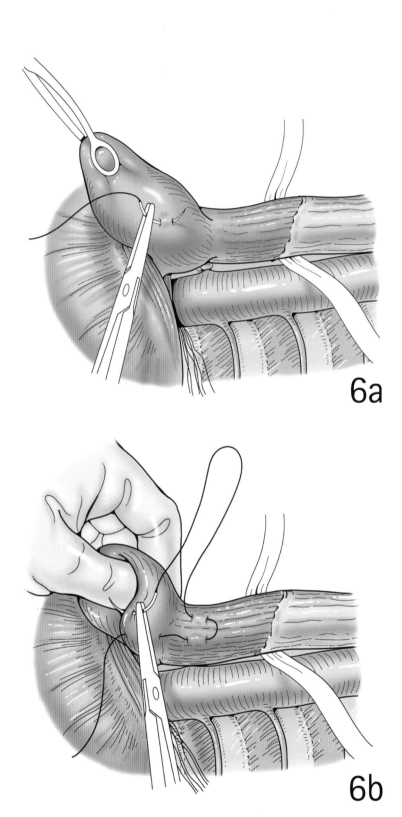

6a

6b

7a,b The sutures, when tied, provide a delicate reapproximation of the tissues and create a first 1.5–2.0 cm fold between the esophagus and stomach.

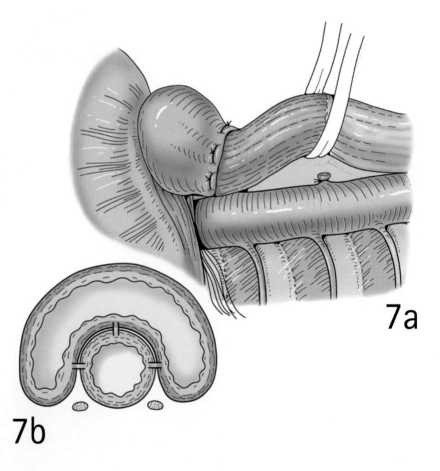

7a

7b

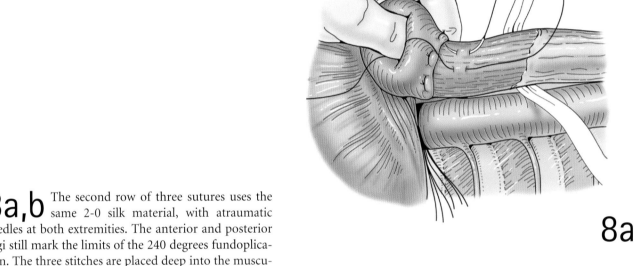

8a

8a,b The second row of three sutures uses the same 2-0 silk material, with atraumatic needles at both extremities. The anterior and posterior vagi still mark the limits of the 240 degrees fundoplication. The three stitches are placed deep into the muscularis of the esophageal wall, without penetrating the lumen. Each suture is then anchored into the seromuscular layers of the fundus using the same precautions.

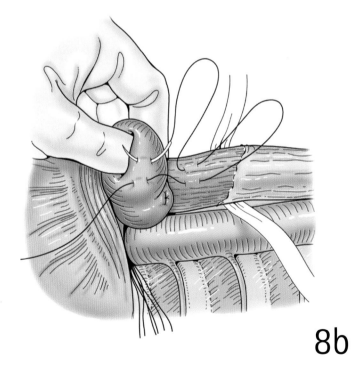

8b

9 The second row of sutures reapproximates once more the fundus against the esophageal wall and the sutures are tied, completing the effects of the fundoplication. The partial wrap is ready to be reduced in an abdominal position.

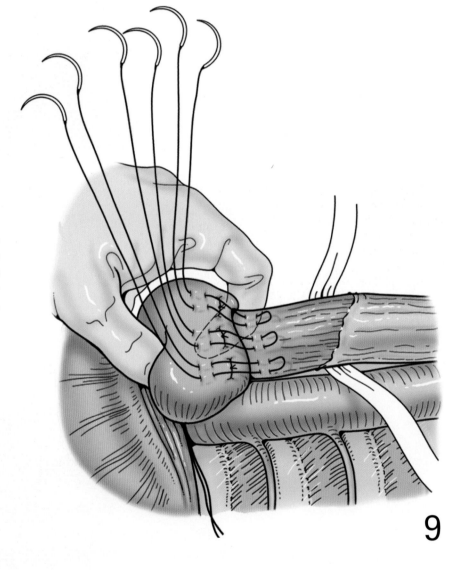

9

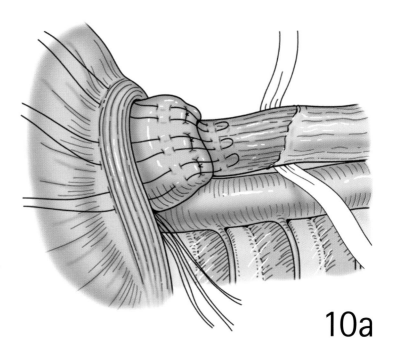

10a

10a,b The two needles at the extremities of each silk suture are now placed through the diaphragmatic hiatus, peritoneal side first, to emerge through the pleura on the thoracic side of the muscle. The first suture is positioned immediately behind the pericardial reflexion, through the fibrous portion of the diaphragm. The second suture is also placed in the tendinous portion of the diaphragm at its junction with the muscle of the hiatus, while the third suture traverses the tendinous part, juxtaposed to the last suture reapproximating both crura behind the esophagus.

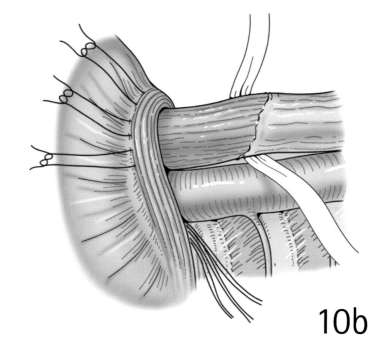

10b

11 The reconstructed esophagogastric junction is reduced under the diaphragm by pushing on the cardia while delicately tugging on the transdiaphragmatic sutures. Snug apposition of the fundus on the undersurface of the diaphragm is insured. The repair must be completed without any tension.

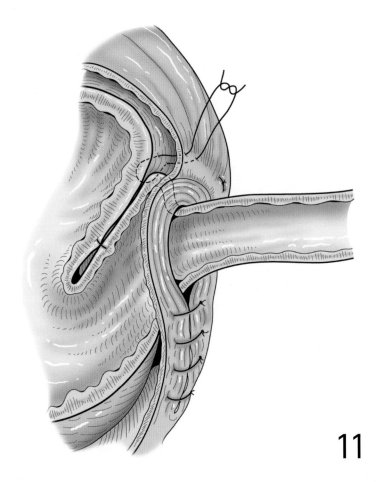

11

Any stress on the repair should alert the surgeon to the requirement of a lengthening procedure, as illustrated in Figure 12.

The uncut elongation gastroplasty with total fundoplication

The entire esophagogastric junction lies within the chest. A number 50 tapered bougie is positioned in the esophagus and stomach. The bougie is held snug against the wall of the lesser curvature, and the gastroplasty is created using a linear stapler. Three techniques are available to create an elongation gastroplasty in association with a total fundoplication.

12a The uncut elongation gastroplasty is made by applying a 3 cm linear stapler with 4.8 mm staples to appose the anterior and posterior walls of the fundus around the bougie held against the lesser curvature. Pushing through the pin of the stapling device results in small anterior and posterior gastric perforations, which are closed with separate monofilament resorbable sutures.

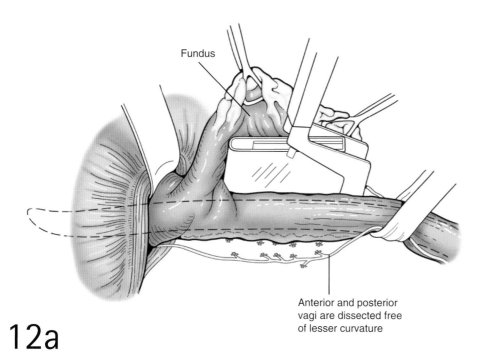

Fundus

Anterior and posterior
vagi are dissected free
of lesser curvature

12a

12b The fundus, extensively mobilized, is manipulated to bring the anterior and posterior walls together to surround the entire length of the uncut gastroplasty while the intraesophageal bougie remains in place. The fundoplication is completed with the vagi safely retracted away from the gastroplasty.

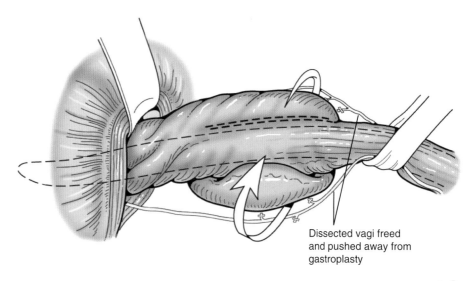

Dissected vagi freed
and pushed away from
gastroplasty

12b

12c 2-0 silk sutures are used to tie the free fundus to a line immediately anterior to the staple line. Fixation of the sutures on the neoesophagus is optional. The entire length of the gastroplasty is then covered by the wrapped fundus. The bougie is removed, and a nasogastric tube is positioned under direct guidance.

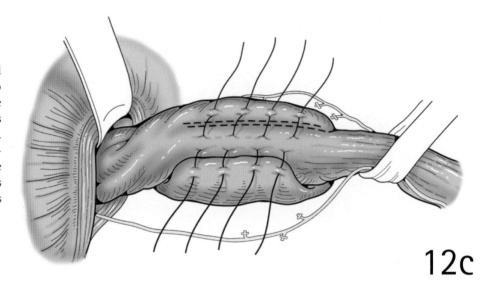

12c

3 anchoring sutures passed through esophagus, top of fundoplication and through diaphragm

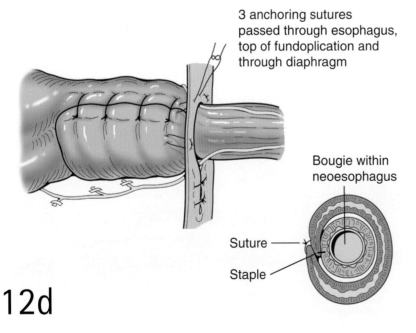

12d

Bougie within neoesophagus

Suture

Staple

12d A second row of silk sutures buries the first series of sutures, and the repair is reduced under the diaphragm. Using a double needle, three 2-0 prolene sutures are positioned on the apex of the gastroplasty tube, passed through the apex of the fundoplication, and tied. Both needles are then passed separately through the diaphragm from below to above, and the sutures are tied on the pleural side of the diaphragm. The repair is reduced and fixed under the diaphragm.

The cut elongation gastroplasty with total fundoplication (Orringer–Henderson)

13a The anterior and posterior proximal lesser curvatures are free. Both vagi have been dissected away from the gastroplasty tube. With the endoluminal bougie held against the lesser curvature, the GIA stapling device is applied, creating a 5 cm gastroplasty around the bougie.

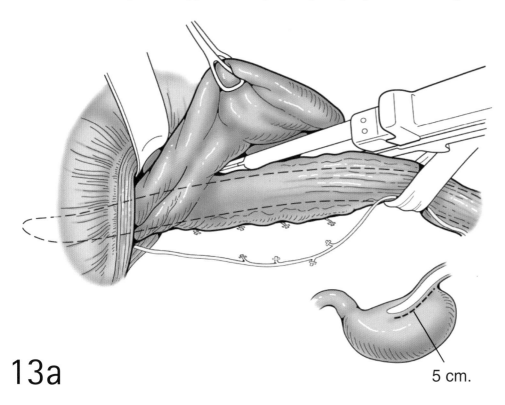

5 cm.

13a

13b The gastric tissue has been transected between the staple lines. Both suture lines are scrutinized for hemostasis and suture integrity. The fundus remains attached by its base to the gastric body.

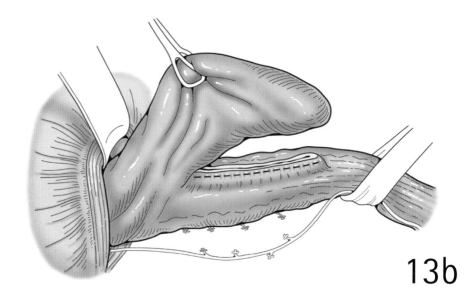

13b

13c The tip of the fundus is brought around the elongation gastroplasty to create a total fundoplication. The fundic wrap is sutured anterior to the gastroplasty suture line and to the wrap itself, completing a 360 degrees fundoplication that covers both suture lines.

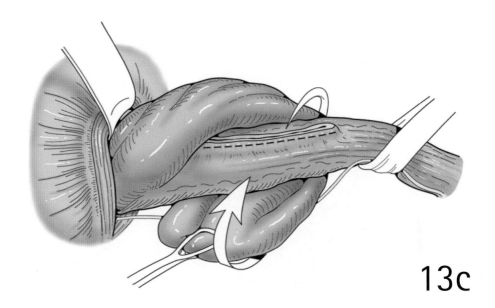

13c

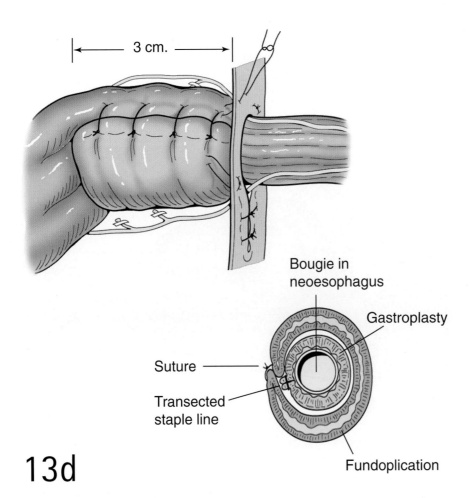

3 cm.

Bougie in neoesophagus

Gastroplasty

Suture

Transected staple line

Fundoplication

13d

13d The elongation gastroplasty covered by the fundoplication is reduced under the diaphragm. The anchoring sutures are passed from the apex of the gastroplasty through the apex of the fundoplication and through the diaphragm to be tied above the diaphragm. The crural sutures are then tied behind the esophagus, leaving enough space to pass an index finger between the last suture and the esophageal wall.

The cut elongation gastroplasty with transverse fundoplasty and total fundoplication (Jeyasingham)

14a A second type of cut gastroplasty may be useful to repair a shortened esophagus. The GIA stapler with 4.8 mm staples is applied to appose and divides the anterior and posterior stomach walls around the number 50 bougie held against the lesser curvature of the stomach.

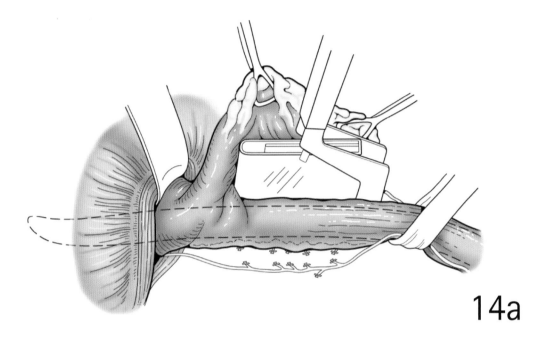

14a

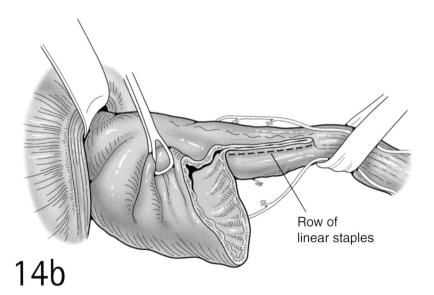

14b

Row of
linear staples

14b The fundus on the side of the stapler is transected open. This results in a closed 3 cm elongation gastroplasty and a wide-open gastrotomy. The fundus is positioned for transverse closure to provide a widened fundus for the subsequent fundoplication.

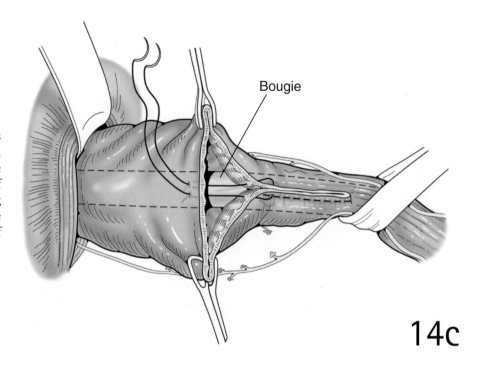

14c The fundoplasty line is made symmetrical, and a "u" stitch apposes the middle of the fundic tissue to the distal extremity of the staple line. Separate inverting resorbable sutures are used to close the fundoplasty line on both sides of the middle suture.

Bougie

14c

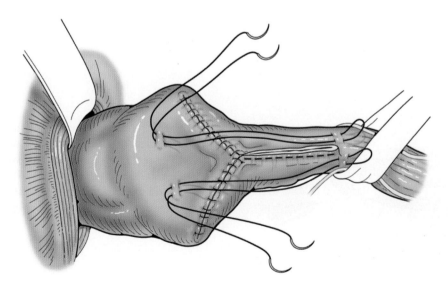

14d

14d The remaining fundus and the extensively mobilized greater curvature are then brought up to completely cover the gastroplasty suture line. The new fundus is applied symmetrically to cover the gastroplasty and is held in place by two sutures positioned on each side of the proximal gastroplasty.

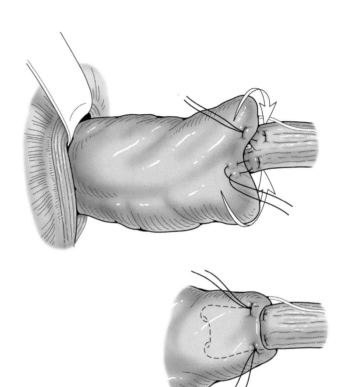

14e A standard total fundoplication is created, with the sutures anchored on the lesser curvature side, away from the gastroplasty line; this makes the transverse fundoplasty part of the total fundoplication wrapping the gastroplasty.

14e

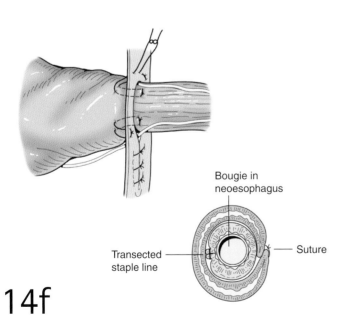

Bougie in neoesophagus

Transected staple line

Suture

14f The 3 cm total fundoplication is reduced under the diaphragm, and three or four anchoring sutures are passed from the apex of the gastroplasty to the apex of the fundoplication and then through the diaphragm.

14f

Elongation gastroplasty with partial fundoplication (Pearson)

15 When a lengthening procedure is required with a partial fundoplication as a wrap around the gastroplasty, the same technique can be used to create the elongation of the esophagus. The 240 degrees wrap around the gastroplasty uses exactly the same method as for the Belsey mark IV repair, using both vagi as the anterior and posterior limits of the fundic wrap. The transsection line of the gastroplasty is completely covered by the partial fundic wrap. The primary indicator for this type of repair is an acquired shortening of the esophagus as occurs with massive paraesophageal hernias, especially if poor propulsion or poor contraction strength has been documented in the esophagus.

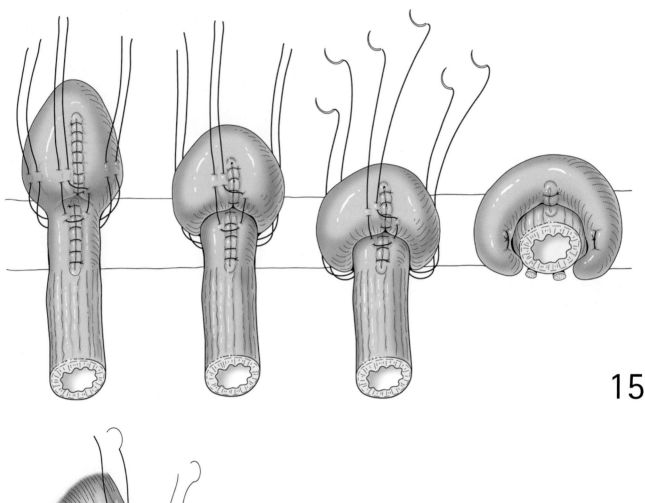

15

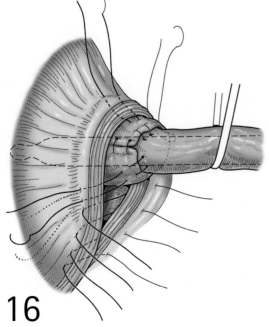

16

16 Standard partial or total fundoplication or elongation gastroplasties with their fundoplication are reduced into the abdomen in the same way as illustrated in the Belsey repair. The heavy silk sutures reapproximating the left and right crura are then tied.

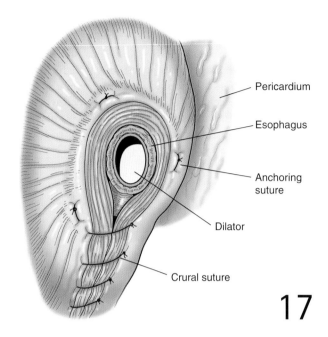

17 With the repair reduced and anchoring completed, an index finger should pass easily between the esophageal wall and the last crural suture.

Pericardium

Esophagus

Anchoring suture

Dilator

Crural suture

17

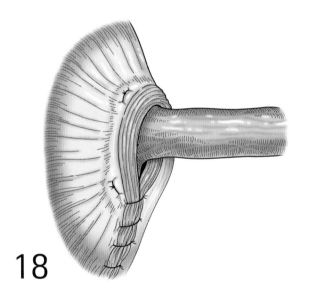

18

18 The final result should be a tension-free repair and a closed hiatus.

Surgical closure

The peripheral diaphragm, when opened, is closed with 2-0 interrupted silk sutures. A number 28 chest tube is installed in a posterolateral position to allow proper re-expansion and drainage. The chest wall is closed in the usual manner.

POSTOPERATIVE CARE

Pain relief

Most patients undergoing repair by means of a thoracotomy for a simple hiatus hernia or for the complications of gastro-esophageal reflux receive an epidural analgesia catheter before the operation starts. Impressive comfort is afforded by the technique supplemented by nonsteroidal anti-inflammatory medication or morphine derivatives.

Respiratory care

Optimal care is obtained by early ambulation and active physiotherapy favoring full diaphragmatic excursion. The chest tube installed after the repair is left in place until drainage decreases to less than 200 ml in a 24-hour period. The epidural is discontinued after the chest tube is removed.

Gastric drainage

A double-lumen nasogastric tube is installed and verified for its position in the gastric cavity at the end of the repair. This type of tubing favors the use of continuous low-grade suction without mucosal occlusion of the drainage ports. Early return of active peristalsis and the absence of significant gastric retention prevents undue distension and pressure on the repair. The repair is verified radiologically once the nasogastric tube has been removed.

Infection and thromboembolic prophylaxis

When the esophagus or esophagogastric junction is opened, prophylactic antibiotics (a third generation cyclosporin with metronidazole) are provided before the operation starts and are given for the initial 24 hours after the operation.

Subcutaneous heparin (5000 IU) is administered every 8 hours until the patient leaves the hospital. Discharge is usually within 5–6 days.

OUTCOME

The Belsey mark IV operation provides a good early control of reflux symptoms for 95% of the patients treated. When followed up for over 20 years the failure rate increases by 1% per year.

The elongation gastroplasty proposed by Collis in 1957, and subsequently modified by Orringer in 1976 and Henderson in 1977 to include a total fundoplication, provides excellent results for over 90% of patients treated. The uncut Collis–Nissen repair has shown favorable results in 94% of patients.

FURTHER READING

Allison P. Reflux esophagitis, sliding hiatal hernia and anatomy of repair. *Surgery Gynecology and Obstetrics* 1951; **92**: 419–31.

Chen LQ, Nastus D, Hu C-Y, Chughtai TS, Taillefer R, Ferraro P, Duranceau A. Results of the Collis–Nissen gastroplasty in patients with Barrett's esophagus. *Annals of Thoracic Surgery* 1999; **68**: 1014–21.

Collis JL. Gastroplasty. *Thorax* 1961; **116**: 197–206.

Ferraro P, Duranceau A. Elongation gastroplasty with total fundoplication (Collis–Nissen operation). *Operative Techniques in General Surgery* 2000; **2**: 24–37.

Hiebert CA. Surgical management of esophageal reflux and hiatal hernia. *Annals of Thoracic Surgery* 1991; **52**: 159–60.

Pera M, Deschamps C, Taillefer R, et al. The uncut Collis–Nissen gastroplasty: early functional results. *Annals of Thoracic Surgery* 1995; **60**: 915–21.

Stipa S, Belsey R. La Chirurgia dell'esofago. Indicazioni e techniche Piccin Editore, Padova.

Skinner DB, Belsey R. *Management of esophageal disease*. Philadelphia: WB Saunders, 1988: 576–99.

43

The uncut Collis–Nissen procedure

VICTOR F. TRASTEK MD
Professor of Surgery, Consultant Division of General Thoracic Surgery, and Chair, Board of Governors Mayo Clinic Arizona, Scottsdale, Arizona, USA

FRANCIS C. NICHOLS MD
Assistant Professor of Surgery and Consultant Division of General Thoracic Surgery, Mayo Clinic College of Medicine, Rochester, Minnesota, USA

HISTORY

The repair of diaphragmatic hiatal hernia began with reduction of the hernia and reapproximation of the crura. Over time it was appreciated that solely this approach failed to relieve the associated symptoms of gastroesophageal reflux disease (GERD). Increased knowledge of the pathophysiology of GERD led to the development of a surgically created antireflux valve. These procedures included the Nissen fundoplication, the Belsey partial fundoplication, and the Hill repair.

In 1957, Collis described an esophageal lengthening procedure utilizing gastric tissue to create a connecting tube (neoesophagus) between the lower end of the esophagus and the proximal stomach. In 1974, Bingham modified the cut gastrotomy portion of the Collis gastroplasty by utilizing an uncut staple line followed by a 360-degree stomach wrap over the connecting tube (uncut Collis–Nissen procedure). Piehler and colleagues from our institution in 1984 reported results of this procedure showing better relief of symptoms associated with GERD.

PRINCIPLES AND JUSTIFICATION

Lower gastroesophageal sphincter incompetence permits free reflux of gastroduodenal contents into the esophagus. The recognized esophageal consequences of this reflux are directly related to the effects of the secretions on the esophagus and to the esophageal mucosa's response to chemical injury. These consequences include desquamation, erosion, ulceration, inflammation, pain, bleeding, motility disturbances, esophageal shortening, stricture formation, and Barrett's disease (columnar epithelial lining of the lower esophagus). Complications vary from patient to patient, and the patho-logical processes are often reversed by eliminating the exposure of the esophageal mucosa to the corrosive secretions.

Surgical control of the complications of gastroesophageal reflux depends upon restoring gastroesophageal competence. While many different surgical approaches have been utilized to accomplish competence, all have three basic goals in common. First is adequate mobilization of the esophagus resulting in an adequate length of both the esophagus and gastroesophageal junction resting comfortably in the abdomen. Second is proper closure of the esophageal hiatus. Third is restoration of the lower esophageal high-pressure zone. Over the past 15 years, laparoscopic fundoplication has become the most common surgical approach. Recognized benefits of the laparoscopic approach include less morbidity, decreased pain, shorter length of hospital stay, and earlier return to normal daily activities. Nevertheless, laparoscopic fundoplication may not be feasible in certain clinical situations. While not absolute contraindications, some of these situations include: obesity, previous upper abdominal surgery, giant paraesophageal hernia, and failed previous fundoplication. For nearly 30 years, the authors and our colleagues have advocated the uncut Collis–Nissen procedure when an open surgical approach is required. This technique is a modification of Nissen's 360-degree fundoplication and Collis's technique for lengthening the esophagus, to provide a tension-free wrap.

The uncut Collis–Nissen gastroplasty uses a stapling device applied to the stomach to create a 3 cm neoesophagus around which a 360-degree Nissen fundoplication is performed. This restores gastroesophageal competence and provides excellent protection from esophageal reflux. By minimization of the length of the uncut Collis maneuver (3 cm) and the fundoplication (2 cm), a reasonably low rate of dysphagia is possible without sacrificing control of reflux.

PREOPERATIVE ASSESSMENT AND PREPARATION

Preoperative evaluation includes a thorough history, barium upper gastrointestinal swallow, and upper gastrointestinal endoscopy. Esophageal motility and 24-hour pH studies are obtained selectively. Both of these studies are performed in most patients with GERD, particularly in those with complicated or atypical reflux histories. Alternatively, both of these studies are not routinely performed in patients with symptomatic large paraesophageal hernia.

ANESTHESIA

Placement of a thoracic epidural assists in initial management of postoperative pain. Utilization of a double-lumen endotracheal tube collapses the ipsilateral lung leading to a less obtrusive operative field. The patient is placed in the right lateral decubitus position.

OPERATION

Incision

1 A left thoracotomy is performed, and the pleural space is entered through the periosteal bed of the nonresected eighth rib. After a posterolateral thoracotomy, the chest cavity and lung should be thoroughly explored.

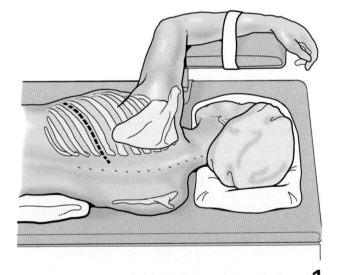

1

Exposure

2a–c The inferior pulmonary vein is divided, and the lung is collapsed, retracted cephalad, and packed away out of the operative field. The esophagus, gastroesophageal junction, stomach, and hernia sac (if present) should be freed from the mediastinum extending from the inferior pulmonary vein to the hiatus. The mediastinal pleura along the pericardium is divided and dissected down through the associated plane to the parietal pleura of the opposite chest cavity. A second incision is made parallel to the aorta through the mediastinal pleura and carried down, which frees the hernia sac and esophagus from the parietal pleura down to the hiatus. The intrathoracic protrusion of proximal stomach and gastroesophageal junction is usually apparent. The esophagus (including the vagal nerves) is then surrounded with a Penrose drain.

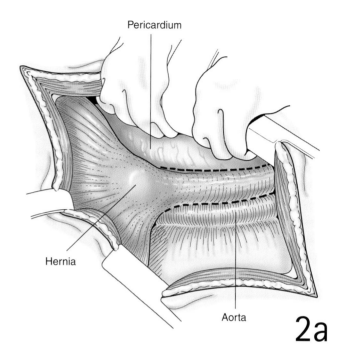

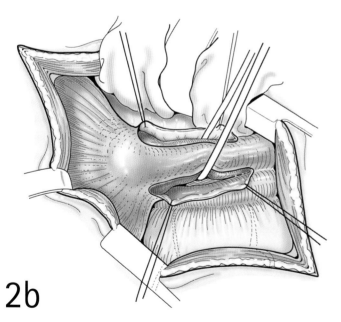

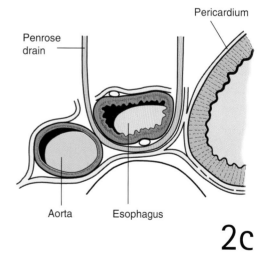

Dissection of the esophageal hiatus

3a–d The posterior or right crus is identified during the exposure of the hiatus, the lesser sac is entered, and the liver edge identified. Anteriorly, the phrenoesophageal ligament should be freed from the anterior or left crus using cautery to increase the portion of sac available for division. The sac is then entered and the phrenoesophageal ligament and sac are resected medially by placing the fingers of the left hand astride the attachments between the gastroesophageal junction and the crura of the diaphragm, dividing the hepatic branches of the vagus nerve, and joining up with the posterior division of the sac made previously. The anterior sac is then divided laterally, stopping at the level of the short gastric vessels. This completely frees the sac circumferentially from all hiatal attachments except the short gastric vessels.

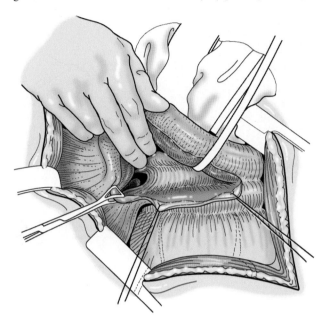

3a

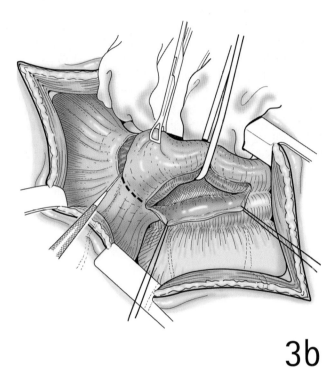

3b

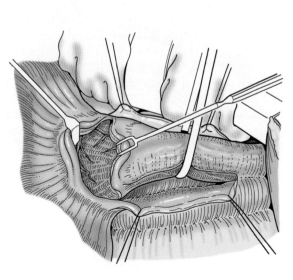

3c

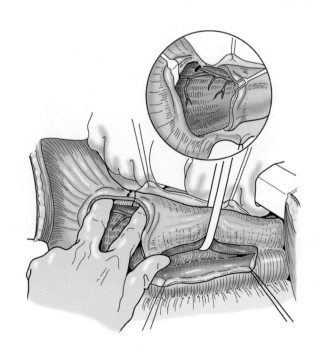

3d

Division of the short gastric vessels

4 A small Richardson retractor is placed in the caudad position and a lung clamp is placed on the stomach in the cephalad direction just below the gastroesophageal junction, and the short gastric vessels are exposed, ligated with 2/0 silk, and divided. If the hernia is large, this task is relatively easy as the short gastric vessels are elongated. If the hernia sac is very small, however, this portion of the operation may need to be completed through a separate radial incision in the diaphragm. The short gastric vessels are divided until the right gastroepiploic arcade is visible. This completes the exposure and mobilization of the esophagus, gastroesophageal junction, and fundus, from the inferior pulmonary vein to midstomach on the greater curve side.

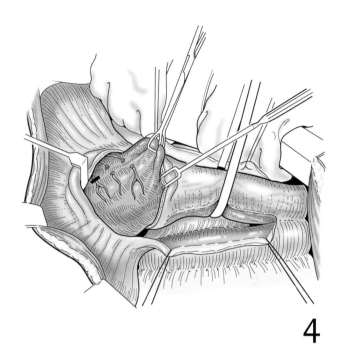

4

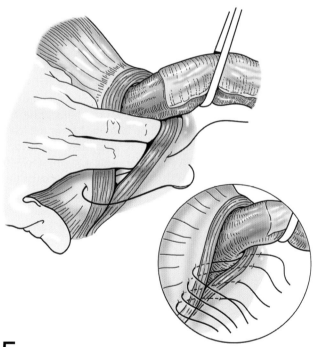

5

Placement of crural sutures for closure of the hiatus

5 The stomach and gastroesophageal junction are reduced to ensure that they will easily go below the hiatus. The need for a lengthening procedure is rare, except in the case of reoperations. At this stage the hiatal crural sutures should be placed and tagged, because they will allow the hiatus to be closed as the last step of the procedure. Figure-of-eight sutures of 1 polypropylene (Prolene) are placed through the right and left crura, taking up the right crus to the insertion of the pericardium but using only half of the left crus. This allows space for the esophagus and gastroesophageal junction when the sutures are tied. Care must be taken that the sutures are not driven within the pericardium and that they do not become twisted during placement.

Removal of the gastroesophageal fat pad

6 The gastroesophageal fat pad is divided in the midline and removed, with the division proceeding cephalad from the stomach to the gastroesophageal junction and esophagus. Both vagal trunks should be carefully preserved. The trunks may be visualized and palpated, but at no time should they be put in jeopardy. The remaining fatty tissue, including the vagus nerves, is allowed to retract and will be included within the wrap. Meticulous cauterization or ligation of multiple gastric nutrient vessels is required to avoid formation of a hematoma. This maneuver clears a portion of the gastric serosa and gastroesophageal junction for the later steps of the operation and exposes sound tissue in which to place the fundoplication sutures.

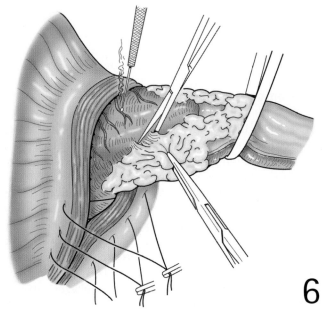

6

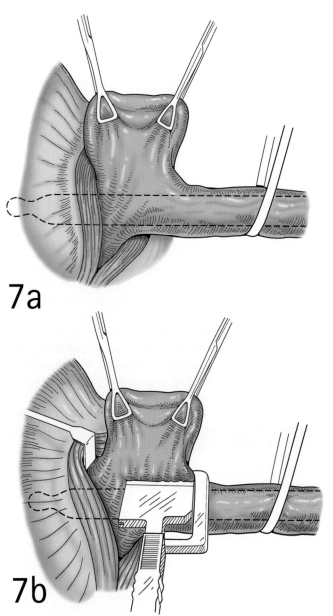

7a

7b

Uncut Collis gastroplasty

7a,b A 50-Fr Maloney dilator is passed by mouth through the gastroesophageal junction into the stomach, for use as a mandrel about which an uncut tubular extension of the esophagus will be fashioned from the lesser curvature of the stomach. This is accurately and simply achieved by applying a TA 30 stapler using 4.8-mm staples to the stomach at the angle of His, parallel to the lesser curvature of the stomach and the indwelling dilator. Because the alignment pin is not used in this application, special care should be taken to ensure that the staples and crimping anvil are accurately aligned.

Nissen fundoplication

8a,b After the staples have been placed and the stapling device removed, the previously mobilized fundus is imbricated 360 degrees around the 30-mm uncut Collis gastroplasty tube or neo-esophagus, following the technique developed by Nissen. The wrap is fashioned loosely with the dilator in place and is maintained with one row of interrupted seromuscular 2/0 silk sutures, which initially approximate the fundus to the Collis gastroplasty tube over a 2-cm length. A second, outer row of 3/0 silk is used to reinforce these sutures, going from stomach to stomach. The vagi are located within the fundal wrap in their normal position. At each step of the procedure injury to these nerves must be avoided – accidental vagotomy is the most common cause of 'gas bloat' syndrome in the postoperative period. It is noteworthy that the fundoplication, as described, avoids placing sutures near the vagal trunks: the anchoring sutures for the plication are all on the stomach, not the esophagus. The purpose of the uncut staple line is to establish a frenula that will prevent the neo-esophagus from telescoping out of the fundoplication and to reduce tension.

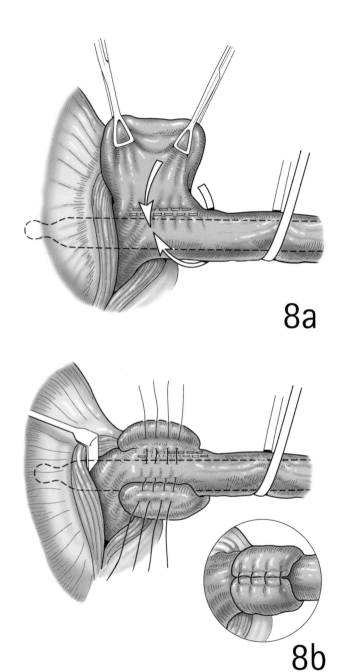

8a

8b

Reduction of the wrap and closure of the hiatus

9a–c Once the fundoplication is complete, the reconstructed area is reduced below the diaphragm and is held in place with three interrupted horizontal mattress sutures of 2/0 polypropylene (Johnsrud sutures). These sutures catch the esophagus just above the gastroesophageal junction, passing through the stomach and underneath the crus and diaphragm. These sutures cover 270 degrees, beginning medially at the level of the last posterior crural suture at the insertion of the pericardium. The second suture should be positioned halfway between the first and third sutures. The final suture should be placed at the last suture of the left or anterior crus. The wrap is then reduced with the dilator in place, and the anchoring Johnsrud sutures are tied and divided. The crural sutures are then tied and divided; the surgeon works from the aorta to the pericardium, ensuring that there is one finger's breadth posteriorly between the esophagus and the crus with each suture tied. If the last suture is too tight, one throw (or an entire suture) should be removed to allow adequate space posteriorly. This ensures a hiatus large enough to prevent dysphagia. At this stage the dilator is removed and a nasogastric tube is passed into the stomach. Hemostasis is secured, a chest tube is placed, and the incision is closed in the usual manner.

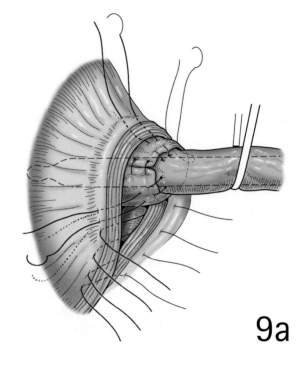

9a

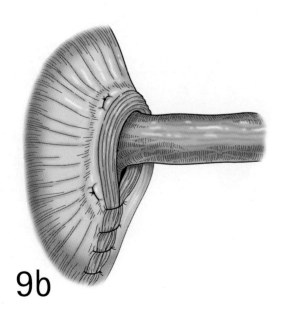

9b

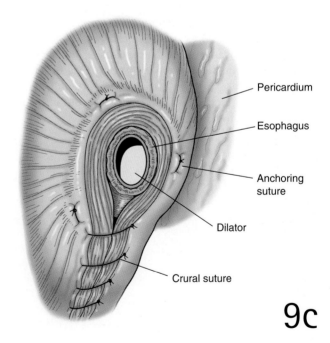

Pericardium

Esophagus

Anchoring suture

Dilator

Crural suture

9c

POSTOPERATIVE CARE

The morning after the day of the operation, the nasogastric tubes may be removed. Oral feeding may begin safely on the next day and progresses from a liquid to a general diet during the next 2–3 days. Chest tubes are removed once drainage has reduced to less than 250 mL. Total hospitalization time is approximately 6 days.

Complications

Minor leakage from any site is usually asymptomatic, localized, and confined. If leakage is suspected, a fluoroscopic study should be performed using a water-soluble medium (Gastrografin). If a leak is observed, chest and nasogastric tubes should remain in place for 5–7 days. After this period, repeat radiographical examination almost invariably shows that the leaks have sealed completely. Oral feeding may be resumed safely after tapering off parenteral feeding and removing all the drainage tubes.

OUTCOMES

The results of the uncut Collis–Nissen procedure have been described extensively in the literature by the authors and their colleagues. Mortality has been extremely low. The reports by Piehler et al (1984), Allen et al (1993), and Deschamps et al (1997) collectively reported on 300 patients who had the transthoracic uncut Collis–Nissen procedure with no operative deaths. Trastek et al in 1998 reported on the first 100 consecutive patients undergoing primary uncut Collis–Nissen procedure by one surgeon. In that series, there were two postoperative deaths (2%) both cardiac in origin and both occurring in the first 25 patients. Morbidity remains acceptable and consistent: Piehler (29%), Allen (30.8%), and Trastek (23%). Similar to so many procedures, Trastek et al (1998) demonstrated a learning curve with the uncut Collis–Nissen procedure. In the first 25 patients there were 10 complications (40%) compared with 13 complications (17%) in the next 75 patients ($p = 0.03$). The leak rate in our series ranged from 0% to 3.9%, with most being contained and never requiring further treatment.

While complete objective follow-up is the gold standard, we at Belsey feel that the patients remain the most sensitive tool for assessing the late results of antireflux surgery. In general, postoperative studies were not routinely performed on totally asymptomatic patients but were often performed to evaluate specific symptoms. Trastek et al (1998) described subjective long-term results for the uncut Collis–Nissen procedure. Median follow-up was 8.3 years. Results were excellent (no symptoms) in 59% of the patients, good (mild reflux without treatment necessary) in 25%, fair (moderate reflux controlled with medication or dilations needed) in 8%, and poor (severe reflux unrelieved with medication, or worse postoperatively, or reoperation required) in 7%. Dysphagia was present in 6%, recurrence of reflux symptoms in 5%, and hiatal hernia recurrence in 3%. This was similar to the findings of Piehler et al – excellent to good results in 84% of patients, fair results in 7.8%, and poor results in 8.4%.

ACKNOWLEDGMENTS

All the illustrations used in this chapter have been redrawn from originals supplied by the Mayo Foundation, for which copyright is held by the Mayo Foundation.

FURTHER READING

Allen MS, Trastek VF, Deschamps C, Pairolero PC. Intrathoracic stomach: presentation and results of operation. *Journal of Thoracic and Cardiovascular Surgery* 1993; **105:** 253–59.

Deschamps C, Trastek VF, Allen MS, Pairolero PC, Johnson JO, Larson DR. Long-term results after reoperation for failed antireflux procedures. *Journal of Thoracic and Cardiovascular Surgery* 1997; **113:** 545–51.

Piehler JM, Payne WS, Cameron AJ, Pairolero PC. The uncut Collis–Nissen procedure for esophageal hiatal hernia and its complications. *Problems in General Surgery* 1984; **1:** 1–14.

Trastek VF, Deschamps C, Allen MS, Miller DL, Pairolero PC, Thompson A. Uncut Collis–Nissen fundoplication: learning curve and long-term results. *Annals of Thoracic Surgery* 1998; **66:** 1739–44.

Trastek VF, Visbal AL. The Collis gastroplasty for gastroesophageal reflux. In: Yang SC, Cameron DE eds. *Current therapy in cardiovascular surgery*. Philadelphia: Mosby, 2004: 410–13.

44

Reoperative antireflux surgery using the thoracic approach

ALEX G. LITTLE MD

Elizabeth Berry Gray Chair and Professor, Department of Surgery, Wright State University School of Medicine, Dayton, Ohio, USA

HISTORY

Although the history of antireflux surgery is relatively brief, a multitude of surgical options are available that have been performed through both thoracic and abdominal routes. Predictably, failure and/or success rates have varied. Globally speaking, however, a long-term success rate of approximately 90% has been the standard. The 10% failure rate may be due either to the recurrence of reflux or the substitution of new symptoms, such as dysphagia or bloating for heartburn.

The limited long-term follow-up of laparoscopic antireflux surgery patients means that neither its failure rate as an initial operation nor its appropriateness as an option for reoperative surgery can yet be determined. Speculatively, the failure rate can be expected to remain relatively unchanged, as laparoscopic surgical technique now appears to be identical to that used in the open approach.

PATHOPHYSIOLOGY

Diagnosis

An antireflux operation may seem to fail because it was an inappropriate procedure. An antireflux procedure performed for a primary motility disorder of the esophagus, for cardiac disease, or for cholecystitis obviously will not succeed. For this reason, before surgical intervention for gastroesophageal reflux disease is undertaken, any doubts regarding the diagnosis should be eliminated, and esophageal function tests, both esophageal manometry and pH monitoring, should be performed if there is any question. Patients with classic heartburn and endoscopically confirmed esophagitis probably do not routinely need this level of testing. However, patients with atypical symptoms, patients with significant dysphagia, and patients without endoscopically identified esophagitis should all be strongly considered for function testing before operation to avoid this type of error.

Surgical technique

Although surgeons differ regarding some aspects of surgical technique, such as the need for division of the short gastric vessels, some principles are clearly essential. These include the need to close the esophageal hiatus posteriorly before construction of a fundoplication, the need to ensure placement of a gastric wrap around the distal esophagus rather than the proximal stomach, and the requirement of performing a fundoplication that is neither too tight nor too long. When these principles are violated, failure is more likely. Closure of the hiatus retards mediastinal dislocation of the wrap, which potentiates its disruption. Wrapping the proximal stomach can result in recurrent reflux or cause obstruction or dysphagia, or both. Finally, either an excessively tight or long wrap can cause both dysphagia and severe bloating.

PREOPERATIVE ASSESSMENT AND PREPARATION

Functional tests

Whereas esophageal function tests should be obtained selectively before primary antireflux surgery, they should routinely be performed in all patients before reoperative surgery. They provide essential information regarding remaining esophageal peristaltic capability and document the presence or absence of recurrent reflux.

Anatomical study

All patients should be studied both with a barium contrast radiological examination and an endoscopic examination. These examinations provide essential information about the relationship of the esophagus and fundus to each other and to the diaphragm. Endoscopy not only supplements the radiographical information but also is used to assess the absence or presence and the severity of esophagitis and the tightness of the wrap.

SURGICAL OPTIONS

Reoperative surgery can be carried out through either an abdominal or a thoracic approach, can utilize either open or minimally invasive techniques, and can consist of either a redo of the standard antireflux procedure, a standard antireflux procedure complemented by an esophageal lengthening technique such as the Collis gastroplasty, or resection of diseased tissue and reconstruction with colon interposition. The author's opinion, based on painful experience, is that the thoracic approach is necessary for many patients. The supradiaphragmatic, virginal esophagus is easily mobilized. After peripheral detachment of the diaphragm, ready access to and exposure of the left upper quadrant is achieved, which allows safe and expeditious lysis of adhesions and mobilization of the necessary structures.

Experience has also shown that patients undergoing their first reoperation can usually be adequately treated with a redo of the standard procedure, with or without a Collis gastroplasty. In patients undergoing their third reoperation, functional deterioration and anatomical compromise are both usually present, and a more reliable outcome can be obtained with resection and interposition of either colon or jejunum. When a patient is undergoing a second reoperation, the surgeon must use judgment as to the wisdom of performing a redo procedure versus resection.

OPERATION

After induction of anesthesia, a double-lumen endotracheal tube is inserted, the stomach is decompressed with a nasal gastric tube, the patient is placed in the right decubitus position, and the operation is performed either through the bed of the resected left seventh rib or in the seventh intercostal space.

1 The inferior pulmonary ligament is divided up to the level of the inferior pulmonary vein, and the lung is collapsed and packed anteriorly and superiorly to provide exposure of the thoracic esophagus. The esophagus is dissected from its mediastinal bed at a location above any inflammatory changes and encircled with a Penrose drain. The esophagus is subsequently mobilized fully from the aortic arch to the esophageal hiatus. The diaphragm is then incised peripherally approximately 2 cm from its insertion into the chest wall. This incision begins at the pericardial fat with avoidance of the phrenic nerve and extends laterally until the spleen is identified and accessible.

The stomach is initially separated from the spleen with division of the short gastric vessels if they were not previously divided. This provides access to the lesser sac. The dissection is then carried superiorly and medially with complete release of the fundus from the diaphragm and retroperitoneum. The stomach and diaphragm are typically nearly fused. Separating them requires patience and persistence. Adhesions between the anterior stomach and the liver are also lysed, and the liver is retracted free. When the adhesions and scar tissue binding the esophagus and stomach to the esophageal hiatus are being divided, it is helpful for the surgeon's left hand to be placed in the hiatus below the diaphragm while the sharp dissection is performed from the thoracic side.

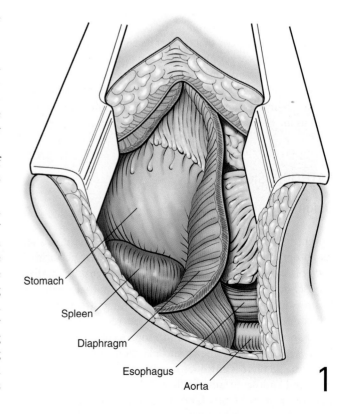

Stomach

Spleen

Diaphragm

Esophagus

Aorta

1

2 With complete freedom of the distal esophagus and the fundus, the anatomy is inspected to determine the cause of failure. This is carried out in the context of the data obtained from the preoperative assessment. Most frequently what is found is either a partial or total disruption of the initial wrap, placement of a Nissen fundoplication around the proximal stomach, or excessive length or tightness of a Nissen wrap. All remnants of the previous wrap need to be dissected free to try to restore normal anatomy. At this point, based on operative assessment of the integrity of the tissues and the preoperative data, the surgeon chooses between the surgical options.

It is always difficult and sometimes impossible to identify and/or preserve the integrity of the vagus nerves. Nonetheless, clinically important problems with delayed gastric emptying are uncommon, and the sequelae of pyloroplasty can be quite unpleasant. Consequently, the author does not routinely perform any type of gastric emptying procedure. This can be done at a later date for the small number of patients who require it.

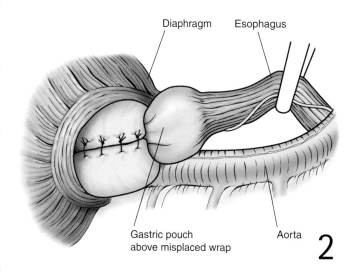

3 When a redo approach is chosen, the same principles as for primary antireflux surgery should be used. In the author's experience, a Nissen fundoplication is usually possible. This is performed with a large bougie in the esophagus and consists of the usual three-stitch-length fundoplication around the distal esophagus with closure of the hiatus posteriorly.

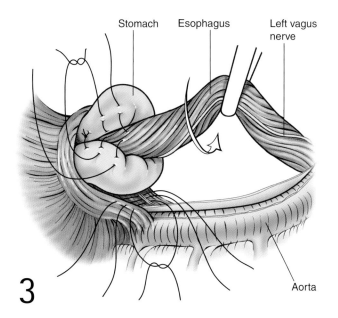

4 When patients are being reoperated for the third time, when the esophagus has been rendered nonfunctional, or when there is loss of tissue integrity with either a nondilatable stricture or an actual chronic fistula, the distal esophagus should be resected and replaced with a segment of healthy colon or jejunum. The author's experience is with the use of a short segment of left colon, which provides good long-term function. This means that for all patients undergoing reoperative surgery, the bowel should be mechanically cleansed preoperatively. At surgery, enough colon is prepared to bridge the short gap between the distal esophagus and the stomach; division of the midcolic vessels is usually not required. The colon is placed in isoperistaltic fashion and sutured in an end-to-side fashion to the posterior fundus.

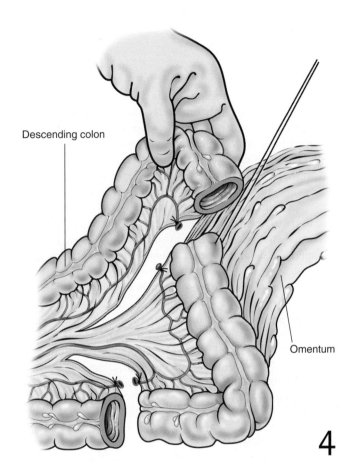

Descending colon

Omentum

4

OUTCOME

The outcome of repeated antireflux surgery is not as good as for primary surgery. Experience shows that after one previous operation and when a redo procedure is performed, 75–85% of patients have a good result with elimination of heartburn and only minor dysphagia or bloating. Although these are good results, they are significantly worse than for primary operations. In patients who have undergone multiple previous operations, it is essential that the surgeon maximize the chances of a good outcome. For this reason the conservative approach of resection and interposition with healthy tissue should be considered in the presence of extensive functional or anatomic compromise.

FURTHER READING

Hunter JG. Approach and management of patients with recurrent gastroesophageal reflux disease. *Journal of Gastrointestinal Surgery* 2001; 5: 451–57.

Little AG, Ferguson MD, Skinner DB. Reoperation for failed antireflux operations. *Journal of Thoracic and Cardiovascular Surgery* 1986; 91: 511–17.

Luketich JD, Fernando HC, Christie NA, et al. Outcomes after minimally invasive reoperation for gastroesophageal reflux disease. *Annals of Thoracic Surgery* 2002; 74: 328-32.

Smith CD, McClusky DA, Rajad MA, Lederman AB, Hunter JG. When fundoplication fails. *Annals of Surgery* 2005; 241: 861–69.

45

Thoracoscopic cardiomyotomy for achalasia

CHRISTOPHER JOHN MARTIN MB BS, MSC, FRACS
Professor of Surgery, University of Sydney; Head of Surgery, Nepean Hospital, Sydney, Australia

HISTORY

Longitudinal myotomy of the distal esophagus through a thoracotomy was first reported for achalasia by Heller in 1914. The morbidity of the thoracotomy wound, both immediate and delayed, led to popularization of distal esophageal myotomy by laparotomy.

Since the early 1990s the procedure has been performed increasingly using a minimally invasive technique such that open operations are now only rarely performed. Initially most operations were performed thoracoscopically rather than laparoscopically. That balance has now changed for several reasons. Firstly, the incidence of persistent dysphagia after thoracoscopy would appear to be higher because an adequate distal extent of longitudinal myotomy is more difficult to achieve. Secondly, the rate of convalescence would appear to be slower after the thoracoscopic approach. Thirdly, the incidence of pathological gastroesophageal reflux is probably higher than initially thought after thoracoscopic cardiomyotomy, and addition of an antireflux procedure is technically difficult by the thoracoscopic but not the laparoscopic approach. At this stage, however, these comparisons have not been made in a randomized study.

Nevertheless there is still a place for thoracoscopic cardiomyotomy. For instance, the laparoscopic approach might be precluded by postoperative adhesions or the operating surgeon might feel more adept operating in the chest rather than the abdomen.

In this section thoracoscopic cardiomyotomy will be described in detail, with limited additional remarks only made to cover the operation performed by thoracotomy.

PRINCIPLES AND JUSTIFICATION

The principal alternative approach to surgery for achalasia is forceful disruption of the lower esophageal sphincter with an endoscopic balloon. The advantages of the surgical approach are a low perforation rate, an ability to recognize and remedy perforation at the time should it occur, and a long-term improvement in quality of swallowing for a higher percentage of patients.

PREOPERATIVE ASSESSMENT

The diagnosis of achalasia is suspected on clinical history of dysphagia, supported by contrast radiology and endoscopy of the esophagus and proven by esophageal manometry. Complications of achalasia, such as gross malnutrition and severe respiratory impairment due to repeated aspiration are rarely seen these days.

PREPARATION

Preoperative discussion with the patient should cover the following issues: intraoperative perforation, incomplete myotomy leading to persistent dysphagia, and postoperative gastroesophageal reflux. Patients should be aware that associated dysfunction of the esophageal body can result, in the long term, in dysphagia, irrespective of the therapy chosen.

The patient is advised to take fluids only in the 24 hours before surgery to ensure that no residual solid matter is left in the esophagus. This interval may need to be adjusted depending upon the amount of food noted at the diagnostic endoscopy after a standard 6- to 8-hour fast.

OPERATION

Anesthesia

Deflation of the left lung during the procedure is achieved after insertion of a double-lumen endotracheal tube.

Positioning

1 The patient is placed in the right lateral decubitus position, slightly prone. The left lateral interspaces are distracted to facilitate port placement by placing a large sand bag under the right lower lateral chest wall.

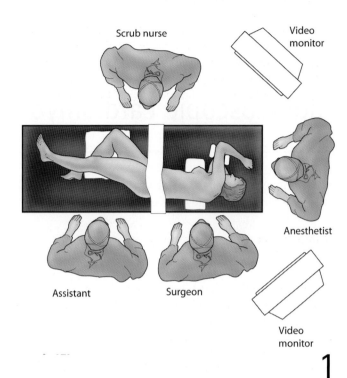

1

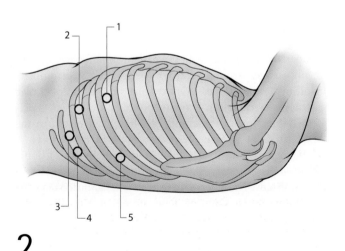

2

Port placement

2 A left pneumothorax is created by blunt dissection in the seventh interspace in the anterior axillary line. Insertion of an 11 mm port allows the insertion of a 30 degree thoracoscope. The remaining ports are inserted under direct vision. Choosing the best site for port insertion is assisted by preliminary palpation of the interspace, while at the same time viewing the interspaces internally with the thoracoscope.

An 11 mm port is placed as caudally as possible in the midaxillary line in the ninth interspace just above the lateral insertion of the diaphragm. This port is used for distal retraction of the left crus with the claws of a laparoscopic Babcock forceps as well as distal displacement of the dome of the left hemidiaphragm with the shaft of the instrument.

An 11 mm port is placed in the tenth interspace, just lateral to the lateral border of the erector spinae muscles. A 5 mm port is also placed in the tenth interspace 3–4 cm anterior to the 11 mm port. After insertion of these ports, the thoracoscope is switched to the 11 mm port in the tenth interspace.

Finally a 5 mm port is inserted in the eighth interspace in the posterior axillary line. This port is used for periesophageal dissection and the cardiomyotomy.

Positioning of staff and monitors

The surgeon stands on the left-hand side of the operating table. The assistant stands just caudad to the surgeon. The scrub nurse stands on the right-hand side of the operating table. Two monitors are placed cephalad to these three persons, one on either side of the operating table. (see Figure 1)

Mobilization of the left lung

3 The patient is tilted head down to assist cephalad displacement of the left lung. A blunt retractor is placed between the diaphragm and the diaphragmatic surface of the left lung to push the lung cephalad and expose the left inferior pulmonary ligament. This ligament is divided in a cephalad direction with scissors inserted through the tenth interspace 5 mm port. The cephalad limit of this dissection is the left inferior pulmonary vein. After this dissection the lower portion of the left lung falls away cephalad.

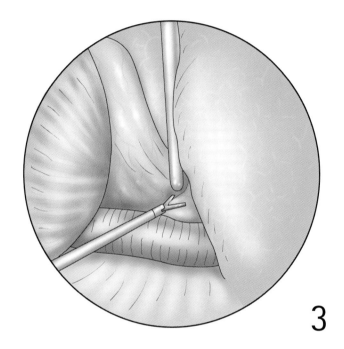

3

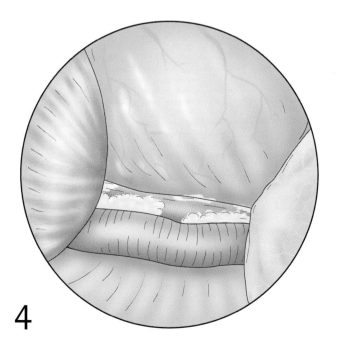

4

Exposure of the esophagus

4 The structures of the mediastinum are identified for orientation. To be defined in a posterior to anterior axis just above the diaphragm are the vertebral bodies, the descending aorta, the triangular space overlying the distal esophagus, and the pericardium. If the position of the esophagus is uncertain at this point, it can be defined by having a flexible endoscope passed into the distal esophagus and prodding its lateral wall with the instrument lighted.

5 The mediastinal pleura overlying the esophagus is picked up and divided in a caudad direction. The incision starts just caudad to the left inferior pulmonary vein and extends to the reflection of mediastinal pleura onto the diaphragm. The scissors are inserted through the eighth interspace 5 mm port. Laparoscopic Debakey forceps inserted in the ninth space 11 mm port and the tenth space 5 mm ports distract the pleura anteriorly and posteriorly respectively. The scrub nurse holds the anterior grasper. The assistant holds the posterior grasper in his left hand and the telescope in his right. This exposes the fibro-fatty tissue overlying the left lateral side of the esophagus, which needs to be divided in a longitudinal direction to expose the longitudinal fibers of the distal esophagus. One or two interconnecting branches between the anterior and posterior vagal trunks may be encountered which need to be divided. There may also be one or two small esophageal branches to the aorta, which need to be coagulated. Once the peri-esophageal plane has been identified it should be opened up both anteriorly and posteriorly by blunt dissection to expose the left lateral wall of the esophagus. The two DeBakey forceps are used to retract peri-esophageal adventitia laterally during this exposure.

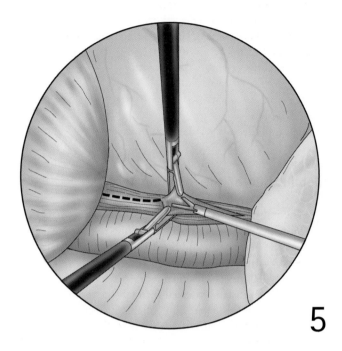

5

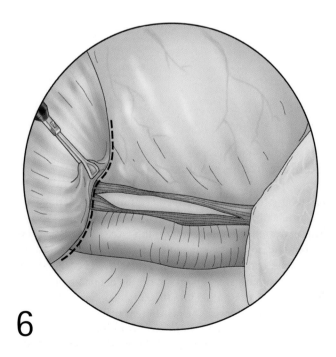

6

6 Once the fleshy fibers of the left crus are encountered, division of the pleura proceeds anteriorly and posteriorly along the line of reflection of mediastinal pleura onto the diaphragm for 1–2 cm in either direction. This allows the muscular left crus where it overlies the esophagus to be firmly grasped with the laparoscopic Babcock forceps. At this point the anterior and posterior vagal trunks should be clearly visible at the anterior and posterior limits of the subcrural dissection. Subcrural dissection is essential to access and divide the circular fibers of the distal esophagus and the uppermost sling fibers of the stomach. The phrenoesophageal ligament is not recognizable as a distinct structure. It amounts to little more than peri-esophageal adventitia slightly more resilient than the adventitia above.

The myotomy

7 The longitudinal myotomy is begun at the level of dilated esophagus as determined endoscopically at the time. In order to find the submucosal plane the muscle is grasped anterior and posterior to the point of commencement of the myotomy and distracted. The plane is soon encountered after several small trial longitudinal cuts. The graspers need to be slightly repositioned at this time to pick up and gently distract the edges of the myotomy.

The submucosal plane is developed caudad by opening the blunt-nosed scissors. The myotomy is extended caudally through mobilized muscularis propria. With each cut of the myotomy the graspers are repositioned further caudad. The mucosa is separated from the muscularis propria over a quarter of the esophageal circumference by blunt lateral dissection through the loose relatively avascular submucosal plane. This allows the disturbingly thin mucosa to bulge laterally with minimal luminal insufflation

The endoscopist determines the end point of the myotomy functionally. It is the point at which the myotomy enables the gastroesophageal junction to pout open with air insufflation alone. The endoscope needs to manipulated very gently as the esophageal mucosa deep to the myotomy might potentially be torn. If necessary the myotomy will need to be extended to achieve this end point. The other guide to the end point is the submucosa itself. In the esophagus it is loose and avascular. At the gastroesophageal junction it becomes less loose and more vascular.

Once the myotomy is complete, it is leak tested by gentle luminal insufflation with the myotomy submerged in irrigation fluid.

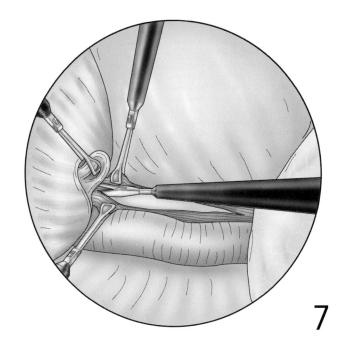

7

PROBLEMS

Bleeding points on the cut muscle can be carefully coagulated, taking great care not to coagulate the mucosa.

The most likely point for perforation is the distal end of the myotomy where the submucosal tissue is less loose. A tiny perforation can be closed by careful mucosa-to-mucosa suture and decompressed with a nasoesophageal tube placed proximal to the myotomy

Closure

A small caliber intercostal catheter is inserted to drain the base of the left pleural cavity. The left lung is then re-inflated. Skin wounds are closed with subcuticular absorbable sutures.

POSTOPERATIVE CARE

The intercostal catheter is usually removed on the first postoperative day. Clear fluids are commenced on the first postoperative day after the integrity of the esophagus is assured by contrast radiology. A pureed diet is usually commenced on the second postoperative day and continued for a week.

OUTCOME

The primary expectation of the patient will be a relief of dysphagia and an ability to eat normally. Whilst a very significant improvement in swallowing is to be expected, the ability to swallow normally never really returns completely. Nevertheless, the usual improvement is so great that patients don't seem to mind that normality has not been quite achieved. Weight gain postoperatively can be very impressive. Regurgitation is likely to disappear and the patient should be able to lie flat without fear of aspiration. Enquiry should be made about heartburn as a possible complication.

THORACOTOMY FOR CARDIOMYOTOMY

Only differences from the thoracoscopic approach are mentioned.

Good access to the lowermost esophagus is possible through a left lateral seventh space thoracotomy. The assistant stands on the right-hand side of the table opposite the surgeon. The wound is distracted with a Finochetti retractor. The instruments used to mobilize the left lung, expose the esophagus, and perform the myotomy will be different, obviously, but the sequence of the surgical steps will be the same.

FURTHER READING

Csendes A, Braghetto I, Henriquez A, Cortes C. Late results of a prospective randomized study comparing forceful dilatation and esophagomyotomy in patients with achalasia. *Gut* 1989; **30**: 299–304.

Patti MG, Pellegrini CA, Horgan S, et al. Thoracoscopic versus laparoscopic modified myotomy for achalasia: efficacy and safety in 87 patients. *Journal of the American College of Surgeons* 1999; **189**: 164–70.

Way LW. Minimally invasive surgery for achalasia. An 8 year experience with 168 patients. *Annals of Surgery* 1999; **230**: 587–94.

46

Esophagogastrectomy for adenocarcinoma of the esophagus and cardia

A. H. HÖLSCHER MD, FACS, FRCS
Professor of Surgery and Chairman, Department of Visceral and Vascular Surgery, University of Cologne, Cologne, Germany

RUDOLF BUMM MD
Associate Professor, Department of Surgery, Technical University of Munich, Munich, Germany

J. RÜDIGER SIEWERT MD
Professor, Director and Chairman, Department of Surgery, Technical University of Munich, Munich, Germany

CLASSIFICATION

1 In this institution the term *adenocarcinoma of the gastroesophageal junction* is used to describe all tumors that have their center within an area 5 cm orad or 5 cm aborad to the lower esophageal sphincter (LOS). Esophageal adenocarcinomas and subcardial gastric carcinomas are included in this category if they infiltrate the cardia, meaning the terminal esophageal musculature. This therefore leads to the following classification for different types of adenocarcinomas at the gastroesophageal junction:

1 Type I: adenocarcinoma in Barrett's esophagus (center of tumor 1–5 cm oral to the LOS)
2 Type II: carcinoma arising from the cardia proper (center of tumor between 1 cm above and 2 cm below the LOS)
3 Type III: subcardial or fundal carcinoma of the stomach that infiltrates the lower esophagus mostly within the submucosa (center of tumor 2–5 cm below the LOS)

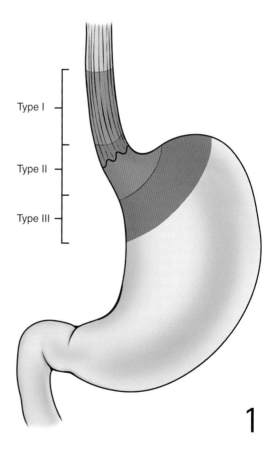

1

PRINCIPLES AND JUSTIFICATION

2a–d Five different procedures are available for the surgical treatment of these types of carcinoma:

For type I carcinomas transthoracic en bloc esophagectomy or transmediastinal (transhiatal) esophagectomy and partial upper gastrectomy can be applied (Figure 2a).

For type II and III carcinomas extended total gastrectomy with distal esophageal resection via a transhiatal approach is appropriate (Figure 2b, d). Splenectomy en bloc with gastrectomy is only performed in case of tumor infiltration of the splenic hilus or overt lymph node metastasis in this area.

Total esophagogastrectomy is a procedure for very advanced type II carcinomas (Figure 2c). This is only applied if tumor free resection margins cannot be achieved by distal esophageal resection in combination with total gastrectomy.

Distal esophageal resection with proximal partial gastrectomy and jejunum interposition represents the so-called Merendino operation.

In this chapter the surgical technique for transmediastinal subtotal esophageal resection and partial upper gastrectomy as well as total esophagogastrectomy is described (Figures 2a, c). Transthoracic en bloc esophagectomy is shown in Chapter 36.

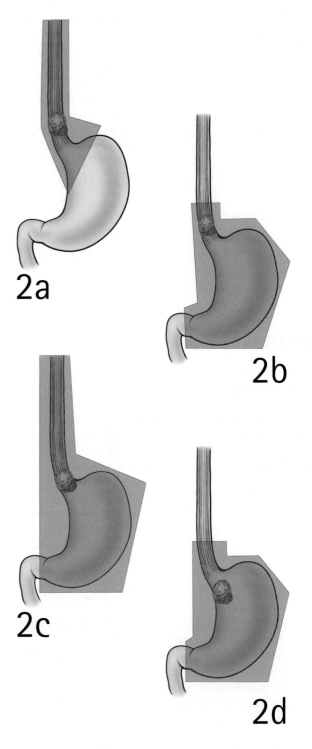

Indications

From the authors point of view transthoracic en bloc esophagectomy and upper partial gastrectomy with gastric pull-up and high intrathoracic anastomosis represents the procedure of choice for type I adenocarcinoma. The justification is the more extended mediastinal lymphadenectomy compared to transmediastinal esophagectomy. This principal is supported by the results of the prospective randomized trial by Hulscher.

Transmediastinal esophagectomy as described in the following can be justified in patients with a disturbed lung function to avoid thoracotomy. For patients with type I or type II mucosal carcinomas which usually have no lymphnode metastasis, a Merendino operation could be appropriate.

PREOPERATIVE ASSESSMENT AND PLANNING

A careful preoperative diagnostic examination is necessary for surgery of adenocarcinoma of the gastroesophageal junction. The tumor is staged by endoscopy, endoscopic ultrasonography, barium swallow, and computed tomographic scan. These investigations give quite exact information for TNM staging. If an advanced tumor of the gastroesophageal junction is present, neoadjuvant chemotherapy or radiochemotherapy may be appropriate. It is also important in preoperative assessment to consider the risk factors that are present. This includes an assessment of pulmonary, cardiac, renal, and hepatic function. In most cases a reconstruction is performed by stomach interposition, but the colon should be prepared before operation by orthotopic bowel lavage and ideally, a colonoscopy, so that an alterna-

tive is available should technical difficulties occur, as described in Chapter 35.

Anesthesia

The operation is performed under routine general anesthesia. In contrast to a transthoracic esophagectomy, a double-lumen endotracheal tube is not necessary. A peridural catheter is recommended.

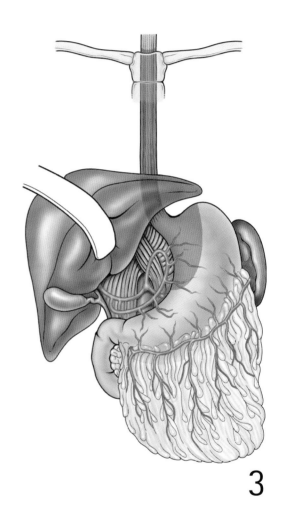

3

OPERATIONS

Transmediastinal esophagectomy and proximal gastrectomy (open technique)

3 Transmediastinal esophagectomy with proximal gastrectomy involves the subtotal removal of the esophagus and proximal stomach by a transmediastinal route (without a thoracotomy) and is performed through an abdominal and cervical approach.

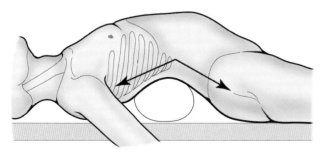

4

POSITION OF PATIENT

4 Transmediastinal esophagectomy is performed with the patient lying supine. A bolster is used to bring the cardia region forward to lessen the depth of dissection.

5 The neck is positioned as for thyroid gland surgery with the head turned to the right to expose the left part of the neck. Sterile draping is placed in such a way that two surgical teams (cervical and abdominal) can work simultaneously. The esophagus is intubated with a large tube to facilitate palpation.

If the cervical dissection is performed endoscopically, the position of the video monitor on the right side of the neck of the patient must be taken into account. In addition, enough space should be available for the movement of the mediastinoscope on the left side of the neck where the surgeon for the cervical approach is positioned.

A suprapancreatic lymphadenectomy is an important part of the operation for adenocarcinoma of the cardia. Therefore, a wide abdominal approach is necessary. The authors perform the operation via a transverse upper abdominal incision with enlargement by an upper midline incision in the direction of the xiphoid process. This approach provides an excellent view of the whole upper abdominal cavity.

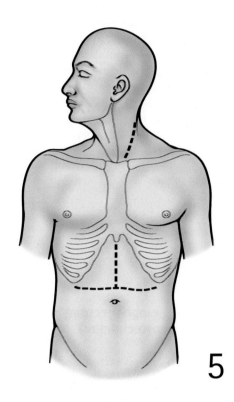

5

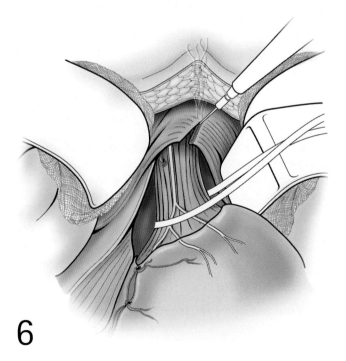

6

PREPARATION OF THE DISTAL ESOPHAGUS

6 The first step in the operation is to divide the left triangular ligament of the liver and to hold the left lobe to the right side using a retractor. The esophageal hiatus is next enlarged. It is crucial to enlarge the hiatus enough. This enlargement is performed in a ventral and slightly left lateral direction and should avoid opening the adjacent pericardium. This dissection of the anterior commissure of the diaphragm is nearly always sufficient. Very rarely an additional division of the left or right diaphragmatic crus is undertaken to improve exposure further. After dissection of the visceral peritoneum, the terminal esophagus is bluntly dissected and a tape is passed around it. The lower mediastinum can now be palpated to decide the resectability of the tumor. If it is removable, attention is turned to the stomach. The preparation of the stomach as an esophageal substitute is described in Chapter 35 on pp. 353–366.

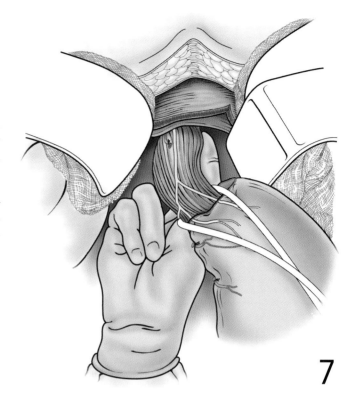

PREPARATION OF THE MEDIASTINAL ESOPHAGUS

7 After the stomach has been mobilized, transmediastinal blunt dissection of the esophagus is performed. Two or three fingers are moved close to the esophageal wall and used to free the esophagus with spreading and circular movements. A 42-Fr bougie is placed within the esophagus to facilitate palpation. All pliable tissue can be dissected bluntly without danger provided the dissection is kept close to the esophageal wall. Direct aortic branches are very rare in the lower part of the mediastinum. The only structures that cannot be bluntly divided by the fingers are the vagal trunks. These are divided with scissors.

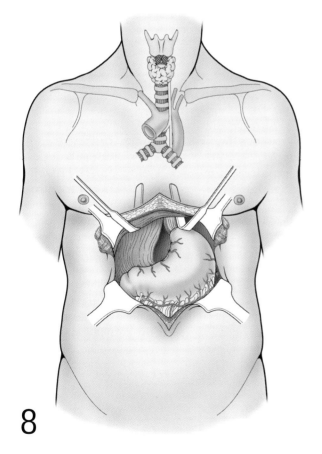

8 The esophageal hiatus can be opened up using two very long hook retractors. This allows the whole posterior mediastinum nearly up to the tracheal bifurcation to be inspected without difficulty. If bleeding occurs in this area, it can be controlled under direct vision. If bleeding is severe, it is not necessary to reposition the patient immediately and perform a thoracotomy because most of the bleeding points can be exposed and stopped through the abdominal approach.

The exposure afforded by this approach allows lymphadenectomy of the lower posterior mediastinum to be performed under direct vision. The ideal plane of dissection is the anterior wall of the aorta. The periesophageal lymphatic tissue between the pericardium and the aorta, as well as between both diaphragmatic bundles, should be removed en bloc with the esophagus. If the tumor is infiltrating the diaphragmatic bundles or the pericardium, these should be included in the resection. Attention has to be paid to the thoracic duct in order to avoid chylus fistula.

PREPARATION OF THE PROXIMAL ESOPHAGUS

9 A second surgical team commences at the same time as the first operative team by opening the neck and exposing the cervical esophagus. The approach is via a skin incision along the anterior edge of the left sternocleidomastoid muscle. The dissection of the cervical esophagus is usually accomplished without difficulty. The recurrent laryngeal nerve is displayed and preserved. The left inferior thyroid artery is dissected, ligated, and divided.

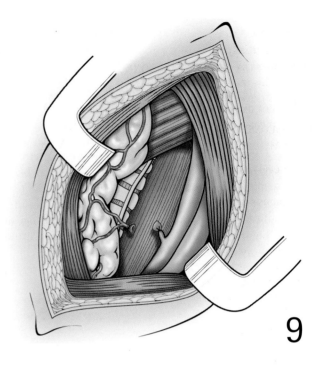

9

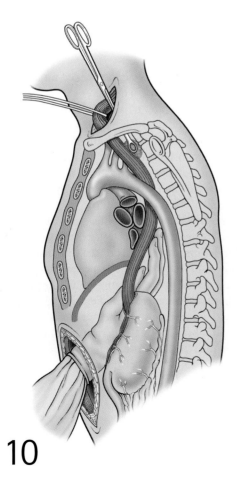

10

10 After circumferential mobilization a tape is placed around the cervical esophagus. Further dissection of the esophagus in the posterior mediastinum is performed bluntly using a sponge on a stick and goes as far as possible in the intrathoracic direction. The last step of the esophageal dissection is performed by the first surgeon, who pushes the right hand from the esophageal hiatus into the posterior mediastinum to meet the left hand or the sponge stick coming from the cervical approach. Often it is not possible to free the esophagus completely by digital dissection, but a short section remains above the tracheal bifurcation that must be dissected blind. It is very important to keep as close to the esophageal wall as possible during dissection to prevent damage to the pars membranacea of the trachea and also the azygos vein.

11 Once mobilization of the esophagus is complete, it is partially pulled up and out of the cervical incision and stapled closed. It is then divided proximal to the staple line. In this manner, a cervical esophageal stump of sufficient length is preserved.

ENDOSCOPIC DISSECTION OF THE CERVICAL AND INTRAMEDIASTINAL ESOPHAGUS

The development of a novel mediastinoscope and suitable instruments has allowed the preparation of the mediastinal esophagus under endoscopic view. Endoscopic dissection of the esophagus has advantages over conventional surgery for several reasons. First, it saves time because simultaneous work with the abdominal surgeon is possible. Second, initial experience suggests that damage to the recurrent laryngeal nerve is significantly less. Third, postoperative pulmonary problems seem to be less frequent. An alternative to the endoscopic cervical approach for mediastinal dissection is the transhiatal laparoscopic approach (see pp. 497–508).

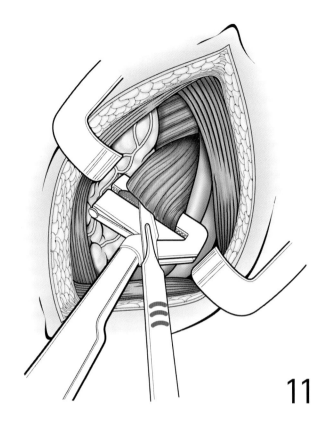

11

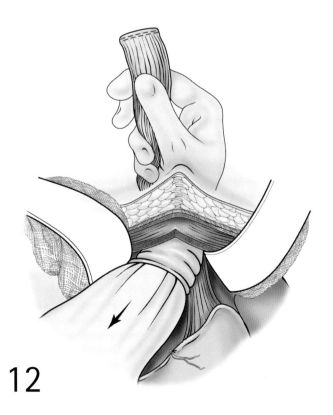

12

TRANSMEDIASTINAL PULL-THROUGH AND EXTIRPATION OF THE ESOPHAGUS

12 After conventional laparoscopic or endoscopic dissection of the esophagus and division in the cervical part, the esophagus can be pulled downward by gripping it as high as possible to avoid tearing it.

13 When the esophagus has been removed, the posterior mediastinum is tamponed with a hot, moist towel, which is left *in situ* for 5–10 minutes. As the stomach has previously been prepared in a typical manner as described in Chapter 35, the esophagus, together with the stomach, can be placed in front of the abdominal cavity. The formation of the gastric tube or the preparation of the whole stomach as an esophageal substitute is now performed using a stapler. Finally, the towel is removed from the posterior mediastinum and the esophageal hiatus is again opened by two long hook retractors. Under vision, the posterior mediastinum is checked for bleeding points. In many cases the mediastinal pleura is inadvertently opened during the dissection on one or even both sides of the esophagus. Closure of the pleura is not necessary, but the insertion of chest tubes is recommended. The esophageal hiatus is narrowed around the gastric tube to avoid internal herniation and also to close the thoracic cavity off from the abdominal cavity. If the reconstruction is undertaken using the retrosternal route, the hiatus is closed completely.

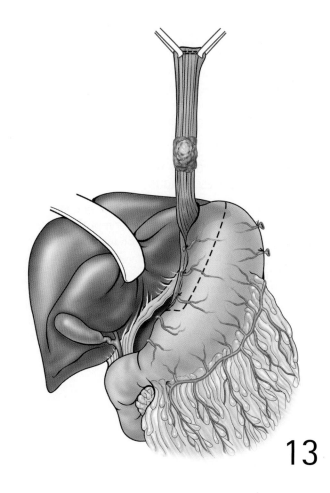

13

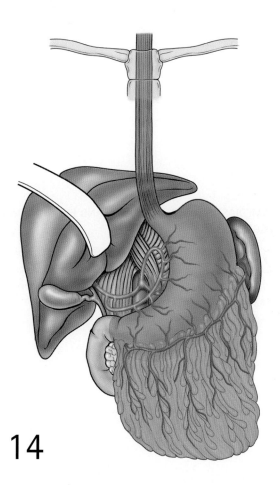

14

Total esophagogastrectomy

POSITION OF PATIENT

The positioning and approach are the same as in transmediastinal esophagectomy.

14 The shading in Figure 14 represents the extent of resection in total esophagogastrectomy. After the surgeon checks the oncological situation in the abdominal cavity with regard to distant metastases and makes sure that the tumor is resectable, the procedure starts with the usual preparation of the stomach for gastrectomy as described for gastric cancer.

15 For this purpose the omentum is dissected from the transverse colon. The right gastro-omental (epiploic) artery and vein, as well as the left gastro-omental (epiploic) vessels are divided between ligatures.

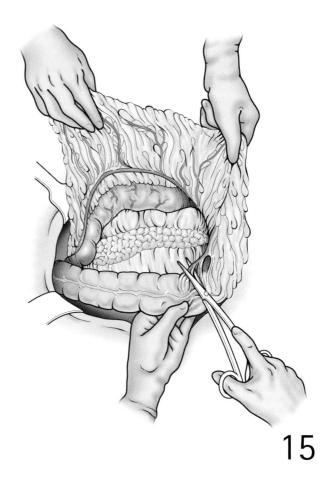

15

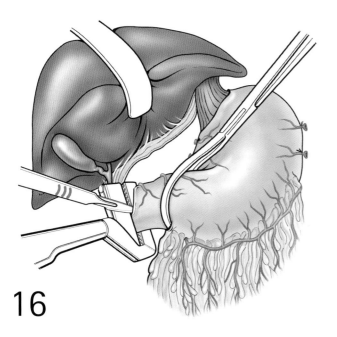

16

16 As the disease is at the cardia, the preparation of the duodenal stump is usually a relatively simple procedure. The duodenum should be closed 2 cm aborad to the pylorus using a TA 55 stapler; it is then divided. Further closure of the duodenal stump using seromuscular interrupted sutures is optional.

17 After the lesser omentum has been divided it is possible to elevate the stomach and to start preparing the tumor. Advanced tumors that initially seem difficult to remove can often be resected if dissection is performed as for a lymphadenectomy of compartment II of cancer of the body of the stomach, using the plane of the adventitia of the common hepatic artery.

The position of the common hepatic artery is usually easy to find if the gastroduodenal artery, which is exposed during dissection of the duodenal stump, is followed in a central direction. An incision in the adventitia of the common hepatic artery is continued from the right side toward the celiac trunk. All tissue in front of the common hepatic artery is removed. Another important step is the dissection of the origin of the splenic artery. Once this has been achieved it is certain that the common hepatic artery has been completely freed and is safely preserved. The coronary (left gastric) vein is divided above the junction of the common hepatic artery and the splenic artery. The left gastric artery is easy to find and is ligated and divided near the celiac trunk. If it is not possible to dissect free the common hepatic artery due to tumor infiltration, it may be sacrificed (Appleby procedure) provided the arterial vascularization of the liver is guaranteed via the gastroduodenal artery or an accessory liver artery. In this way nearly all cardia carcinomas can be dissected from the aortic wall, even if it is necessary to resect some of the diaphragmatic crura to achieve a complete resection. In the authors' experience, carcinomas of the cardia infiltrate the arteries mentioned very infrequently.

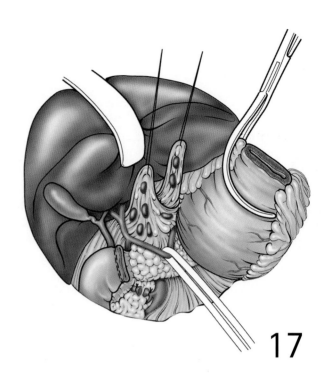

17

EXTRAGASTRIC EXTENT OF RESECTION

RETRODUODENAL AND PARA-AORTIC LYMPH NODES

The authors recommend that the lymph nodes of station 13 – that is, the retroduodenal and retropancreatic lymph nodes – be removed. For this purpose, an extensive Kocher maneuver is performed. The duodenal stump is pulled via some retained seromuscular sutures in a medial and cranial direction to facilitate the lateral mobilization of the duodenum. Lymph nodes in this area are removed. Further mobilization of the cardia tumor is performed from the left side.

PANCREAS-PRESERVING SPLENECTOMY

In advanced cancer, tumor penetration is often found at the back wall of the fundus. If the tumor has not yet infiltrated the pancreas but has led to lymph node metastases at the splenic hilus and along the splenic artery, a 'zone splenectomy' is also recommended. The authors try to avoid left pancreatectomy as it leads to a high postoperative morbidity because of pancreatic fistulae.

Zone splenectomy refers to the meticulous dissection of the splenic artery from the celiac trunk to the splenic hilus to remove the lymphatic tissue of this zone together with the spleen. The splenic artery is suture ligated halfway between the celiac trunk and the splenic hilus, whereas the splenic vein is suture ligated between the pancreatic tail and the spleen. After ligation and division of both vessels the splenectomy is performed en bloc with the cardia cancer.

LEFT PANCREATIC RESECTION

If the tumor is infiltrating the tail or the corpus of the pancreas, a radical resection is possible only by adding a left-sided pancreatectomy. The authors find it helpful to tunnel under the pancreas above the mesenteric vein and to sever the organ at an early stage of the operation. Further on, it is useful to ligate the splenic artery at the origin of the celiac trunk, and the splenic vein is ligated at its junction with the superior mesenteric vein. After severing these vessels, the left hemipancreas together with the spleen can be removed from the retroperitoneum en bloc together with the tumor.

TRANSMEDIASTINAL ESOPHAGECTOMY

18 Transmediastinal esophagectomy is performed by the method described earlier after widely opening the esophageal hiatus. After this procedure is completed, the whole of the stomach, together with the cardia and esophagus, can be removed. A reconstruction is performed using a colon interposition (as described in Chapters 36 and 37).

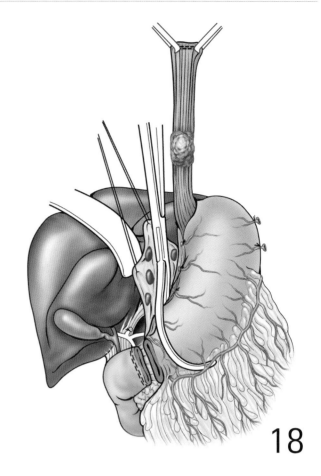

18

POSTOPERATIVE CARE

Usual postoperative care involves artificial respiration in the intensive care unit and afterward a slow change to active respiration and extubation.

Intraoperative and postoperative complications that occur after transmediastinal esophagectomy are shown in **Table 47.1**. Intraoperative complications are quite rare, with bleeding being seen only in exceptional cases. Damage to the trachea also represents a rare situation. During the early postoperative phase pneumothorax often develops if no chest drains have been placed. Chylothorax resulting from damage to the thoracic duct is fortunately also quite rare. Recurrent laryngeal nerve palsy occurs more frequently. The reason for this may be related to the blunt digital dissection of the vagus nerve during the operation, which results in intramediastinal damage to the nerves. The quite high rate of respiratory insufficiency in spite of avoidance of a thoracotomy shows that transmediastinal esophagectomy is not a lesser procedure than transthoracic esophagectomy, and is associated with the same pathophysiological consequences.

OUTCOME

Rentz reported for a series of 945 patients a postoperative mortality or morbidity of 10% and 47% after transthoracic and 9.9% and 49% after transhiatal esophagectomy.

Table 46.1 *Intraoperative and postoperative complications of 1085 transmediastinal esophagectomies* (Orringer 1999)

	Percentage
Intraoperative	
Entry in one or both pleural cavities	77.0
Splenectomy	3.0
Intraoperative uncontrollable mediastinal bleeding and death	0.3
Intraoperative abdominal or mediastinal bleeding	0.5
Membranous tracheal laceration	0.4
Postoperative	
Mediastinal bleeding < 24 h postoperative	0.5
Recurrent laryngeal nerve palsy	7.0
– transient	4.6
– persistent	2.4
Chylothorax	1.7
Cervical anastomotic leakage	13.0

In the largest available series with 1085 patients by Orringer the hospital mortality rate of transmediastinal esophagectomy was 4%. The functional results of 748 cancer patients with an average follow-up of 29 months showed dysphagia in 20%, but 10% needed no treatment. The 5-year survival rate for patients with squamous cell carcinoma in this series was 17% compared to 24% for adenocarcinoma.

In the prospective randomized Dutch trial for esophageal adenocarcinoma the 5-year survival rate after transhiatal esophagectomy was comparable with 27% but after transthoracic resection the 5-year survival rate amounted to 39%. This difference increased to 20% when the cardia cancer cases were eliminated from both arms of the trial. Therefore many esophageal centers today prefer transthoracic compared to transhiatal esophagectomy for adenocarcinoma of the esophagus.

FURTHER READING

Hölscher AH, Bollschweiler E, Bumm R, Bartels H, Siewert JR. Prognostic factors of resected adenocarcinoma of the esophagus. *Surgery* 1995; **118**: 845–55.

Hulscher JBF, van Sandick JW, de Beure AGEM, van Lanschot J. Extended transthoracic resection compared with limited transhiatal resection for adenocarcinoma of the esophagus. *New England Journal of Medicine* 2002; **347**: 1662–9.

Luketich JD, Alvelo-Rivera M, Buenaventura PO, Christie NA, McCaughan JS, Little VR, Schauer PR, Close JM, Fernando HC. Minimally invasive esophagectomy. Outcomes in 222 patients. *Annals of Surgery* 2003; **238**: 486–95.

Orringer MB, Marshall B, Jannettoni MD. Transhiatal esophagectomy: clinical experience and refinements. *Annals of Surgery* 1999; **230**: 392–403.

Siewert JR, Hölscher AH, Becker K, Gössner W. Kardiakarzinom. Versuch einer therapeutisch relevanten Klassifikation. *Chirurg* 1987; **58**: 25–32.

Stein H, Feith M, Müller J et al. Limited resection for early adenocarcinoma in Barrett's oesophagus. *Annals of Surgery* 2000; **232**: 733–42.

Swanström LL, Hanson P. Laparoscopic total esophagectomy. *Archives of Surgery* 1997; **132**: 943–9.

47

Thoracoscopic techniques for the removal of benign esophageal tumors

DAVID IAN WATSON MB, BS, MD, FRACS
Professor and Head, Flinders University Department of Surgery; Senior Consultant Surgeon and Head of Gastrointestinal Services, Flinders Medical Centre, Bedford Park, South Australia, Australia

The application of thoracoscopic techniques to the excision of benign esophageal lesions provides a minimal access approach to these lesions that avoids the need for an open thoracotomy incision. Benign esophageal lesions, which are usually leiomyomata, or less commonly esophageal wall (bronchogenic) cysts, are found within the esophageal wall musculature. In the case of leiomyomata, the tumor can at times be densely adherent to the underlying esophageal mucosa. Thoracoscopic excision entails dissecting the tumor from the surrounding esophageal wall muscle, while at the same time taking care to avoid opening the mucosa if possible. As this is not always feasible, the mucosa, if breached, can be repaired by thoracoscopic suturing.

PREOPERATIVE ASSESSMENT AND PREPARATION

Patients should undergo full cardiorespiratory evaluation, if necessary with the addition of pulmonary function testing and echocardiography. Patients unsuitable for an open thoracotomy approach should not undergo thoracoscopic surgery, as conversion to an open procedure is occasionally necessary if significant intraoperative difficulties are encountered. Computed tomographic scanning and endoscopy provide important information that helps determine the location of the tumor and ascertain the presence or absence of mucosal involvement or ulceration.

1 Unlike traditional open surgical approaches via a left thoracotomy, thoracoscopic excision can be performed through either a right- or left-sided approach to the esophagus. The choice is determined by the anatomy demonstrated preoperatively by computed tomographic scanning (i.e. if the lesion is in the right esophageal wall, then a right thoracoscopic approach is easiest). For example, for the leiomyoma of the esophagus shown in Figure 1, the best access for thoracoscopic excision entailed a right thoracoscopic approach (the arrow shows the direction of access for the endoscopic dissecting instruments). If the tumor is within the anterior or posterior esophageal wall (i.e. potentially suitable for either left or right thoracoscopic resection), the choice of approach is influenced by the proximity of the tumor to the esophageal hiatus. Distal lesions (within 5 cm of the hiatus) may best be approached from the left, as the elevation of the right hemidiaphragm can restrict access from the right. On the other hand, more proximal lesions are often better accessed from the right side, as the heart and aortic arch can restrict access from the left. From the right side, these structures do not encroach on the operative field.

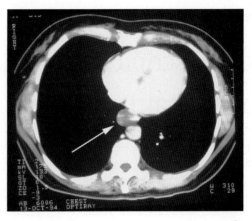

1

OPERATION

Anesthesia and position of patient

2 Two patient positions for thoracoscopic esophageal surgery can be used. Based on open surgical experience, many surgeons position their patients in the lateral position. This necessitates the placement of a double-lumen endotracheal tube to enable the lung to be collapsed. The alternative patient position (which we prefer) is the prone position. This position provides excellent access to the posterior mediastinum and enables thoracoscopic surgery to be performed without the need for lung retraction. In addition, good access to the esophagus can be obtained in this position using low-pressure (6-8 mm Hg) insufflation of the pleural cavity without collapse of the lung. This allows thoracoscopic surgery to be performed while using a single-lumen endotracheal tube if it is known preoperatively that the lung will not need to be collapsed. Low-pressure insufflation rarely creates anesthetic difficulties.

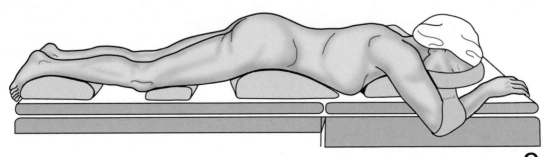

2

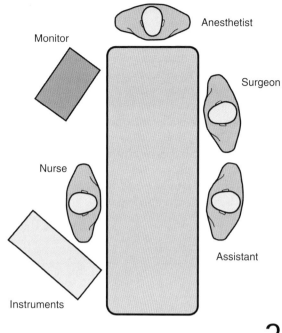

Operating theater set-up

3 When the patient is positioned prone, both the surgeon and assistant stand on the side of the patient that will provide access for thoracoscopy (i.e. right side for right thoracoscopic approach, and left for left thoracoscopy). The video monitor is positioned directly opposite the surgical team. When the lateral position is used, the surgeon and assistant stand in front of the patient, with the video monitor located opposite.

3

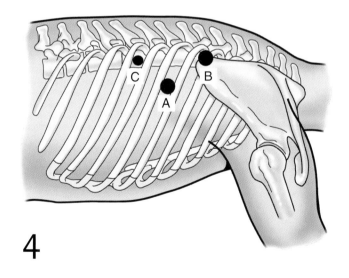

4

Thoracoscopic access

4 For the remainder of this description, a right thoracoscopic approach with the patient positioned prone is assumed. Access to the thoracic cavity is obtained using an open dissection technique. Initially, an 11-mm port is placed through the sixth intercostal space in the midaxillary line to provide access for a conventional 10-mm laparoscope (port A). The port is placed using a blunt dissection technique in which a conventional artery clip is used to open a communication into the pleural cavity before a blunt-ended trocar is passed through the chest wall. The right lung is then collapsed either by using insufflation to a maximum pressure of 5–6 mm Hg or by selectively collapsing the right lung while at the same time letting room air passively enter the pleural cavity.

Three or four ports in total provide access for surgery. All of these are placed using blunt dissection. The passage of sharp trocars should be avoided, as the intercostal vessels can be easily lacerated, which results in troublesome hemorrhage. Placement of the secondary trocars is facilitated by thoracoscopic vision. Two 5-mm ports (port C) are sited in the posterior axillary line in the fifth and seventh intercostal spaces to provide access for dissecting instruments. A further 10-mm port can be placed in the ninth intercostal space in the posterior axillary line to enable the assistant to retract structures and to facilitate specimen retrieval. If only three ports are used, then one of the 5-mm ports must be exchanged with an 11-mm port (port B) to facilitate retrieval of the specimen at the completion of the procedure, unless a 5-mm laparoscope is available.

Thoracoscopic dissection

Providing the thoracoscopic approach is from the same side of the esophagus that the tumor arose from, it can usually be easily seen through the intact mediastinal pleura. If it is not immediately visible, then it will likely become apparent after initial esophageal dissection. Alternatively, intraoperative endoscopy can be used to localize the tumor accurately.

5 The mediastinal pleura is divided to expose the tumor and adjacent esophagus. Full esophageal mobilization is unnecessary unless the tumor arises from the esophageal wall on the opposite side to the operative field.

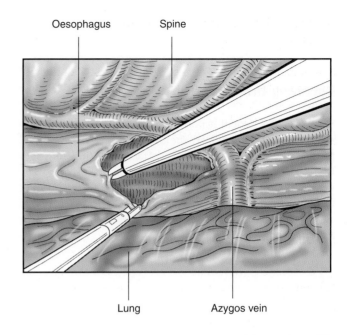

Oesophagus   Spine

Lung   Azygos vein

5

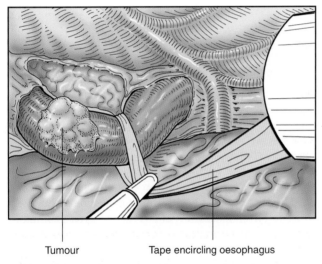

Tumour   Tape encircling oesophagus

6

6 If, however, the esophagus is fully mobilized, exposure of the tumor can be assisted by passing a tape behind the esophagus. This is used to elevate the esophagus from its bed.

7 Because benign esophageal tumors usually arise within the muscle wall of the esophagus and often do not involve mucosa, dissection close to the tumor, by separating it from adjacent muscle and the underlying mucosa, will usually be successful. Dissection is performed using a combination of diathermy hook and endoscopic scissor dissection.

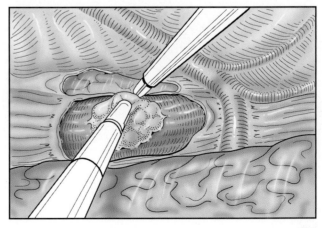

7

Determination of the integrity of esophageal mucosa

It is important to ensure that the underlying esophageal mucosa is intact. Leakage of luminal contents may not occur during thoracoscopic surgery, particularly if positive pressure insufflation is used. Hence, a high index of suspicion is essential to avoid postoperative problems from esophageal leakage. The mucosa should be carefully inspected visually. If there is any doubt about its integrity, careful intraoperative endoscopy with a flexible gastroscope can reveal whether the mucosa is intact.

Repair of esophageal mucosa

8 Perforation (deliberate or inadvertent) of esophageal mucosa is repaired by suturing the mucosal edges. This is performed using standard laparoscopic suturing methods (with intracorporeal or extracorporeal knotting). The author's preference is to use interrupted sutures, placed using a small needle attached to 4/0 polypropylene suture material, with the knots tied intracorporeally.

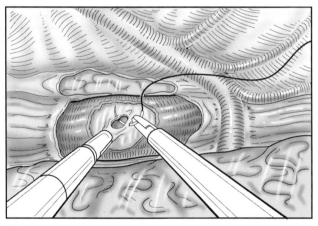

8

Specimen retrieval and closure

The dissected specimen is placed in a specimen retrieval bag, which is introduced through one of the 10-mm ports, and is delivered through this port wound. Use of a bag is essential to prevent wound seeding of the tumor. Small tumors can be removed without the need to enlarge the wound. Larger tumors can only be removed after widening the wound to an appropriate extent.

An intercostal drain is placed with its tip near the excision site to drain any possible mucosal leak.

POSTOPERATIVE CARE

Patients are not allowed oral intake until after a radiological contrast examination has been performed on the first postoperative day. If mucosal integrity is confirmed, oral fluids are commenced and the drain is removed. A vitamised diet is commenced on the second postoperative day. Patients are discharged after the second postoperative day and are maintained on a soft food diet for 2 weeks.

OUTCOME

Surgery for benign esophageal tumors is uncommon. For this reason, most reports of thoracoscopic techniques are limited to small case series or case reports. In general, these reports describe technical success and good short term outcomes. The postoperative recovery appears to be substantially faster than following thoracotomy, and the hospital stay is shorter. It is therefore reasonable to attempt the removal of benign esophageal tumors using the thoracoscopic approach, although the operating surgeon should not hesitate to convert to an open thoracotomy if the procedure is difficult.

FURTHER READING

Elli E, Espat NJ, Berger R, Jacobsen G, Knoblock L, Horgan S. Robotic-assisted thoracoscopic resection of esophageal leiomyoma. *Surgical Endoscopy* 2004; **18:** 713–16.

Roviaro GC, Maciocco M, Varoli F, Rebuffat C, Vergani C, Scarduelli A. Videothoracoscopic treatment of oesophageal leiomyoma. *Thorax* 1998; **53:** 190–2.

Taniguchi E, Kamiike W, Iwase K, Nishida T, Akashi A, Ohashi S, Matsuda H. Thoracoscopic enucleation of a large leiomyoma located on the left side of the esophageal wall. *Surgical Endoscopy* 1997; **11:** 280–2.

von Rahden BH, Stein HJ, Feussner H, Siewert JR. Enucleation of submucosal tumors of the esophagus: minimally invasive versus open approach. *Surgical Endoscopy* 2004; **18:** 924–30.

Watson DI, Britten-Jones R. Thoracoscopic excision of bronchogenic cyst of the oesophagus. *Surgical Endoscopy* 1995; **9:** 824–5.

48

Thoracolaparoscopic esophagectomy for malignancy

DAVID IAN WATSON MBBS, MD, FRACS
Professor and Head, Flinders University Department of Surgery; Senior Consultant Surgeon and Head of Gastrointestinal Services, Flinders Medical Centre, Bedford Park, South Australia, Australia

GLYN G. JAMIESON MS, MD, FRACS, FRCS, FACS
Dorothy Mortlock Professor and Chairman, Department of Surgery, University of Adelaide, Royal Adelaide Hospital, Adelaide, South Australia, Australia

The recent advent of laparoscopic and thoracoscopic surgical techniques now makes esophagectomy using minimal-access techniques feasible. Some initial reports suggest that the use of totally endoscopic techniques may reduce morbidity and improve initial surgical outcomes, particularly when combined with laparoscopic gastric mobilization.

Our preferred open approach for esophageal carcinoma involving the middle or lower third of the esophagus is an Ivor Lewis esophagectomy, performed by two surgical teams working synchronously. Tumors of the upper third of the esophagus are usually dealt with by either a cervico-thoraco-abdominal approach or cervicoabdominal 'blunt' esophagectomy. When 'endoscopic' esophagectomy was commenced, the same procedures performed at open surgery were replicated. The procedure begins with induction of general anesthesia and the placement of a double-lumen endotracheal tube to enable single-lung ventilation during the thoracoscopic phase (if required), and the choice of technique influences the order in which the various components of the procedure, i.e. laparoscopic, thoracoscopic, and open cervical, are performed. The exact combination and sequence of these steps is discussed later.

OPERATION

Laparoscopic gastric mobilization and distal esophageal dissection

POSITIONING FOR LAPAROSCOPIC GASTRIC MOBILIZATION

1 The patient is positioned in the reverse Trendelenburg position, with the table tilted 20–30 degrees head up and the legs extended in stirrups, with minimal hip flexion. This enables the surgeon to stand between the patient's legs for the laparoscopic phase.

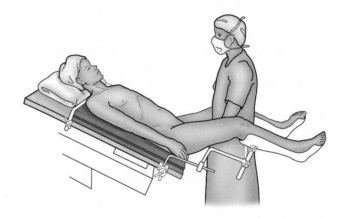

1

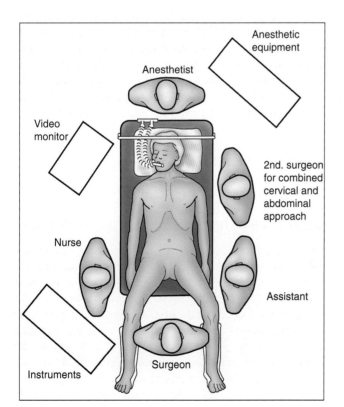

2

2 An assistant stands on the patient's left, and the scrub nurse on the right. A single video monitor is placed at the head end of the operating table adjacent to the patient's right shoulder.

TROCAR PLACEMENT

3 A 12 mm port (port A) is placed initially through a periumbilical incision, and the abdomen is insufflated to a pressure of 12 mm Hg. A 30- or 45-degree laparoscope is used for laparoscopic vision. Two further ports are placed: a 12 mm port (port B) below the left costal margin in the midclavicular line and a 5 mm port (port C) in the left flank. A 5 mm incision (incision D) is made in the epigastrium for the placement of a large Nathanson liver retractor (Cook Medical Technology, Eight Mile Plains, Queensland, Australia).

HAND-ASSISTED TECHNIQUE

A hand-assisted laparoscopic technique facilitates this phase, although the same steps can be performed using a totally laparoscopic technique. The latter approach is more time consuming, and an incision will still be necessary at some stage for specimen retrieval. A 7 to 8 cm transverse incision is made after fully insufflating the peritoneal cavity and placing all laparoscopic ports. This is sited 3–5 cm above the level of the umbilicus and centered over the right midclavicular line (incision E). The incision is deepened through all layers of the abdominal wall, using a muscle-splitting approach, to allow the placement of a sleeve that enables the surgeon's left hand to be introduced into the peritoneal cavity while a pneumoperitoneum and laparoscopic exposure are still maintained. There are now several devices available which are suitable for this approach.

The assistant controls the laparoscope and assists with a grasping instrument placed through the left flank port (C), while the surgeon uses the left hand for manipulation and

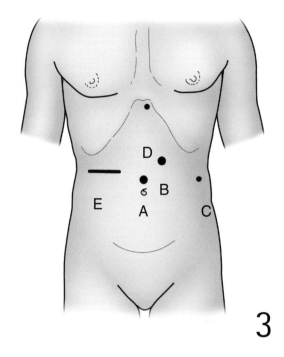

3

dissection, and manipulates laparoscopic instruments through the left-sided 12 mm port (B). The use of the left hand greatly facilitates the initial abdominal dissection phase, simplifying the surgeon's task of preserving the gastroepiploic arcade, creating a gastric tube, and dissecting the distal esophagus from within the abdomen. The same muscle-splitting incision is used at the completion of the procedure for specimen retrieval.

MOBILIZATION OF THE GREATER CURVE OF THE STOMACH

4 Gastric mobilization begins with dissection along the greater curve of the stomach. The lesser omentum is opened initially through its avascular portion using blunt finger dissection. This enables the surgeon's left hand to enter the lesser sac and lift the stomach forward, which places the gastrocolic omentum under appropriate tension to facilitate dissection of the greater curve. The entire length of the greater curve of the stomach is dissected from distal to proximal, with the right gastroepiploic artery and the gastroepiploic arcade preserved. We do this with ultrasonically activated coagulating shears, which cut and coagulate vessels and tissue, and thus eliminate the need for metal clips for small vessels.

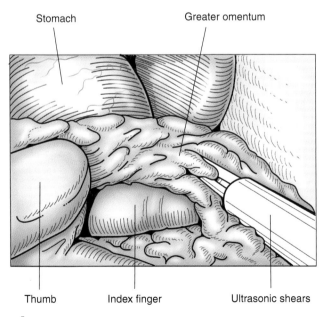

Stomach   Greater omentum

Thumb   Index finger   Ultrasonic shears

4

5 The short gastric blood vessels are also divided with the ultrasonic shears, and dissection is extended to the hiatus. Identification and preservation of the gastric blood supply, particularly when the gastrocolic omentum is fatty, is facilitated by manipulation of the stomach with the left hand and palpation of the arterial pulsations of the gastroepiploic arcade.

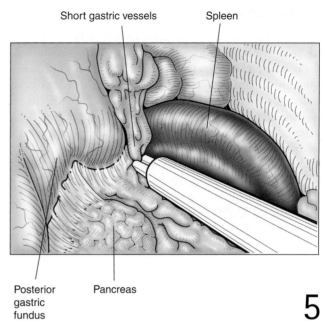

Short gastric vessels   Spleen

Posterior gastric fundus   Pancreas

5

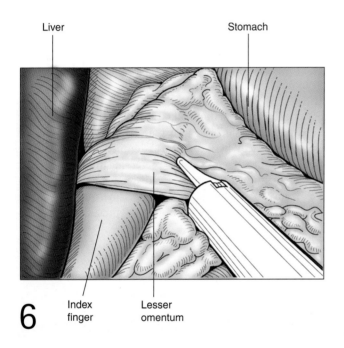

Liver   Stomach

Index finger   Lesser omentum

6

DISSECTION OF THE HIATUS, MOBILIZATION OF THE LESSER CURVE, AND DIVISION OF THE LEFT GASTRIC PEDICLE

6 The division of the lesser omentum is completed by dividing it at a distance from the lesser curve of the stomach, where the omentum is predominantly avascular. The hepatic branch of the anterior vagus nerve is divided. The hiatus is then dissected, and the gastroesophageal junction and the distal esophagus fully mobilized.

7 At this stage the only remaining structure tethering the stomach is the left gastric vessels. This pedicle is dissected from its surrounding adventitial and nodal tissue, and the pedicle is divided close to the origin of the left gastric artery with a single application of an endoscopic linear cutting stapling device. This secures the vascular pedicle with a triple rows of staples on either side of the cutting blade.

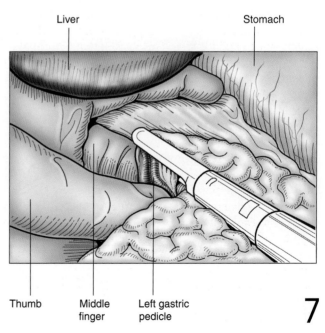

Liver   Stomach

Thumb   Middle finger   Left gastric pedicle

7

MOBILIZATION OF THE DUODENUM

The first, second, and proximal third part of the duodenum are readily mobilized by using a combination of division of the peritoneal attachments of the duodenum with the ultrasonic shears and digital dissection to lift the duodenum and pancreatic head forward and to the left. This mobilization is continued until the pylorus is fully mobilized. The pylorus can then be left intact or can be disrupted by a pyloroplasty or pyloromyotomy, depending on the surgeon's preference. A pyloromyotomy is achieved using a combination of scissors and diathermy hook dissection. Pyloroplasty requires the creation of a gastroduodenostomy using cutting electrocautery, and suture repair using interrupted sutures.

TRANSHIATAL DISSECTION OF THE DISTAL ESOPHAGUS

Dissection of the lower intrathoracic esophagus is performed next. This is facilitated by widening the esophageal hiatus by dividing the muscle of the right, and sometimes the left, hiatal pillar using the ultrasonic shears. The distal esophagus (and the esophageal tumor if it is in the distal esophagus) can be mobilized as far as possible under vision, with exposure and dissection being facilitated and guided by the surgeon's left hand. Blind digital dissection is unnecessary as the esophageal dissection is completed thoracoscopically.

CONSTRUCTION OF THE GASTRIC TUBE

The choice of technique for construction of a gastric tube depends on whether the anastomosis will be performed in the thoracic cavity or in the neck.

TUBE CONSTRUCTION FOR THORACOSCOPIC ANASTOMOSIS

8 If a thoracic anastomosis is planned, a gastric tube is fashioned intracorporeally using multiple applications of an endoscopic linear cutting stapling device; stapling commences at the lesser curvature and moves progressively in a cephalad direction, toward the gastric fundus. This is more easily achieved if the laparoscope is placed through the left upper 12-mm port and the stapling instrument is introduced through the periumbilical port. Complete division of the gastric tube from the pathological specimen is withheld. By leaving a small portion of the division incomplete, the surgeon is able to pull the gastric tube into the chest during the thoracoscopic phase. The extent to which the stomach is tubularized or left intact is determined by the location of the tumor, its histological type, and the presence or absence of macroscopic involvement of the lesser curvature lymph nodes.

Once this step is completed, the thoracic phase can commence. Our preference is to reposition the patient in the prone position for thoracoscopic dissection and anastomosis. At the end of the thoracoscopic part of the procedure, the resected specimen is placed in the abdomen in the vicinity of the esophageal hiatus. The patient is then repositioned supine, and the specimen is retrieved through the previously made muscle-splitting incision. Reinflation of the abdomen is not necessary for this step. An alternative method of specimen retrieval is through the chest wall. This requires a small thoracotomy incision, however, which is avoided by use of the technique described.

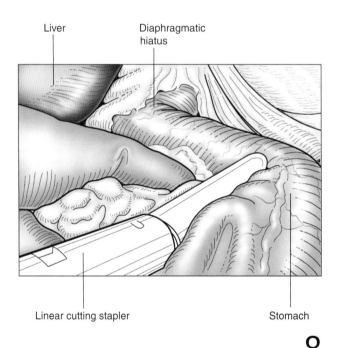

Liver — Diaphragmatic hiatus

Linear cutting stapler — Stomach

8

TUBE CONSTRUCTION FOR CERVICAL ANASTOMOSIS

If a cervico-thoraco-abdominal procedure is performed, then the first stage of the operation is to place the patient in the prone position and carry out a thoracoscopic mobilization of the esophagus. The patient is then repositioned supine for the second stage, which is gastric dissection and construction of the gastric tube. (On the other hand, if a cervicoabdominal procedure is performed, the esophagus is fully mobilized using a laparoscopic transhiatal dissection technique, and a thoracoscopic phase is avoided.)

9 Once the patient has been repositioned for the second stage, a second surgeon undertakes an open cervical approach synchronously with the abdominal dissection. The esophagus is divided in the neck, and a long tape is tied to the end to be removed. The mobilized stomach and esophagus are then delivered through the small abdominal incision used for the introduction of the surgeon's left hand. Because the sleeve used to maintain the pneumoperitoneum may need to be removed to allow exteriorization of the esophagus and stomach, all of the laparoscopic components of the procedure should be completed before this step.

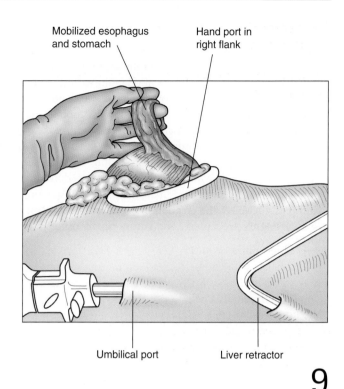

Mobilized esophagus and stomach

Hand port in right flank

Umbilical port

Liver retractor

9

Exteriorized stomach

Open surgical linear cutting stapler

10

10 The long cotton tape attached to the end of the esophagus maintains access to the mediastinum from the neck through to the fully mobilized esophagus and stomach as they are brought out through the abdominal wall. The gastric tube is then constructed extracorporeally using conventional open surgical techniques, and the resected specimen of esophagus and proximal stomach are then removed. The apex of the gastric tube is then pulled up into the neck, aided either by attaching it to the cotton tape, which helps direct its course, or by connecting it to the mouth of a Mousseau-Barbin tube, which when connected to suction allows a more gentle passage of the gastric tube to the neck.

JEJUNOSTOMY

At the conclusion of the procedure, irrespective of the esophagectomy technique used, a feeding jejunostomy is constructed for early postoperative nutrition. Using conventional surgical techniques and working through the abdominal incision, the surgeon places a 14 Fr T tube in the proximal jejunum approximately 20 cm distal to the duodenojejunal flexure and secures the tube with two purse-string sutures. This tube is pulled through either the periumbilical or left upper quadrant port wound and secured. The muscle-splitting incision is closed in layers, and all skin wounds are sutured to complete the abdominal phase of the procedure.

Thoracoscopic esophageal mobilization and intrathoracic anastomosis

POSITIONING FOR THORACOSCOPIC ESOPHAGEAL MOBILIZATION

The patient is positioned in the prone position for the thoracoscopic portion of the procedure. This position places the esophagus uppermost in the pleural cavity, and the right lung falls forward, which eliminates the need for lung retraction. With the patient in this position, bleeding also tends to run away from the operative field.

TROCAR PLACEMENT FOR THORACOSCOPIC DISSECTION OF THE ESOPHAGUS

11 Three ports (two 11 mm, one 5 mm) are placed, usually through the fifth, seventh, and ninth intercostal spaces in the posterior axillary line, using a blunt dissection technique. It is helpful if the anesthetist deflates the right lung just for this initial access. Another 5-mm port can be placed if additional access is needed for the assistant surgeon. Access to the posterior mediastinum is achieved either by collapsing the right lung in association with a gasless laparoscopic exposure technique or by insufflating the right thoracic cavity to a pressure of 5–6 mm Hg. Insufflation may be essential if unilateral lung collapse is poorly tolerated.

ESOPHAGEAL DISSECTION AND DIVISION OF THE AZYGOS VEIN

12, 13 Esophageal mobilization is performed using either ultrasonic shears or electrocautery dissection with scissors and a diathermy hook.

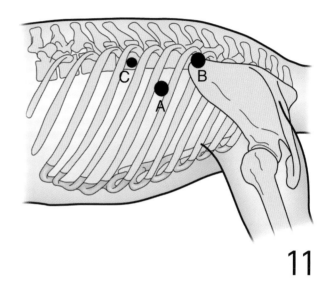

11

Spine

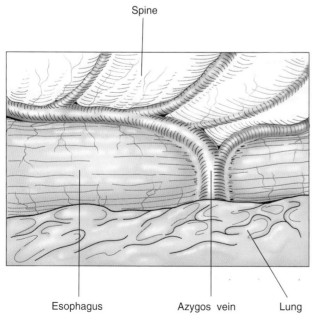

Esophagus   Azygos vein   Lung

12

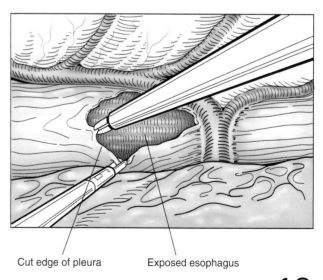

Cut edge of pleura   Exposed esophagus

13

14 This step is facilitated by using a curved instrument to place a tape around the esophagus at an early stage, which allows the esophagus to be lifted away from the posterior mediastinum. The tape is brought out through one of the thoracoscopic port wounds, alongside rather than through the port. A combination of tension on the tape controlled extracorporeally and thoracoscopic manipulation using a grasping instrument enables the esophagus to be more easily manipulated and thereby fully mobilized.

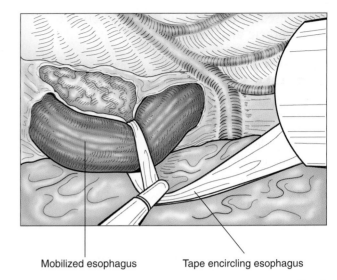

Mobilized esophagus   Tape encircling esophagus

14

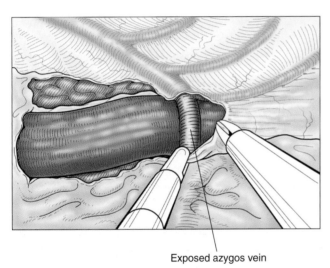

Exposed azygos vein

15

15, 16 The azygos vein is divided to enable mobilization of the upper esophagus. This is achieved either by using an endoscopic stapling device to ligate and divide the vein, or by ligating the vein in continuity and then transfixing it using laparoscopic suturing. Following our practice with the open technique, we usually do both. Dissection of the esophagus is continued to the apex of the thorax if a cervical anastomosis is planned. Alternatively, if an intrathoracic anastomosis is to be performed, dissection continues to a point at least 10 cm above the proximal visible extent of the tumor.

THORACOSCOPIC ESOPHAGEAL ANASTOMOSIS

If an intrathoracic anastomosis is planned, laparoscopic gastric mobilization will have been performed already (see earlier). The esophagus is divided at a level that enables both adequate tumor clearance and a tension-free anastomosis to the mobilized gastric tube. This division can be performed using the ultrasonic shears, which tends to 'weld' the mucosal and muscle layers of the esophageal wall together and thus prevent the retraction of muscle seen in the open technique. This helps with subsequent suturing of the anastomosis. The distal esophagus is now used to pull the gastric tube fully into the chest, with care taken to avoid rotating and twisting the tube. Provided the laparoscopic preparation of the gastric tube has been adequate, division of the tube from the specimen requires only a single application of the endoscopic stapling instrument. The resection specimen is placed elsewhere in the right hemithorax while the esophagus is anastomosed to the gastric tube.

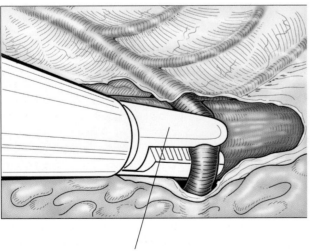

Endoscopic linear cutting stapler

16

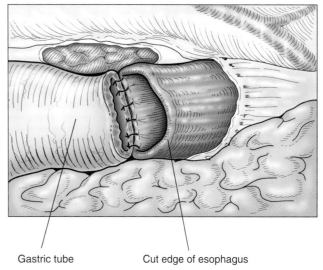

17 An end-to-side thoracoscopic hand-sewn anastomosis between the upper esophagus and the gastric tube is fashioned, using a single layer of interrupted monofilament sutures. Stapling techniques are also feasible but do not replicate our preferred open surgical technique. The posterior layer of sutures is placed first by suturing the gastric wall with seromuscular sutures to the full thickness of the posterior wall of the open esophagus.

Gastric tube   Cut edge of esophagus

17

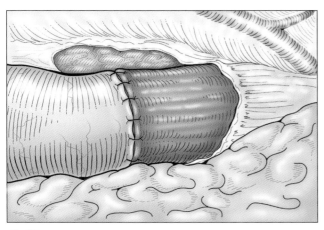

18

18 The gastric wall is then opened adjacent to the suture line, and the anastomosis is completed by suturing the full thickness of both stomach and esophagus anteriorly. Our experience has been that between 15 and 20 interrupted sutures are required for this phase. A nasogastric tube is guided across the anastomosis before its completion. The integrity of the join is checked by instilling water through the nasogastric tube and observing for leakage intraoperatively.

The resection specimen is then pushed back through the esophageal hiatus into the abdomen for subsequent retrieval. Two drains are placed into the chest through the port wounds: a large underwater-seal drain to the apex of the right hemithorax and either a second underwater-seal drain or a low-pressure suction drain to the area of the anastomosis. The remaining port is removed and the skin is closed.

Cervical dissection and esophageal anastomosis in the neck

If a cervico-thoraco-abdominal procedure is performed, the gastric tube is pulled up to the neck and a conventional hand-sewn esophagogastric anastomosis is performed using a standard open surgical technique.

Overview of endoscopic esophagectomy techniques

The choice of anastomotic site determines the sequence of the steps described earlier. If a cervico-thoraco-abdominal procedure is to be performed, thoracic mobilization, with the patient positioned prone, should be performed first. The patient is then positioned in the reverse Trendelenburg position for the laparoscopic and cervical phases of the procedure. These can be performed concurrently if two surgeons are available. Cervicoabdominal (transhiatal) esophagectomy is performed entirely in the reverse Trendelenburg position.

If a laparoscopic/thoracoscopic Ivor Lewis procedure is performed, the operation commences laparoscopically to enable gastric mobilization, construction of a gastric tube, and dissection of the lower intrathoracic esophagus. The patient is then repositioned in the prone position for thoracoscopic esophageal mobilization and anastomosis. The abdominal wounds are covered by a sterile occlusive dressing before repositioning. Once the thoracoscopic phase is completed, the patient is repositioned supine for specimen retrieval.

POSTOPERATIVE CARE

Patients are usually extubated immediately after surgery and managed initially in a high-dependency or intensive care unit. Pain relief is provided by either a patient-controlled analgesia machine, administration of morphine, or thoracic epidural analgesia. The apical drain is removed on the second postoperative day. Jejunostomy feeding commences on the first or second postoperative day, and a barium swallow examination is performed on the fifth to seventh postoperative day to check anastomotic integrity. If this examination demonstrates no leakage, the nasogastric tube and anastomotic drain are removed, and oral intake is commenced. Discharge is allowed once the patient is ambulatory and is maintaining an adequate oral intake. The jejunostomy tube is removed 2 weeks later at the first postoperative visit.

OUTCOME

Our experience with this technique has evolved, and some of our initial experience led to poor outcomes due to problems with the technique used or poor patient selection or both. Because we settled on the techniques described here, our results have been similar to the results achieved in the open setting. In other words, the hoped-for advantages in avoiding the incisions of open surgery have not yet convincingly materialized. However, we still believe it is possible that, as our experience with the technique grows and as operating times shorten, the advantages of minimal-access surgery noted for other procedures will become manifest for thoracolaparoscopic esophagectomy.

FURTHER READING

Cuschieri A, Shimi S, Banting S. Endoscopic oesophagectomy through a right thoracoscopic approach. *Journal of the Royal College of Surgeons of Edinburgh* 1992; **37**: 7–11.

DePaula AL, Hashiba K, Ferreira EAB, de Paula RA, Grecco E. Laparoscopic transhiatal esophagectomy with esophagogastroplasty. *Surgical Laparoscopy and Endoscopy* 1995; **5**: 1–5.

Dexter SPL, Martin IG, McMahon MJ. Radical thoracoscopic esophagectomy for cancer. *Surgical Endoscopy* 1996; **10**: 147–51.

Luketich JD, Alvelo-Rivera M, Buenaventura PO, Christie NA, McCaughan JS, Litle VR, Schauer PR, Close JM, Fernando HC. Minimally invasive esophagectomy: outcomes in 222 patients. *Annals of Surgery* 2003; **238**: 486–94.

Martin D, Bessell JR, Watson DI. Thoracoscopic and laparoscopic oesophagectomy – initial experience and outcomes. *Surgical Endoscopy* 2006 – In Press.

Smithers BM, Gotley DC, McEwan D, Martin I, Bessell J, Doyle L. Thoracoscopic mobilization of the esophagus. A 6 year experience. *Surgical Endoscopy* 2001; **15**: 176–82.

Watson DI, Davies N, Jamieson GG. Totally endoscopic Ivor Lewis oesophago-gastrectomy. *Surgical Endoscopy* 1999; **13**: 293–97.

Watson DI, Jamieson GG, Devitt PG. Endoscopic cervico-thoraco-abdominal oesophagectomy. *Journal of the American College of Surgeons* 2000; **190**: 372–8.

Index